Practical Neurotology and Skull Base Surgery

Practical Neurotology and Skull Base Surgery

Seilesh Babu, MD

PLURAL PUBLISHING
INC.
SAN DIEGO
OXFORD
MELBOURNE

PLURAL PUBLISHING INC.

5521 Ruffin Road
San Diego, CA 92123

e-mail: info@pluralpublishing.com
Web site: http://www.pluralpublishing.com

Typeset in 10½/13 Palatino by Flanagan's Publishing Services, Inc.
Printed in Malaysia by Four Colour Print Group

Cover image courtesy of Daniel Pieper.

NOTICE TO THE READER
Care has been taken to confirm the accuracy of the indications, procedures, drug dosages, and diagnosis and remediation protocols presented in this book and to ensure that they conform to the practices of the general medical and health services communities. However, the authors, editors, and publisher are not responsible for errors or omissions or for any consequences from application of the information in this book and make no warranty, expressed or implied, with respect to the currency, completeness, or accuracy of the contents of the publication. The diagnostic and remediation protocols and the medications described do not necessarily have specific approval by the Food and Drug administration for use in the disorders and/or diseases and dosages for which they are recommended. Application of this information in a particular situation remains the professional responsibility of the practitioner. Because standards of practice and usage change, it is the responsibility of the practitioner to keep abreast of revised recommendations, dosages, and procedures.

Library of Congress Cataloging-in-Publication Data

Practical neurotology and skull base surgery / [edited by] Seilesh Babu.
p. ; cm.
Includes bibliographical references and index.
ISBN-13: 978-1-59756-511-0 (alk. paper)
ISBN-10: 1-59756-511-3 (alk. paper)
I. Babu, Seilesh.
[DNLM: 1. Otologic Surgical Procedures. 2. Skull Base—surgery. 3. Neurosurgical Procedures.
4. Otorhinolaryngologic Neoplasms. 5. Skull Base Neoplasms. WV 200]

617.5'14—dc23

2012042890

Contents

Foreword

In 1986, the Michigan Ear Institute was established. Dr. T. Manford McGee had been in otologic practice in the greater Detroit area for over 20 years, and it was during these years that he established a very strong and loyal relationship with Providence Hospital in Southfield, Michigan.

My otologic career had taken me from a solo private practice in Victoria, British Columbia, Canada, to membership in the House Ear Clinic in Los Angeles, California, and then to faculty membership in the Department of Otolaryngology/Head and Neck Surgery at the University of Michigan in Ann Arbor. I had the privilege to practice in both private practice and academic sections of otology and witnessed the strengths and weaknesses of both.

As time passed, both Dr. McGee and I had envisioned the concept of an "Ear Institute" with all the resources and services appropriate for such a preeminent center. This "proposal" included a medical office building, fully equipped with audiologic and vestibular evaluation capabilities. At the hospital, three operating rooms dedicated to otologic, neurotologic, and skull base surgery, with specialized, dedicated surgical nurses, appropriate otologic surgical instruments, intraoperative monitoring equipment, surgical microscopes, and audiovisual equipment was designed. Providence Hospital would also fund a fellowship program in otology, neurotology, and skull base surgery, as well as provide a temporal bone surgical dissection laboratory and complete audiologic and vestibular testing facilities; this truly provided a unique opportunity.

We jointly decided to proceed, and in 1986 t he Michigan Ear Institute was established. While Dr. McGee had a career in otosclerosis and stapes surgery, it was decided with the rapid emergence of neurotologic diagnosis and surgery that the practice would be devoted to otology, neurotology, and skull base surgery, and future associates would be young, fellowship-trained individuals in this broader field.

Thus, in rapid succession doctors Jack Kartush, Dennis Bojrab, and Michael LaRouere joined the original faculty. Later, several Michigan Ear Institute fellows remained on faculty as well: doctors John Zappia, Eric Sargent, and Seilesh Babu.

It is with great pride that I introduce this book (and its companion, *Practical Otology for the Otolaryngologist*), edited by Dr. Seilesh Babu and contributed to by many other members of the Michigan Ear Institute and their former fellows. This book reflects 25 years of experience in clinical otology, neurotology, and skull base surgery, an experience rich in contributions in diagnosis, evaluations, electrophysiologic monitoring, and surgical technique innovations and modifications.

As I reflect upon the past 50 years of clinical otology, the changes that have occurred during those decades are nothing less than amazing.

In otosclerosis surgery the fenestration operation had just given way to the stapes mobilization procedure. Soon refixation of the stapes became apparent and the total stapedectomy operation became popular. With time this has been replaced generally by the small footplate fenestra techniques.

In chronic ear and cholesteatoma surgery, canal wall-down techniques were standard when the intact canal wall procedure was proposed. The controversy that ensued was clearly apparent every 4 years when proponents of each technique shared their views at the Shanbaugh-Shea workshops, often in heated exchanges of opinion. Now surgeons are equally adept at either procedure as dictated by the disease process at hand.

In 1957, vestibular surgery was limited to the oval window labyrinthectomy, and later transmastoid labyrinthectomy provided complete unilateral ablation.

Facial nerve surgery at this earlier time was limited to transmastoid decompression. It was believed that one should not incise the facial nerve sheath for fear of disturbing the endoneural fluid compartments. With increasing surgical exposures within the temporal bone we have learned that facial nerve decompression and mobilization from the geniculate ganglion and even more proximally, into the parotid gland, is possible, often without paresis of the facial nerve.

Glomus tumors of the temporal bone, while described earlier by Rosenwasser, were not clearly differentiated into glomus tympanicum or glomus jugulare, a distinction of great importance when surgical removal is entertained.

Transtemporal acoustic tumor surgery was in its infancy in the 1960s. Dr. William House of Los Angeles, California, was evolving the surgical approaches that we routinely use today. In these early days, operative morbidity and mortality were still high. Now mortality rates are less than 1% and postoperative cerebrospinal fluid leaks, meningitis, and facial paralysis are markedly reduced. The concepts of planned subtotal tumor removal, staged removal of large tumors, and leaving a minute fragment of tumor on the facial nerve to preserve function have all evolved. The routine use of facial nerve monitoring in acoustic tumor surgery as pioneered by Dr. Jack Kartush has revolutionized dissection and manipulation of the facial nerve during acoustic tumor surgery.

Cochlear implant surgery is now regularly performed upon the profoundly deafened individual. Surgery is performed as young as 1 year of age and this age continues to become younger. The implant devices are multiple-channeled and reliable. Speech and language acquisition in these early implanted infants are most impressive.

Bone-anchored hearing systems (BAHA) pioneered in Sweden have assumed a useful place in hearing amplification. These devices were not available several decades ago.

Finally, mention must be made concerning temporal bone and cranial imaging techniques, now so crucial in the diagnosis of many otologic and neurotologic conditions. Prior to 1974, the only temporal bone imaging were plain x-rays. To evaluate the posterior fossa and internal auditory canal, pantopaque had to be introduced into the lumbar subarachnoid space and with fluroscopic assistance guided into posterior cranial fossa.

In 1974, the EMI scan, the predecessor of the CT scan, was introduced. Early designs were crude-we now have elegant image capabilities of the temporal bone. However, even with the addition of contrast material, resolution for acoustic tumors is limited to those lesions larger than one centimeter.

However, in the early 1980s the MRI scan was introduced. Initially, this was not a great benefit without contrast. Soon, gadolinium was introduced to MRI imaging, and now allows the greatest resolution of even the smallest lesions, a truly invaluable evaluation tool for the inner ear and adjacent structures.

In summary, I congratulate most sincerely Dr. Babu and his collaborators as they present these most contemporary surgical and practical texts in the field of otology, neurotology, and skull base surgery. It is my hope that by highlighting (be it even so briefly) the state of our otologic subspecialty some 50 years ago, the reader will truly appreciate the progress and advances summarized in these volumes.

Malcolm D. Graham, MD
Department of Otolaryngology—
Head and Neck Surgery
Emory University, Atlanta, Georgia

Preface

The field of neurotology and skull base surgery is evolving. Not so long ago, the morbidity and mortality of the surgical approaches to resect tumors of the skull base were high enough to render these approaches unwarranted and risky. Nowadays, with improved anesthesia, surgical techniques, intraoperative monitoring, and a team approach, these tumors can be successfully resected. Minimally invasive and endoscopic approaches also reduce the morbidity involved with these resections. With the addition of stereotactic radiotherapy, many lesions can now be managed with alternatives to surgery with excellent outcomes.

Fellowships in neurotology do an excellent job of training residents in the complex anatomy and physiology of the temporal bone, as well as the diagnosis and management of skull base lesions. Many of our fellows have discussed wanting a practical book to review for the procedures that are seen daily in the office setting and operating room. This book was developed with this in mind: to provide the student, resident, neurotology fellow, and practicing neurotologist a diagnostic and management textbook describing the practical application of knowledge for patients suffering from skull base pathology. Our goal was to have the reader be able to use this book to capitalize on the breadth of experience and knowledge from experts in the field and apply their experience in an approach that would benefit them on a day-to-day basis.

Introduction

This book is designed for you! Whether a neurotology fellow, ENT resident, medical student, physician assistant, nurse practitioner, physical therapist dealing with dizziness, or a practicing otolaryngologist or neurotologist, this book is for you. Neurotology and skull base surgery is a branch of general otolaryngology dealing with tumors such as acoustic neuroma, paraganglioma, meningioma, petrous apex lesions, petroclival tumors, and issues such as intraoperative monitoring and radiotherapy.

Many of our rotating ENT residents and neurotology fellows continually ask for a recommendation for a concise book covering the disorders of the temporal bone that is up-to-date and clinically and surgically oriented. This book was thus created to attempt to improve residents' and fellows' comfort with diseases and skull base surgeries involving the temporal bone. With this in mind, a practical approach to the clinical management of skull base tumors and lesions and approaches was devised. It is the culmination of countless hours of hard work by numerous authors who are clinically as well as surgically experienced.

Covering the pertinent details for daily practice, this book discusses topics ranging from surgical approaches described from a neurosurgeon perspective to stereotactic radiotherapy. Clinical and surgical pearls abound in this text that all practitioners will find beneficial from authors known for large clinical volume of experience and surgical acumen.

Chapters are organized starting with surgical approaches being described from a neurosurgeon's perspective in Chapter 1 and a neurotologist's perspective in Chapter 2. The unique perspective from our neurosurgeon clarifies the skull base approaches and nomenclature that is used between the two specialties. Chapter 3 discusses the minimally invasive and endoscopic skull base approaches. The next few chapters (Chapters 4–7) cover specific tumors and the described surgical approach to resect them. These chapters cover acoustic neuroma, meningioma, neurofibromatosis, petrous apex lesion, and petroclival tumors. Chapter 8 discusses temporal bone malignancies with description of surgical resection. Chapter 9 covers unusual temporal bone lesions such as Paget's disease, fibrous dysplasia, and osteopetrosis. Chapter 10 describes stereotactic radiotherapy for various types of skull base pathology. The final chapter discusses the importance, benefit, and interpretation of intraoperative monitoring.

The hope for this book is to provide an easy-to-understand format that blends the complexity of diseases of the skull base so that diagnosis, testing and interpretation, and imaging can be combined in a practical way with the surgical approaches for all levels of expertise. The teaching pearls available in this book can be assimilated into the reader's practice, assisting them in daily rounds, patient care, and board preparation.

Acknowledgments

This book required numerous dedicated authors from around the country who devoted a great amount of time and effort to make this a success. It would not be possible without their guidance and assistance and I am deeply appreciative. I also would like to thank my gifted teachers, mentors, friends, and associates who have guided me throughout my medical journey, especially at Northeastern Ohio Universities College of Medicine (NEOUCOM), Henry Ford Health System, and the Michigan Ear Institute (MEI). My colleagues, office staff, and operating room personnel at MEI make it truly enjoyable to come to work and care for patients in a comfortable, caring, and educational manner. I thank them for this as they make it a joy to come to work every day.

I must acknowledge my parents and siblings for their continuous support. My parents (Lakshman and Renuka Babu) sacrificed immensely in order to provide the gift of opportunity through education for my siblings (Niharika Wunnava and Mayukh Babu) and myself. Their dedication has guided each of us to success with our careers and with our families. I would also like to extend my gratitude to my in-laws (Mark and Jan Crooks) for adding to my life and for their generous support.

Of course, I must thank my loving and extraordinary wife, Abbey, who provided support and guidance throughout this project. Even my three sons (Kavan, Kethan, and Karun) and daughter (Kareena) helped by asking when my "story was going to be done?"—thus making sure I would stay on task! I love my children for providing the fun, excitement, and laughter that shows us what makes life so enjoyable and extraordinary on a daily basis.

I would personally like to extend sincere thanks to Cheryl Thrushman at Providence Hospital and Alison Devine at MEI. Their tireless effort and early morning meetings allowed many of the images and text to be created for the book. Their attention to detail and prompt response on project deadlines allowed things to be done in a timely fashion.

Contributors

Gregory Artz, MD
Assistant Professor
Department of Otolaryngology—Head and Neck Surgery
Division of Neurotology/Skull Base Surgery
Thomas Jefferson University
Philadelphia, Pennsylvania
Chapter 3

Seilesh Babu, MD
Otology, Neurotology, and Skull Base Surgery
Michigan Ear Institute
Farmington Hills, Michigan
Clinical Assistant Professor
Department of Otolaryngology
Wayne State University
Detroit, Michigan
Chapters 2, 7, 8, and 9

Brent J. Benscoter, MD
Neurotology and Skull Base Fellow
Michigan Ear Institute
Chapter 10

Dennis Bojrab
Michigan Ear Institute
Chief, Department of Otolaryngology
Wm Beaumont Hospital
Chief, Department of Skull Base Surgery
Providence Hospital
Clinical Professor, Department of Otolaryngology and Neurosurgery
Wayne State University
Chapter 10

Rodney C. Diaz, MD
Assistant Professor
Otology, Neurotology and Skull Base Surgery
Department of Otolaryngology—Head and Neck Surgery
University of California, Davis Medical Center
Sacramento, CA
Chapters 2, 4, and 5

James Evans, MD
Associate Professor
Department of Neurosurgery
Thomas Jefferson University
Philadelphia, Pennsylvania
Chapter 3

Yoav Hahn, MD
Otology, Neurotology, and Skull Base Surgery
Dallas Ear Institute
Chapter 10

Michael Hoa, MD
Neurotology Fellow
House Ear Institute
Chapter 9

Jack M. Kartush, MD
Otology, Neurotology, and Skull Base Surgery
Michigan Ear Institute
Farmington Hills, Michigan
Clinical Assistant Professor
Department of Otolaryngology
Wayne State University
Detroit, Michigan
Chapter 11

Alice Lee, MD
Department of Head and Neck Surgery
Kaiser Permanente Riverside Medical Center
Riverside, California
Chapter 11

Christopher Linstrom, MD
Professor of Otolaryngology—Head and Neck Surgery
Professor of Neurological Surgery
The New York Medical College
Valhalla, New York
Surgeon Director, Otology and Neurotology
The New York Eye & Ear Infirmary
New York, New York
Adjunct Professor of Audiology

The Graduate Center/ Health Sciences Doctoral Program
City University of the City of New York
New York, New York
Chapter 6

Jeremy D. Meier, MD
Resident Physician
Department of Otolaryngology—Head and Neck Surgery
University of California, Davis
Chapter 5

Raj Murali, MD, FRCSE, FACS, FRCSC
Professor and Chairman
Department of Neurosurgery
The New York Medical College,
Valhalla, New York
Chapter 6

Daniel Pieper, MD, FACS
Chief of Skull Base Surgery, William Beaumont Hospital
Michigan Head and Spine Institute
Chapters 1 and 3

Marc Rosen, MD
Associate Professor
Department of Otolaryngology—Head and Neck Surgery
Thomas Jefferson University
Philadelphia, Pennsylvania
Chapter 3

Dan Sdrulla, MD, PhD
Neurotology Fellow
Michigan Ear Institute
Chapter 6

Wayne Shaia, MD
Otologist/Neurotologist
Balance and Ear Center
VCU Health Systems Clinical Assistant Professor
Department of Otolaryngology—Head and Neck Surgery
Richmond, Virginia
Chapter 7

Sean Wise, MD
Neurotology Fellow
Michigan Ear Institute
Chapter 7

John Zappia, MD
Michigan Ear Institute
Farmington Hills, Michigan
Clinical Assistant Professor
Department of Otolaryngology
Wayne State University
Detroit, Michigan
Chapter 8

This book is dedicated to the mentors and teachers that have come before us and led the way to the formation of the Michigan Ear Institute, especially Dr. T. Manford McGee and Dr. Malcolm Graham. They have provided insight and experience that has been passed down to training otologists for decades. Dr. McGee completed tens of thousands of stapedectomies, providing an immense knowledge base about otosclerosis and its surgical treatments. Dr. Graham, having been with the great Drs. William House and Howard House in Los Angeles, California, for many years, brought many of the teachings from the House Ear Institute to the Midwest. Here, it continued to be fostered, cultivated, and expanded.

Much of our current success can be directly attributed to these great doctors and their wonderful contributions to the field of otology and skull base surgery, which has been passed on from one generation to the next with participation in preceptorships and fellowships.

All of us in our current field owe our otologic forefathers a great deal of gratitude for their exquisite teachings and hope that we too will learn the ability to teach effectively and to share experiences with others in a similar fashion, so as to continue to share and expand on our knowledge base for the betterment of patient care.

CHAPTER 1

Skull Base Approaches: Neurosurgical Perspective

Daniel Pieper

INTRODUCTION

One of the most significant challenges to the skull base surgeon in training is learning the different approaches to the skull base. The vast array of approaches and the varying nomenclature lends to this confusion when describing the surgical procedure.

Realizing that each of the skull base approaches are extensions of the basic approaches of cranial surgery, the surgeon can better understand each technique's application. The extensions are nothing more than the addition of an osteotomy (ie, cranio-orbito-zygomatic) or a combination of two or more smaller approaches (ie, transpetrosal) (Figure 1–1). Understanding the improved access gained by an additional osteotomy, as well as its limitation, provides the ability to choose the appropriate approach for the anatomic region of interest. Additionally, the surgeon must also understand the unique differences inherent to different pathologies affecting the same anatomic location.

This chapter is not intended to be an in-depth technical description of the various exposures, but an overview of the more common approaches utilized in skull base surgery, their utilities, and limitations. In a number of the approaches described, different authors throughout the literature have attributed various names to similar procedures. To minimize this confusion this chapter refers to each surgical approach in anatomic terms alone. Many of these approaches are described in further detail in the following chapters of this textbook.

TRANSFACIAL APPROACHES (see Figure 1–1)

Several transfacial approaches have been described for accessing the skull base.[1–17] The risks for these anterior approaches are infection, dental malocclusion, and cosmetic issues (Figure 1–2). Because of the increased risk of infection due to violation of contaminated areas, the use of broad spectrum antibiotics is recommended. When limited to the nasopharynx and/or paranasal sinuses, antibiotics for gram-positive and gram-negative coverage typically are sufficient; however, if the oropharynx is also violated, the addition of anaerobic organism coverage is necessary. Additionally, the use of vascularized flaps and meticulous, multilayered, watertight closure techniques are utilized to minimize the risk of ascending infections, cerebrospinal fluid leaks/fistulas, and osteomyelitis/mal-union of the osteotomies.[18] Three categories of anterior approaches are divided into the transsphenoidal, transmaxillary, and transmandibular.

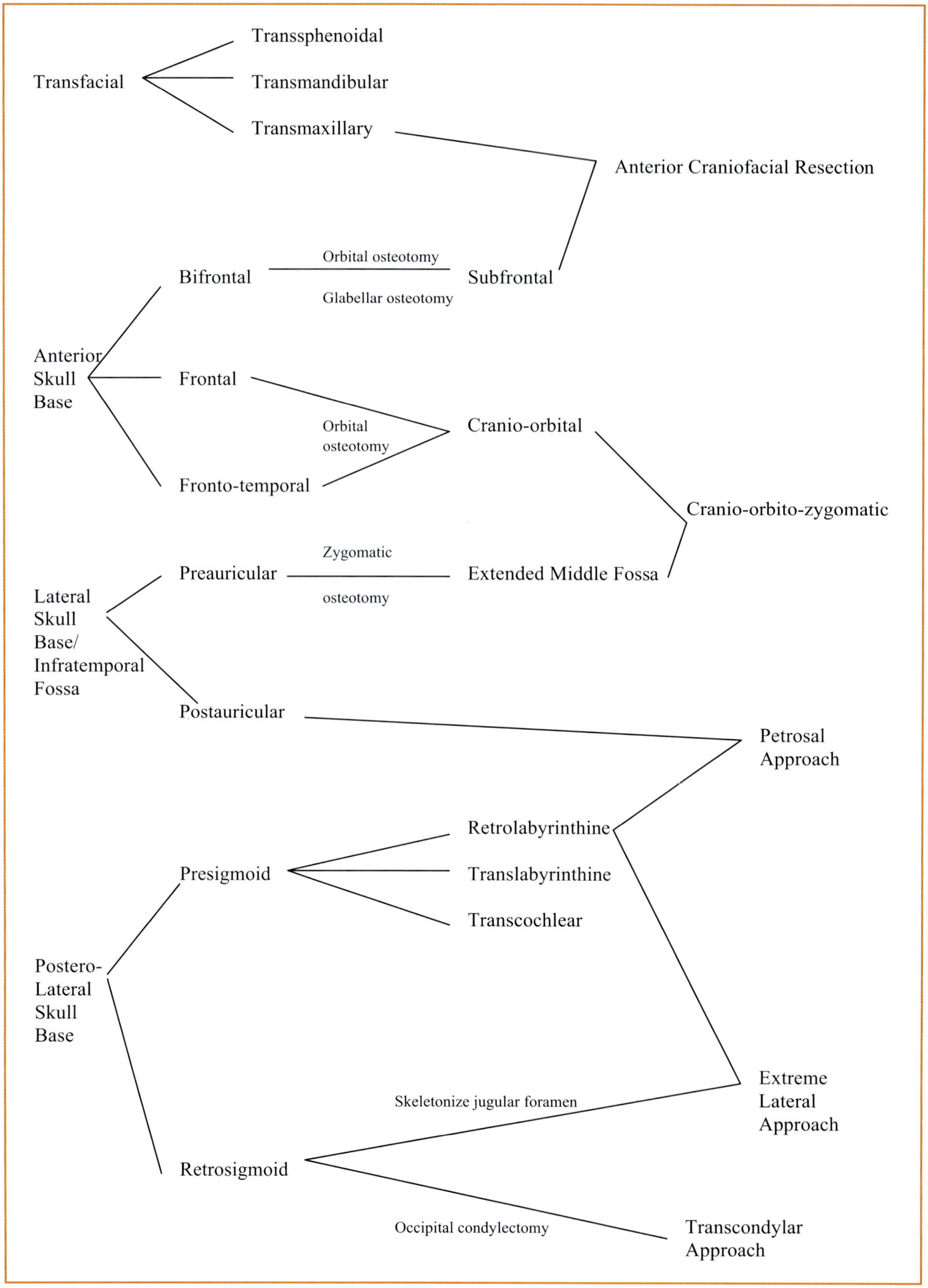

Figure 1–1. Various approaches to skull base with relationships of each approach.

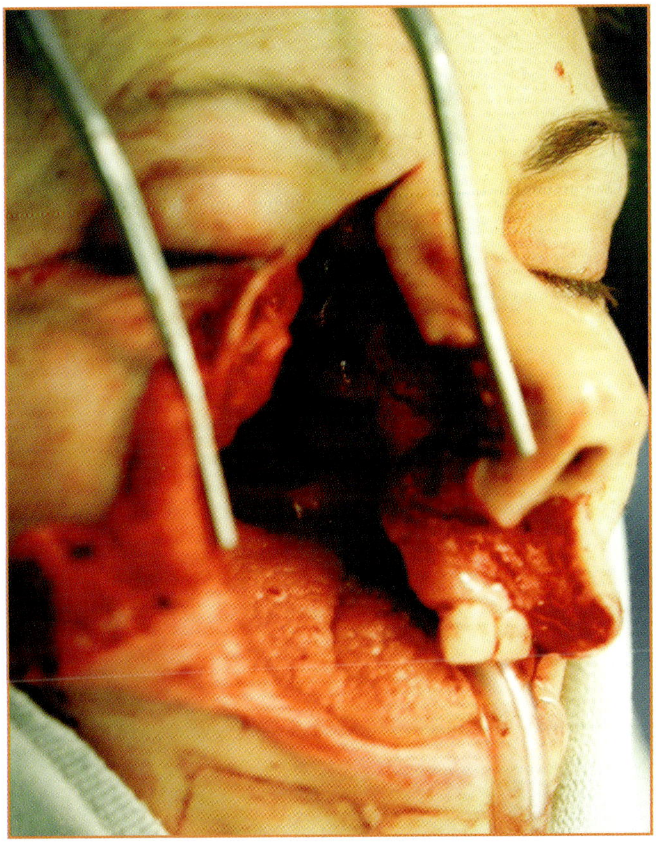

A

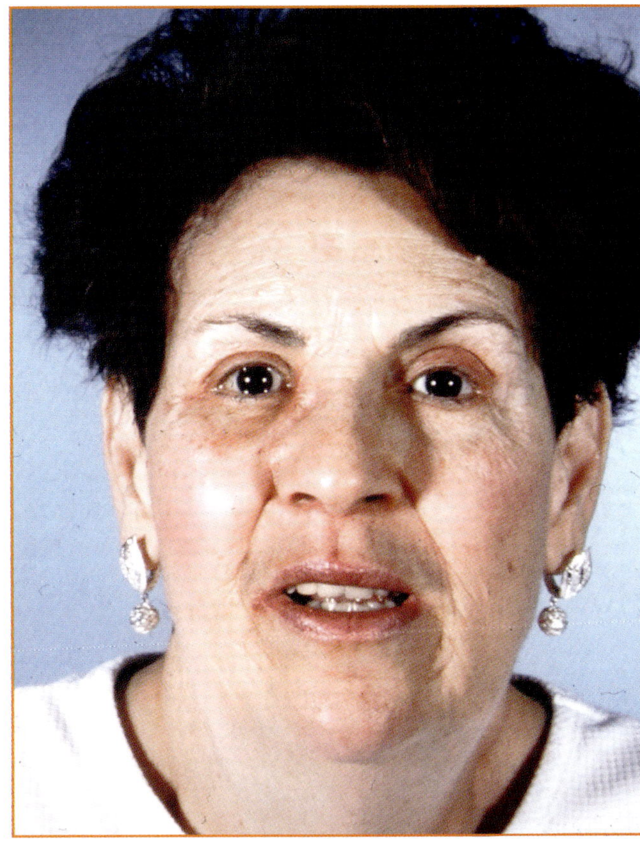

B

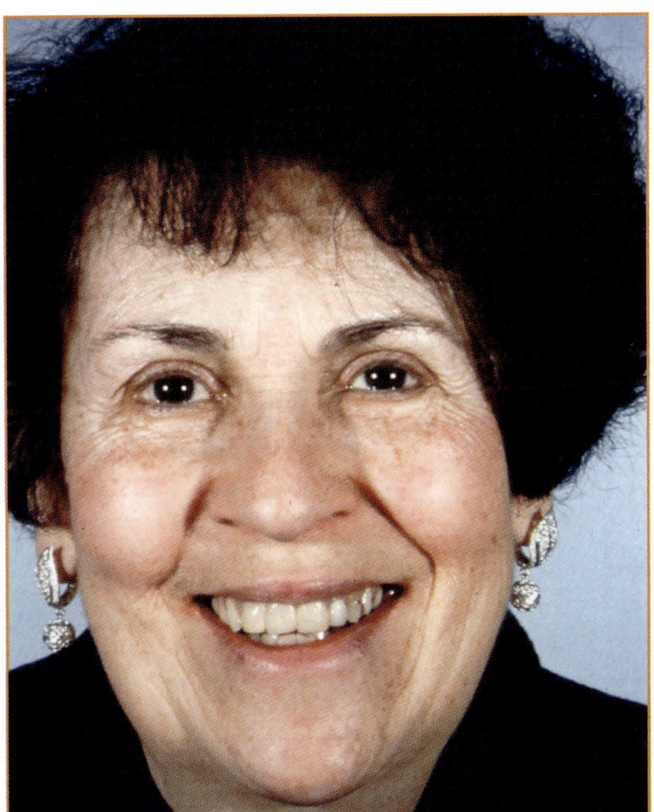

C

Figures 1–2. Cosmesis following the transfacial approach. **A**. Intraoperative. **B**. 3 months postoperative. **C**. 1 year.

Transsphenoidal Approach

Since the original description of the transsphenoidal approach by Cushing in 1912 and the subsequent introduction of the operating microscope in the mid-1960s this approach has remained a mainstay of intrasellar surgery, primarily for use in pituitary adenomas[19,20] (Figure 1–3). The more recent introduction of transnasal endoscopy has further enhanced the utility of this approach to expand the transsphenoidal approach to include not only tumors limited to the sella, but to include many tumors of the skull base that are in direct continuity with the sphenoid sinus (Figure 1–4). Midline pathology extending from the planum sphenoidale superiorly to the superior third of the clivus inferiorly can be accessed. The optic nerve and the anterior loop of the internal carotid artery are typically the anatomic limiting factors laterally. Accessing lesions extending intradurally are limited superiorly by the optic nerves/chiasm and anterior cerebral artery complex, the basilar artery posteriorly, and the cavernous sinuses laterally.

Transmaxillary Approach

James and Crockard[8] were the first to describe the use of the extended maxillotomy to access the upper cervical and inferior skull base. The use of the Le Fort I maxillotomy increased visibility providing access

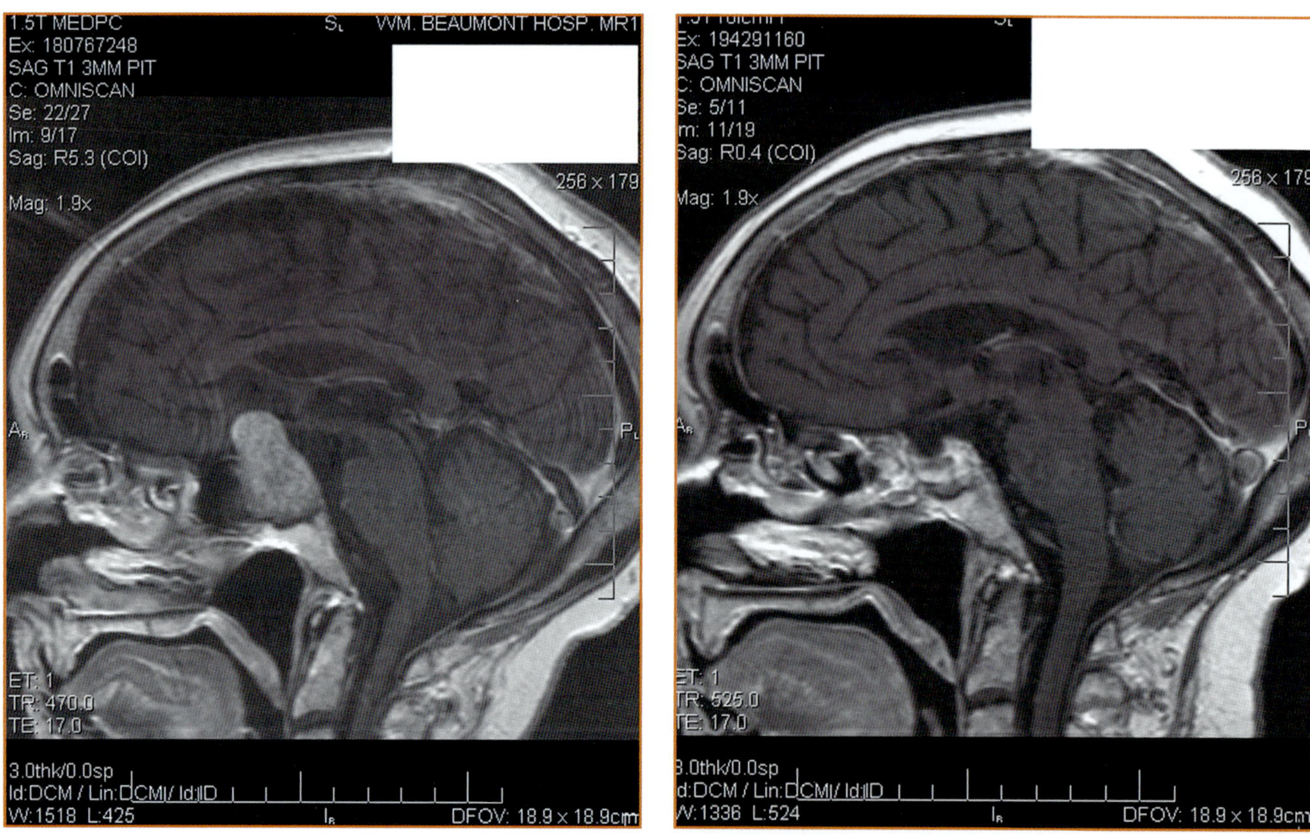

Figure 1–3. Pituitary macroadenoma with extension into the suprasellar space resected through an endoscopic transnasal transsphenoidal approach. **A.** Preoperative MRI sagittal T1 with gadolinium. **B.** Postoperative MRI sagittal T1 with gadolinium showing complete resection of the tumor.

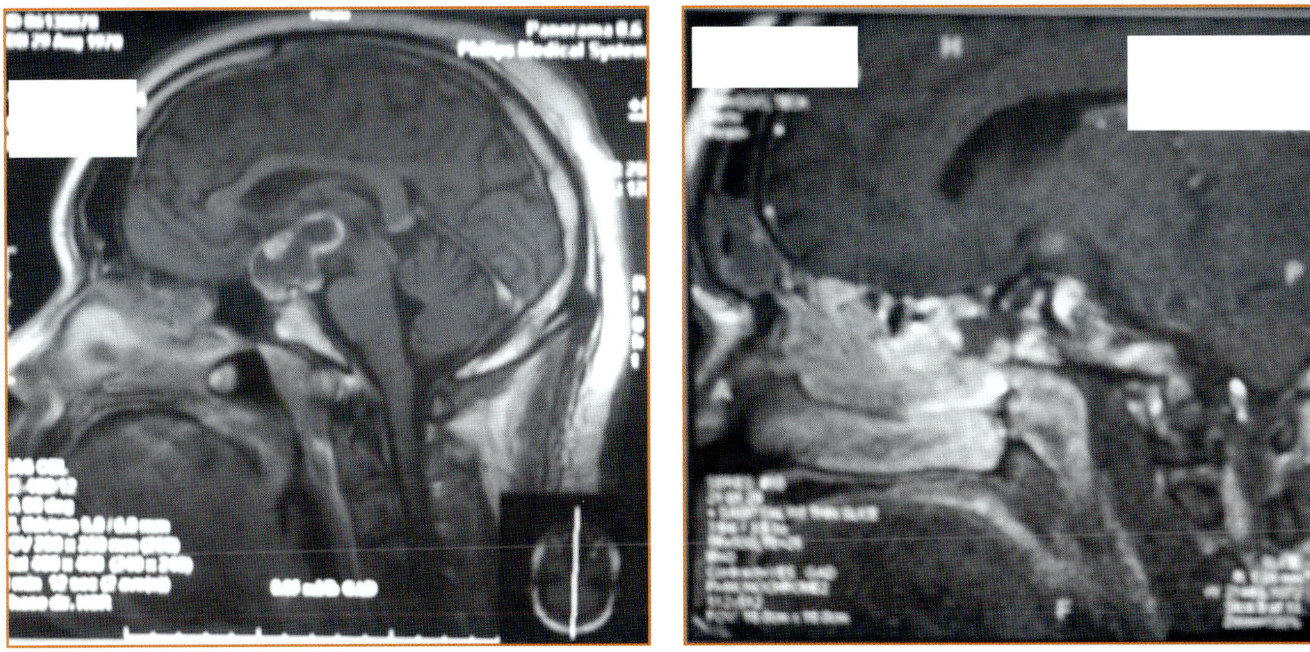

A B

Figure 1–4. Craniopharyngioma of the suprasellar space extending into the third ventricle and interpeduncular cistern. The tumor was accessed via an endoscopic transnasal transsphenoidal approach through the planum sphenoidale. **A.** Preoperative MRI sagittal T1 with gadolinium. **B.** Postoperative MRI sagittal with gadolinium.

to lesions involving the clivus. However, the downward displacement of the maxilla anteriorly caused the posterior aspect of the hard palate to elevate thereby limiting the visibility of the mid-clivus. The addition of a hemi-Le Fort III maxillotomy allows the entire maxilla and inferior orbit to be mobilized and displaced laterally which allows visualization of the entire clivus from the sella to the foramen magnum[16,17] (Figure 1–5). As with the transsphenoidal approach, the limitation laterally, at the level of the sphenoid sinus, is from the internal carotid arteries, optic nerves, and cavernous sinus. In the mid-clivus, the lateral extent is limited by the petroclival synchondrosis and Dorello's canal. Inferiorly, the jugular bulb is the limiting structure laterally. With the mobilization of the orbital floor, access to the inferior half of the orbit and retrobulbar regions is possible. Additionally, the medial aspect of the infratemporal fossa can be accessed to the level of the pterygopalantine fossa. As previously described, lesions extending intradurally are not prohibitive; however, a meticulous, multilayered watertight closure is essential. If necessary, a lumbar drain should be placed at the time of surgery; however, the occurrence of over drainage and tension pneumocephalus must be closely monitored and avoided.

Transmandibular Approach

Since introduced by Spiro, the mandibular swing has been utilized for its wide exposure of the oropharyngeal and infratemporal fossa.[21] The approach allows for a shortened working distance and postoperative rehabilitation with little long-term cosmetic morbidity (Figure 1–6). A mandibular osteotomy is made either between the central incisors or paramedially between the lateral incisor and canine tooth. The anterior belly of the digastric muscle is incised to allow lateral rotation of the hemimandibulotomy.

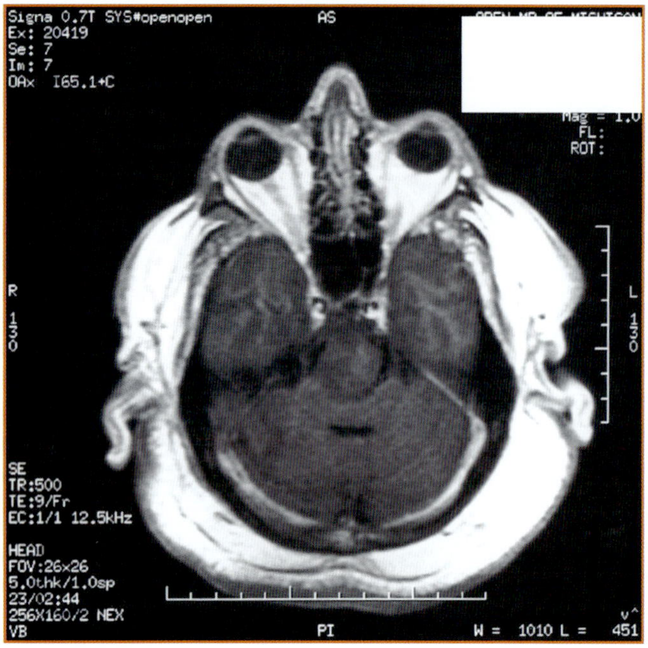

A

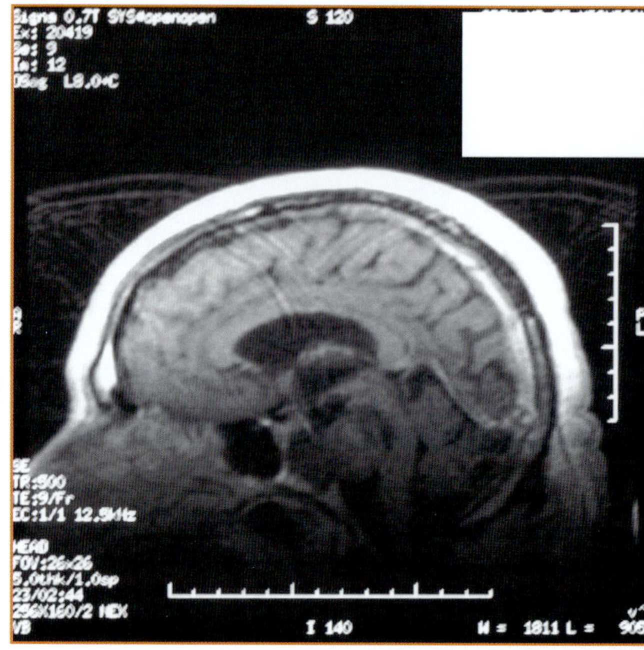

B

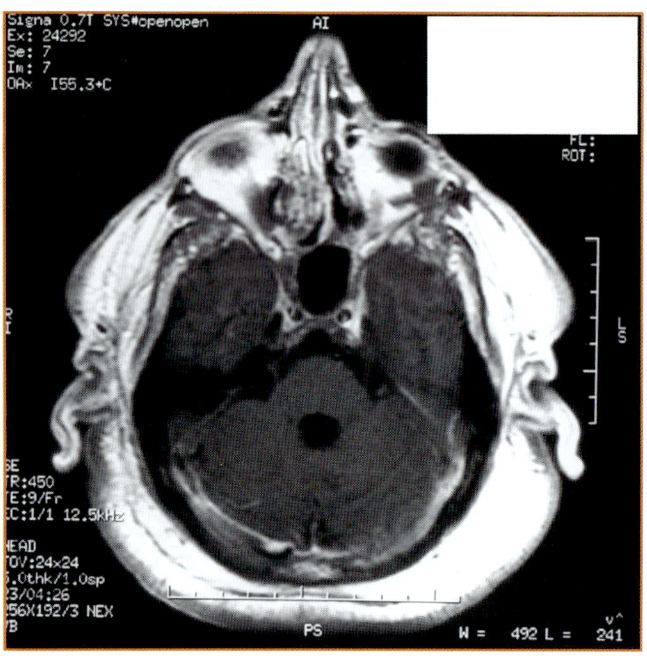

C

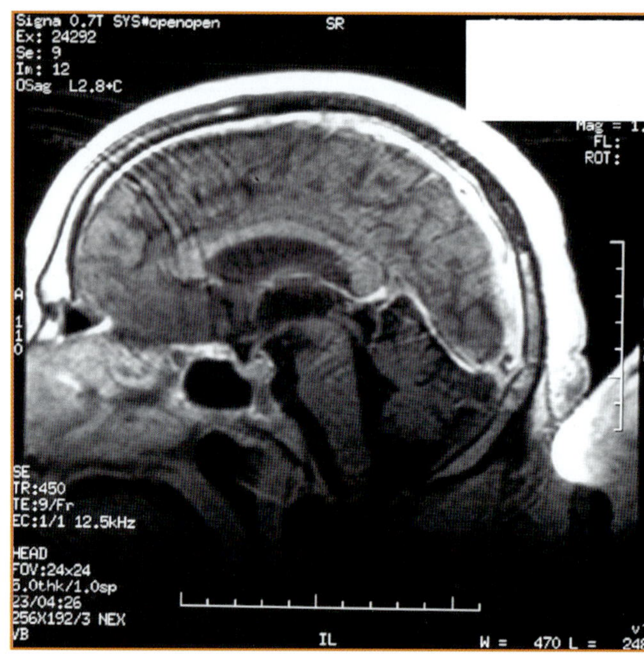

D

Figure 1–5. Clival chordoma with intradural extension and displacement of the brainstem. Preoperative MRI (**A**) axial T1 and (**B**) sagittal T1. Postoperative imaging shows complete resection following a transmaxillary approach. Postoperative MRI (**C**) axial T1 and (**D**) sagittal T1.

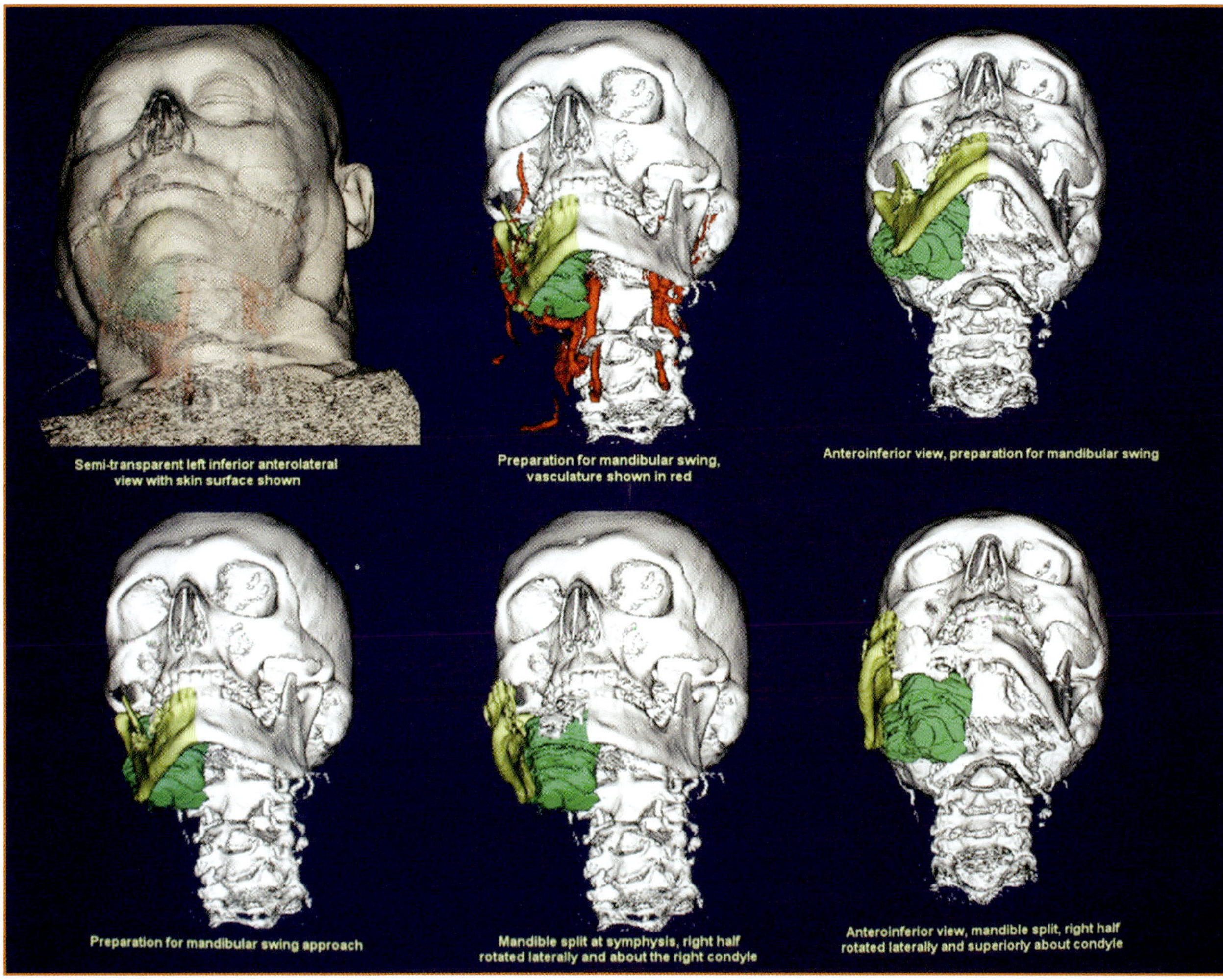

A

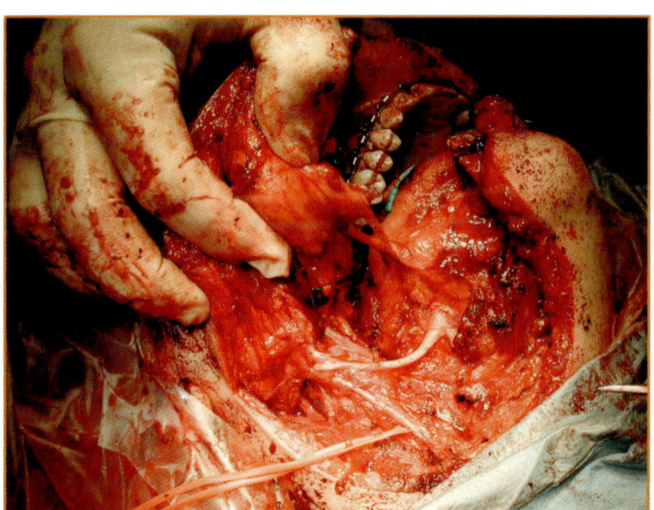

B

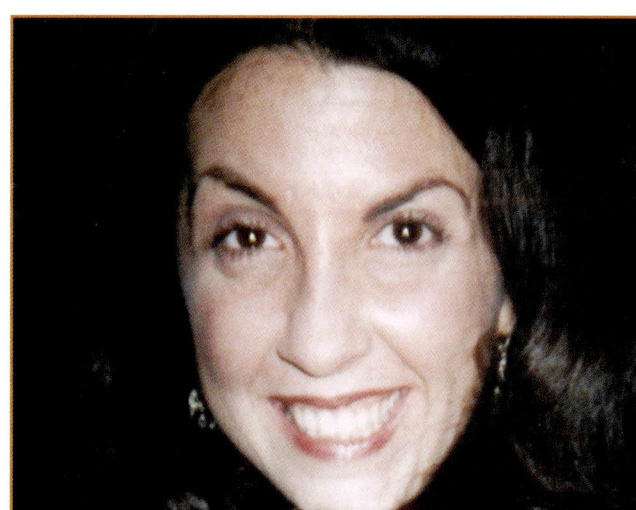

C

Figure 1–6. A. Preoperative 3-D imaging showing an acinic cell carcinoma (green) located in the right parapharyngeal/infratemporal fossa space. **B.** Intraoperative photo of the transmandibular approach and dissected anatomy. Note the lingual nerve which has been mobilized. **C.** Postoperative photo (1 year) of a patient following the transmandibular approach for a carotid body tumor extending superiorly along the vertical portion of the petrous internal carotid artery.

This maneuver allows access to the oropharynx, parapharyngeal space, and base of the tongue. By dividing the medial pterygoid muscle and sphenomandibular ligament the pterygomandibular space and infratemporal fossa medially to the cervical carotid artery complex can be accessed all the way to the petrous bone superiorly. The styloid process can be identified and used to identify the facial nerve to avoid injury. Identification of the lingual nerve and mental nerves are necessary to avoid injury, as well.[17]

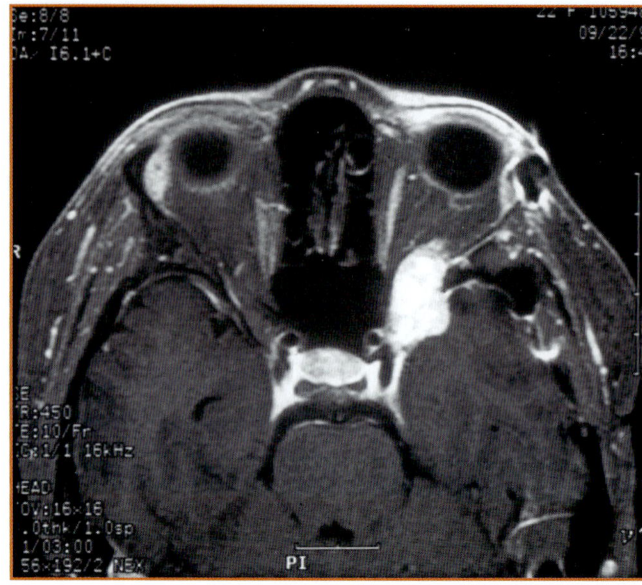

Figure 1–7. Axial T1 with gadolinium MRI image showing a meningiomas involving the right superior orbital fissure and extending into the orbit.

Anterior Skull Base Approaches (see Figure 1–1)

Orbital Osteotomy

The basis for the access to the anterior skull base is either a bifrontal or frontotemporal (pterional) craniotomy. The addition of an orbital osteotomy, first described by McArthur[22] and Frazier[23] is the basis for the cranio-orbital approach (CO). The CO provides a lower frontal approach to the anterior skull base as well as additional access to the orbit superiorly and laterally, the frontal sinus and the ethmoid air cells medially, the inferior and superior orbital fissures, and anterior clinoid process. By providing a lower trajectory to the anterior skull base, retraction of the frontal lobe is unnecessary which reduces the risk of inadvertent injury of the olfactory nerves.[24–59]

With the superior and lateral walls of the orbit removed, the medial, superior, and lateral rectus muscles are accessible, as is the levator palpebra. This allows access to the medial and lateral intraorbital compartments when pathology exists in this region (Figure 1–7). Skeletonization of the superior and inferior orbital fissures provides access to the anterior clinoid process (ACP). Continued removal of the ACP can be performed extradurally providing access to the subclinoid portion of the internal carotid artery. The superior orbital fissure allows access to cranial nerves III, IV, V1, and VI.

Glabellar Osteotomy

In cases where resection of the anterior skull base is also necessary, the incorporation of the glabella, with or without the nasion, along with bilateral superior orbital osteotomies provides wide visualization of the entire anterior skull base posteriorly to the tuberculum sella without frontal lobe retraction (Figure 1–8). This provides excellent access for the removal of the entire floor of the anterior skull base. Extending the osteotomy to include the nasion, the cranio-orbital-nasal approach, provides the widest corridor and decreases the working distance allowing access inferiorly along the clivus to the foramen magnum[60] (Figure 1–9).

Removing the floor of the anterior skull base usually requires sacrifice of the olfaction system, either unilaterally or bilaterally, depending on the extent of the cribriform plate to be sacrificed. When transection of the olfactory bulb is required the stump must be oversewn to avoid a postoperative CSF leak. Reconstruction of the anterior skull base is generally performed using a vascularized pericranial, galeopericranial, or rotational temporalis flap. Combining the subfrontal approach with the transmaxillary approach provides the basis for the anterior craniofacial resection, as shown in Figure 1–8.

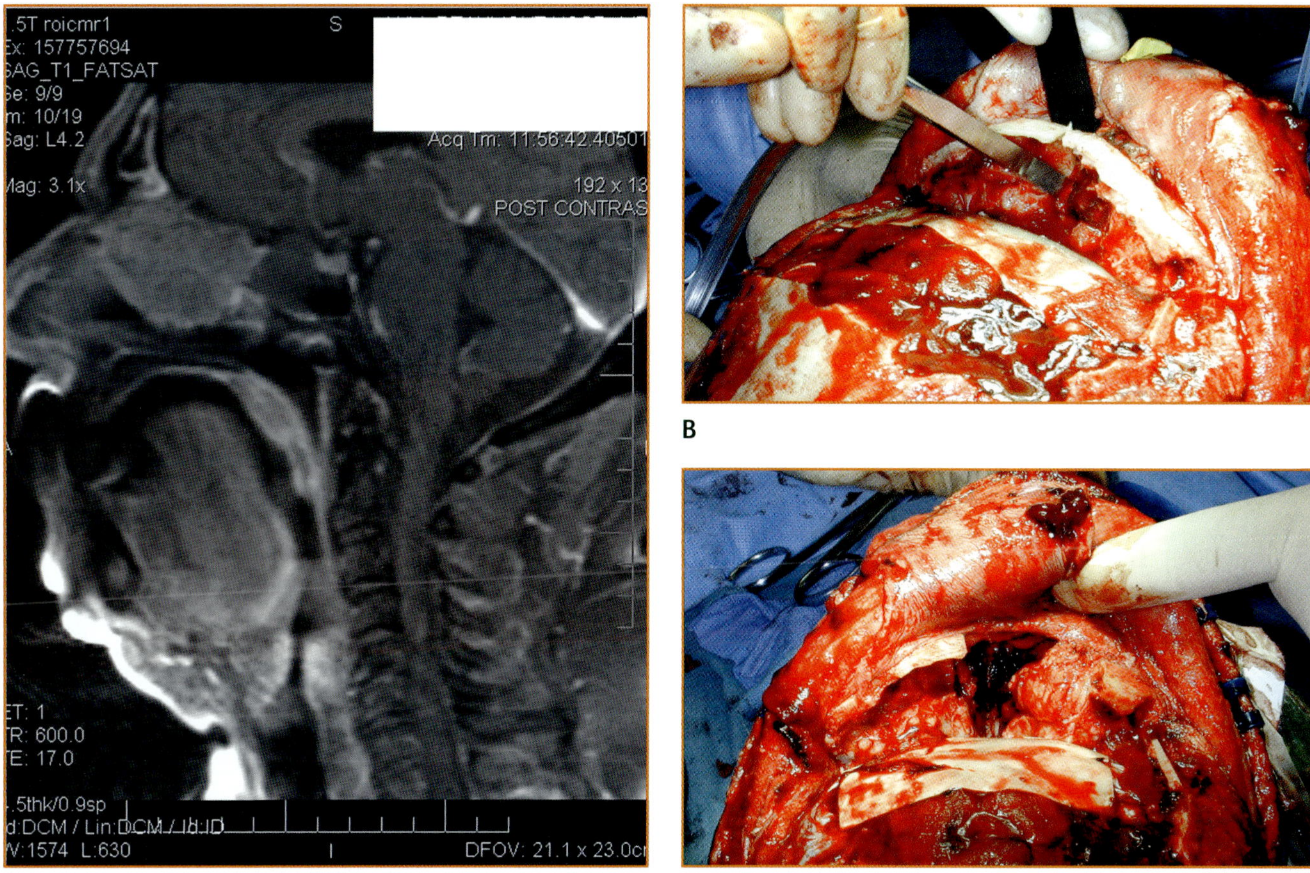

A B C

Figure 1–8. Subfrontal approach. **A.** Preoperative imaging: sagittal T1 with gadolinium showing the presence of a paranasal sinus carcinoma (inverted papilloma with carcinoma in situ) extending through the anterior skull base. **B.** Intraoperative photo showing the removal of the floor of the anterior skull base. Note that the frontal lobes have fallen posteriorly and do not require traction. **C.** The right superior orbital rim and glabella have been removed allowing visualization of the entire anterior skull base and paranasal sinuses. The tumor has been removed at this point.

LATERAL SKULL BASE APPROACHES (see Figure 1–1)

Approaches to the lateral skull base are centered on the auricle and external auditory canal (EAC). As the lateral skull base extends anteriorly from the superior orbital fissure to the transverse/sigmoid junction and roof of the mastoid posteriorly, a single trajectory is generally not possible to allow visualization of the entire area. As such, access to the lateral skull base is subdivided into two types: (1) preauricular and (2) postauricular.

Preauricular Approach

The preauricular approach provides access from the superior orbital fissure anteriorly to the level of the internal auditory canal (IAC) posteriorly (Figure 1–10). Laterally the middle meningeal artery at the foramen spinosum is the first major structure

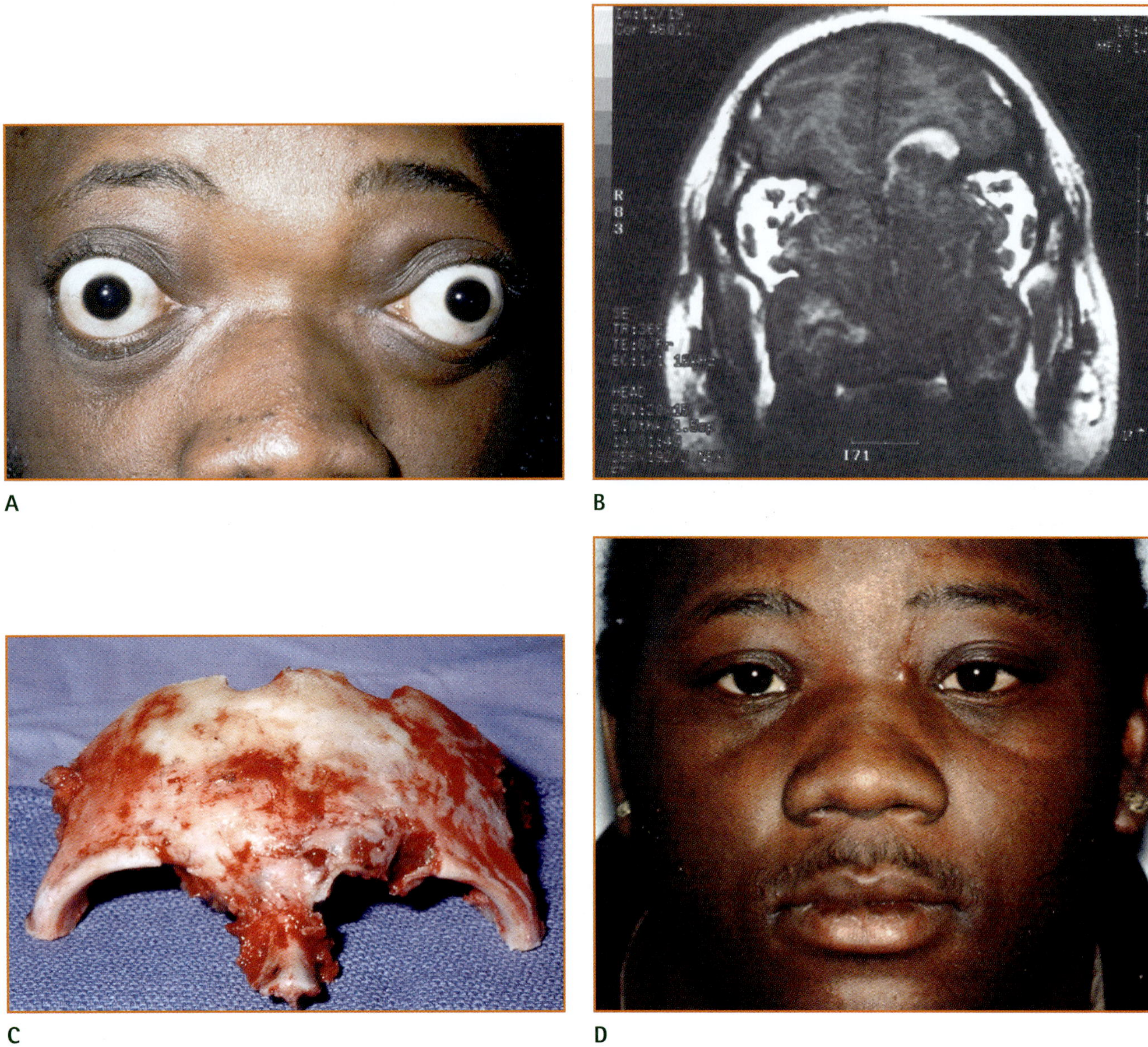

Figure 1–9. Cranio-orbital-nasal approach in which the nasion is also removed providing wider access to the anterior skull base, orbits and paranasal sinuses. **A.** Preoperative photograph of patient as he presented with progressive loss of vision. **B.** Preoperative MRI coronal T2 showing large destructive mass involving the paranasal sinuses, medial orbits and anterior skull base. **C.** Intraoperative photograph of the bone flap. **D.** Postoperative photograph (6 months) following resection.

encountered. Just anteriorly and medially to this is the foramen ovale trasmitting the mandibular branch of the trigeminal nerve (CN V3). At the same depth posteriorly, the facial hiatus with the exiting greater and lesser superficial petrosal nerves (GSPN, LSPN) can be identified as they exit the geniculate ganglion. Care must be taken to identify the GSPN and avoid unnecessary traction as this can cause inadvertent injury to the facial nerve (CN VII). Parallel and deep to the course of the GSPN, posteriorly to foramen ovale, lies the horizontal portion of the petrous part of the internal carotid artery (ICA).

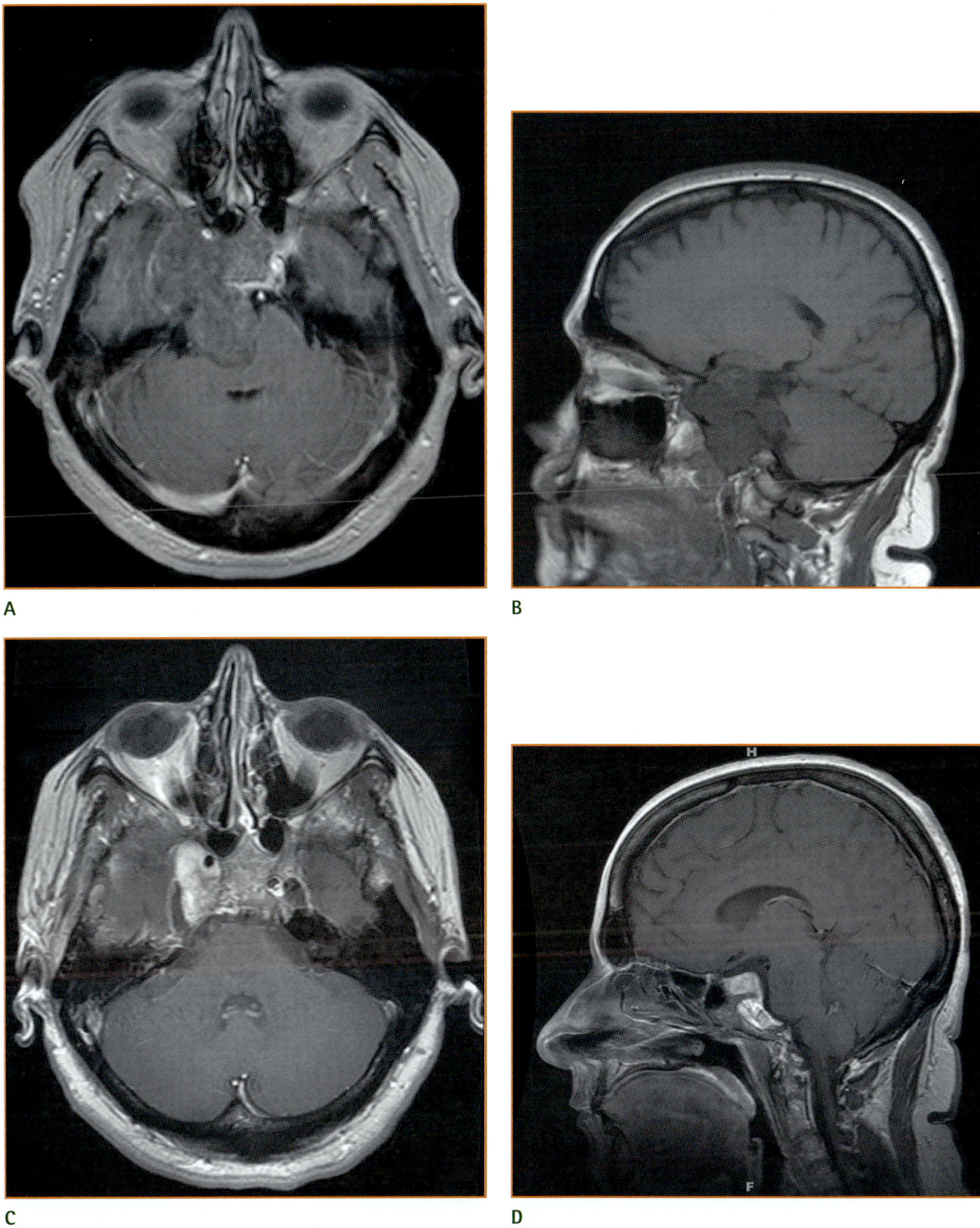

Figure 1–10. Petrous apex chondrosarcomas extending posteriorly with displacement of the brainstem accessed via preauricular middle fossa approach. Preoperative MRI T1 (**A**) axial and (**B**) sagittal. Postoperative MRI T1 with gadolinium (**C**) axial and (**D**) sagittal showing a near complete removal with residual localized to the left cavernous sinus.

The bone over the ICA around foramen ovale is generally dehiscent and care must be taken to avoid injury to the exposed ICA as it traverses the foramen lacerum entering the cavernous sinus. Parallel and lateral to the course of the petrous ICA lies the eustachian tube.[61,62]

Further anteriorly at a similar depth to ovale is the foramen rotundum transmitting the maxillary branch of the trigeminal nerve (CN V2). The lateral aspect of the sphenoid sinus can be approached by removing the bone between ovale and rotundum. Removal of bone medial to the petrous ICA, posteriorly to ovale and anterior to facial hiatus is generally safe; however, care must be taken to identify the superior semicircular canal (SSCC) to avoid inadvertent injury. The arcuate eminence should be identified; however, it is not a consistent landmark for determining the location of the SSCC. Once the SSCC is identified, the surgeon can safely begin to increase the depth of drilling to the level of the IAC.

Zygomatic Osteotomy (Extended Middle Fossa Approach)

The addition of a zygomatic osteotomy to the preauricular middle fossa approach provides access to the infratemporal fossa medial to the parotid, anterior to the cervical carotid artery complex, and posterolateral to the pterygoid plates and lateral wall of the maxillary sinus and is referred to as the extended middle fossa approach.[63] By mobilizing the zygoma, the temporalis muscle can be displaced inferiorly allowing access to the floor of the middle fossa with minimal temporal lobe retraction (Figure 1–11). The zygomatic osteotomy can be incorporated with the orbital osteotomy as a single piece or as a separate osteotomy. Generally, the osteotomies are made at the malar eminence and zygomatic root allowing the ach to be displaced inferiorly with the attached masseter muscle. In order to remove the zygoma, the masseter muscle must be dissected from its insertion and reattached at the conclusion of the case. Regardless of whether the zygoma is removed or remains attached to the masseter, secure fixation of the zygomatic arch anteriorly and posteriorly at the time of closure are necessary. Poor fixation of the zygoma can result in prolonged postoperative temporomandibular joint pain. Combining the extended middle fossa approach to the cranio-orbital approach is the basis for the cranio-orbito-zygomatic approach (COZ).[64]

Postauricular Approach

The postauricular approach has some degree of overlap with the preauricular approach. Anteriorly, the

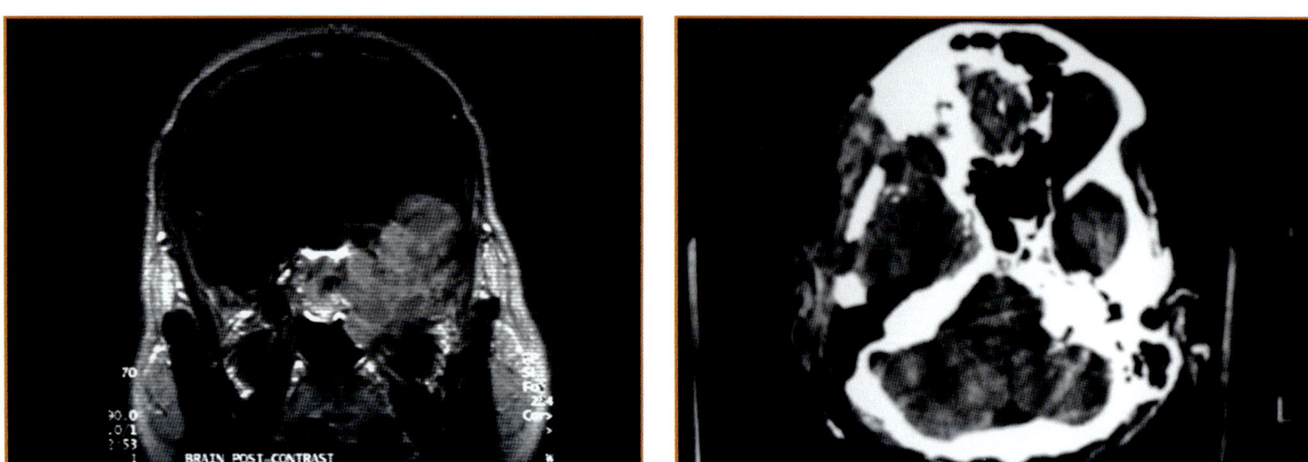

A

B

Figure 1–11. Large recurrent meningiomas extending into the infratemporal fossa and sphenoid sinus. **A.** Preoperative MRI coronal T1 with gadolinium. **B.** Postoperative axial CT showing removal of the middle fossa skull base.

postauricular approach can gain access to the facial hiatus, but provides limited access to the petrous ICA, foramen ovale, or foramen spinosum. The postauricular approach also provides excellent access to the IAC. Posteriorly, this approach can extend access posteriorly to the level of the transverse/sigmoid junction making this an ideal approach for lesions extending from the floor of the middle fossa into the mastoid. As it provides access to both the IAC and mastoid it is generally preferred for accessing lesions involving the facial nerve (CN VII) at the level of the geniculate ganglion.

POSTEROLATERAL SKULL BASE (see Figure 1–1)

The focal point of the posterolateral approaches is the sigmoid sinus (SS). As the SS generally cannot be sacrificed safely, the skull base approaches are based on its preservation. These approaches provide access to one of the most difficult and potentially devastating regions of the skull base. In the area demarcated by the tentorium superiorly and the foramen magnum inferiorly the region is composed of 9 of the 12 pairs of cranial nerves, the brainstem, arteries of the posterior circulation, and a substantial volume of the brain's venous outflow. With these approaches, intraoperative electrophysiological monitoring is recommended.[65,66] There are two major subdivisions of the posterolateral approaches: (1) presigmoid and (2) retrosigmoid.

Presigmoid Approaches

These approaches are posterior and lateral to the sigmoid sinus. This entire area is limited by the floor of the middle fossa and superior petrosal sinus superiorly, the EAC laterally, the jugular bulb and foramen inferiorly, and the sigmoid sinus medially. Essentially, the entire working corridor is the solid bone of the mastoid, which contains the semicircular canals, the cochlea, the vertical segment of the facial canal, and the vertical segment of the petrous ICA. Therefore, removing bone in this region risks these structures. Therefore, these approaches are further divided into hearing preservation and hearing loss. The hearing preservation approach is limited to the retrolabyrinthine approach. The remaining approaches, the translabyrinthine and transcochlear approaches require sacrifice of hearing ipsilaterally. Due to the large amount of bone removed this ultimately can lead to a significant dead space. Second, when opening of the dura is necessary it is usually not possible to obtain a watertight dural closure, it is recommended to fill this space with autologous fat, with care taken to avoid overpacking.

Retrolabyrinthine Approach

Although this approach saves hearing, its utility is extremely limited as it provides a very limited working corridor with poor intradural visibility. It may be useful when lesions are confined to the mastoid, the facial canal, or in combination with the postauricular middle fossa approach. For lesions of the middle fossa extending into the mastoid cavity (ie, encephaloceles) this provides visualization of the entire defect and access to the middle ear structures. Intradurally, this approach, combined with the postauricular middle fossa approach allows for the mobilization of the transverse sigmoid junction by sacrificing the superior petrosal sinus. The petrosal approach, first described by Al-Mefty,[67] provides wide access to the incisura by transecting the tentorium. This provides access from CN III at the level of the midbrain to the jugular foramen (CN IX–XI) at the pontomedullary junction and medially to the midline of the clivus (Figure 1–12).

Translabyrinthine Approach (TL)

Since this procedure was first described by William House in 1960, this approach has served as a mainstay for the surgical treatment of vestibular schwannoma (acoustic neuromas).[68,69] The hallmark of the approach is the removal of the labyrinth to provide wide access to the IAC, porus acousticus, and cerebellopontine angle (CPA) while minimizing retraction of the cerebellum. However, its utility is limited superiorly by the entrance to Meckel's cave and CN V and inferiorly by the jugular foramen. These anatomic restrictions, as well as the sacrifice of the

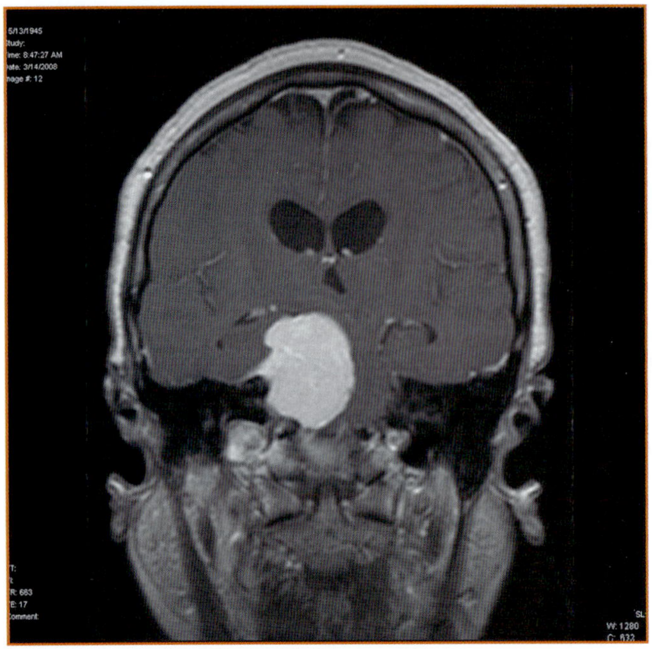

A

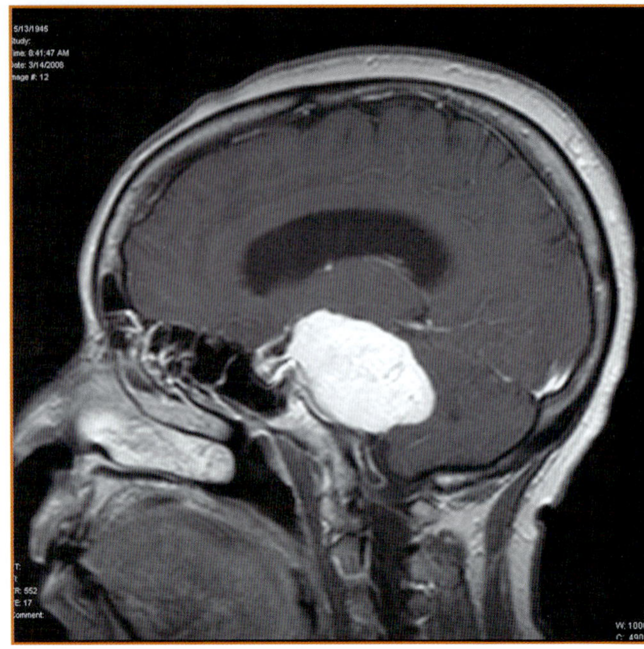

B

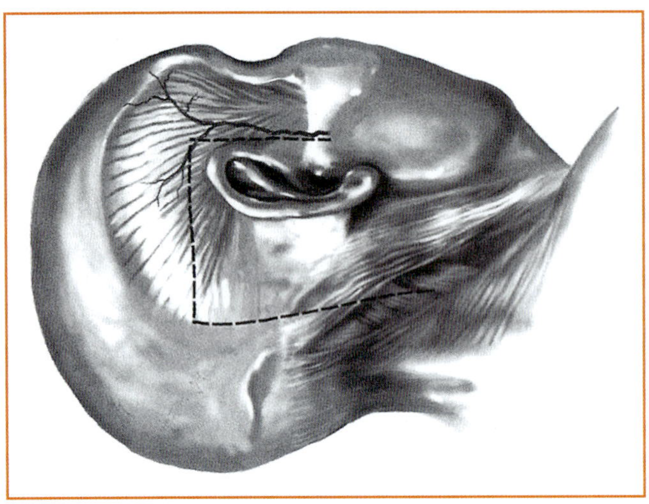

C

Figure 1–12. The petrosal approach. Preoperative MRI of a petroclival meningiomas **(A)** coronal T1 and **(B)** sagittal T1 with gadolinium. **C.** Standard incision for the petrosal approach.

vestibular and auditory function, limit its utility to lesions of CN VII and VIII, and lesions of the CPA that do not involve or extend above the tentorium or below the jugular foramen.

Transcochlear Approach

As anterior exposure is necessary, the cochlea and EAC are sacrificed.[70,71] By removing the cochlea, the entire posterior aspect of the petrous bone can be removed. This provides access to the vertical segment of the petrous ICA and the clivus and its surrounding structures while significantly reducing retraction of the cerebellum. Combining this with an anterior petrosectomy via the preauricular middle fossa approach, a complete petrosectomy can be achieved which is occasionally required for temporal bone malignancies[72] (Figure 1–13).

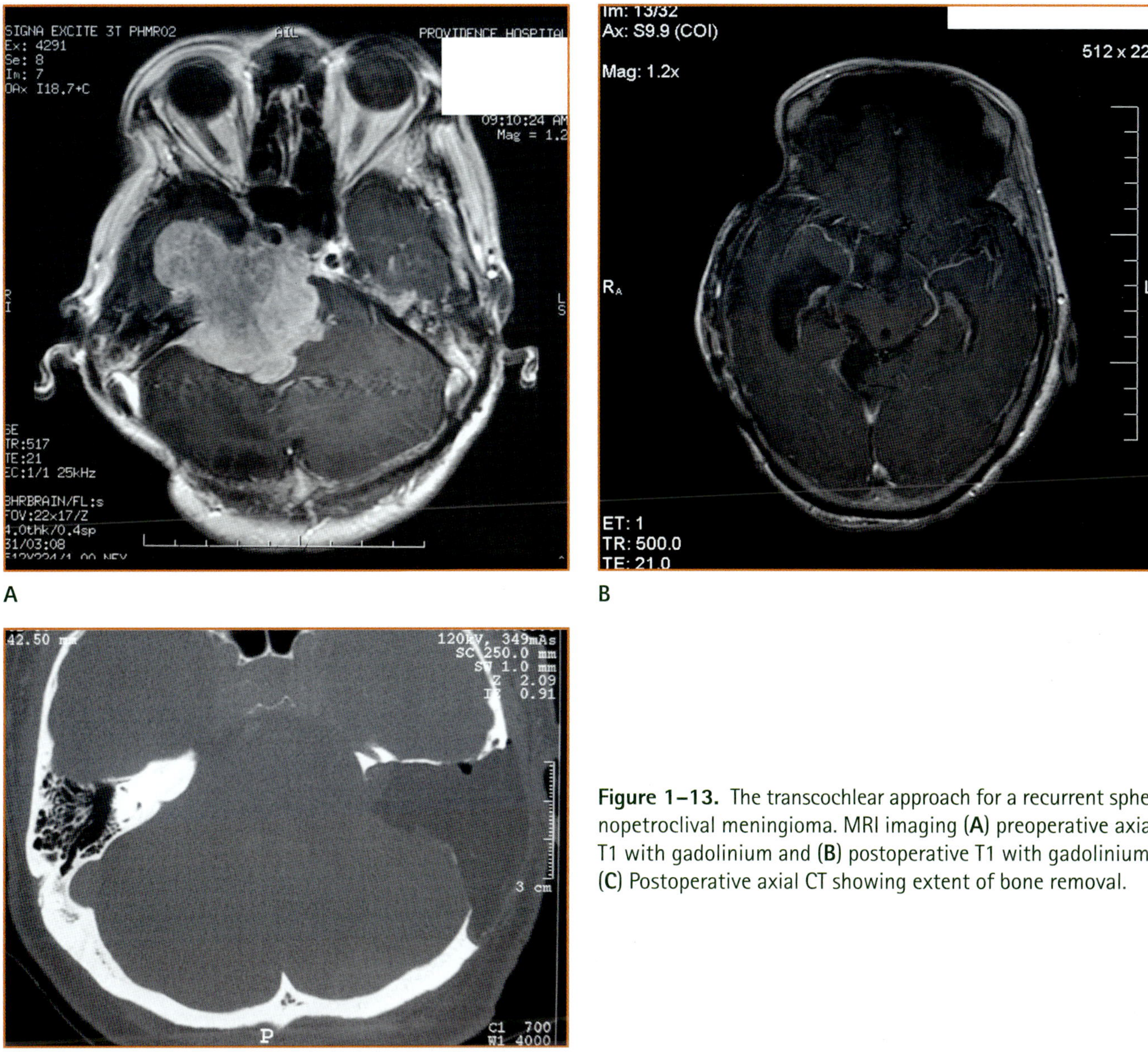

A B C

Figure 1–13. The transcochlear approach for a recurrent sphenopetroclival meningioma. MRI imaging (**A**) preoperative axial T1 with gadolinium and (**B**) postoperative T1 with gadolinium. (**C**) Postoperative axial CT showing extent of bone removal.

Retrosigmoid Approaches

Unlike the presigmoid approaches, the retrosigmoid approaches are all located medially to the sigmoid sinus. They are limited by the transverse sinus which lies at the level of the tentorium superiorly, the sigmoid sinus and jugular bulb laterally, and the foramen magnum inferiorly. These approaches provide a wide array of surgical applications to the posterolateral skull base. As the approach directly overlies the lateral cerebellar hemisphere it is ideally suited for lesions involving the CPA (Figure 1–14). Unlike the presigmoid approaches, the retrosigmoid approaches require mobilization and retraction of the cerebellum in order to access the CPA. Accessing the arachnoid cisterns and removing CSF at the level of the cisterna magna or the supracerebellar cistern generally provides sufficient relaxation to

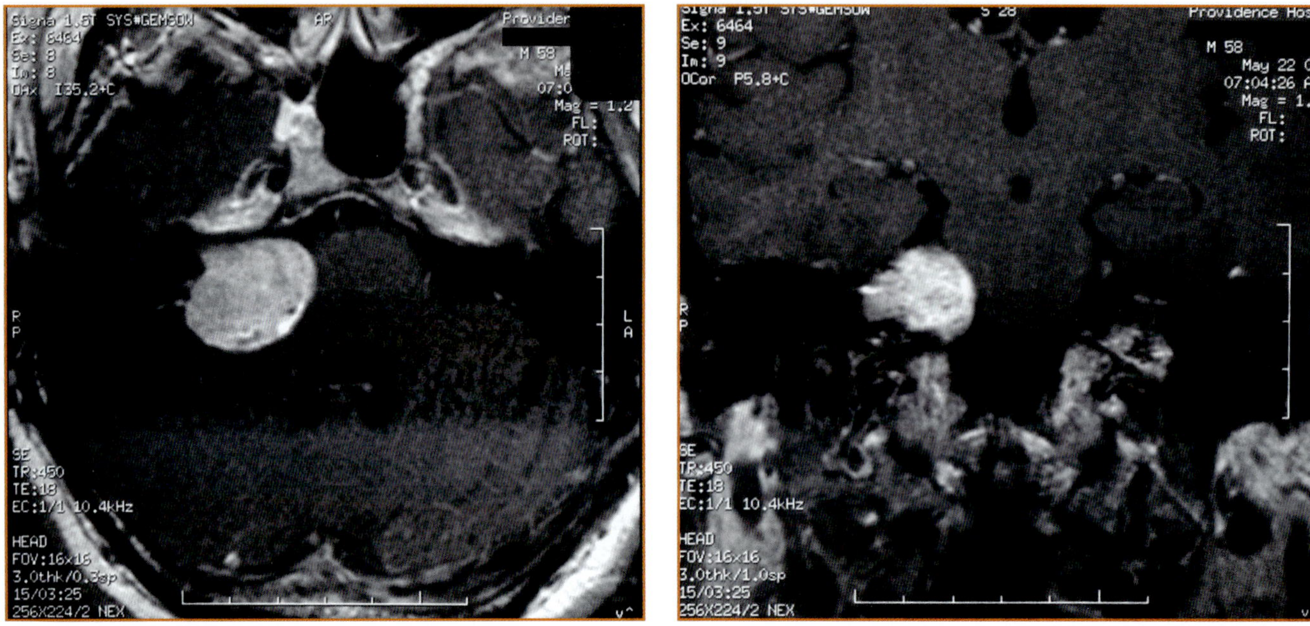

A B

Figure 1–14. Indications for retrosigmoid approach. Vestibular schwannoma with excellent hearing preoperatively. The tumor has limited extension into the internal auditory canal. Preoperative MRI **(A)** axial T1 and **(B)** coronal T1 with gadolinium.

the cerebellar hemisphere, minimizing the extent of retraction required. Because of the enhanced superior-inferior access to the CPA these approaches can be combined with the presigmoid approaches to provide wide access with minimal retraction.

Extreme Lateral Approach

The extreme lateral approach is a further extension of the retrosigmoid approach. This is generally combined with the presigmoid retrolabyrinthine approach described above to provide access to the entire jugular foramen. This approach is ideally suited for lesions that involve the jugular bulb (ie, glomus jugulare) of the jugular foramen (lower CN schwannoma) (Figure 1–15). As a large number of these lesions will affect the venous outflow, a preoperative study to determine patency of the jugular bulb generally is recommended. If, however, there is any question as to the patency of the sinus, care should be taken to preserve it as sacrifice of an otherwise flowing sinus can lead to a fatal outcome.

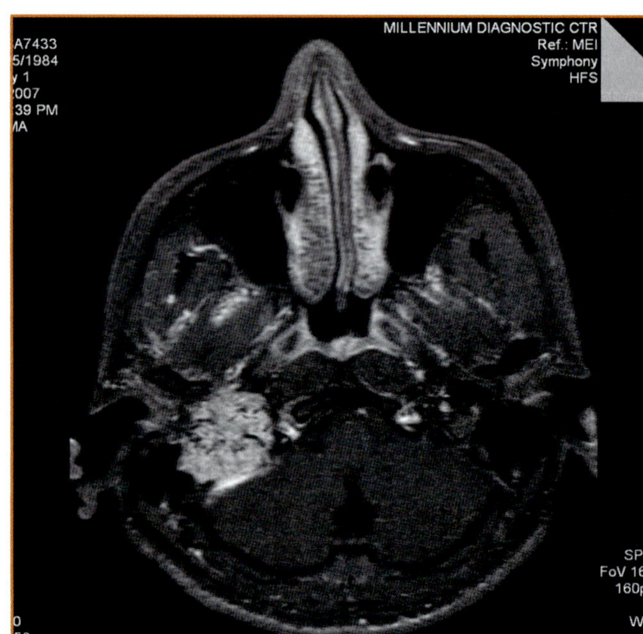

Figure 1–15. Indication for extreme lateral approach. Glomus jugulare extending anteriorly to the level of the vertical segment of the petrous internal carotid artery.

Additionally, due to the functional aspect of the lower cranial nerves (CN IX to XI) a thorough preoperative examination is recommended. An in-depth discussion with the patient and their family about the possibility of postoperative dysphagia and dysphonia requiring either prolonged enteral assistance or tracheostomy is also recommended.

In cases where the lesion extends distally to the jugular bulb or jugular foramen an additional lateral neck dissection may be necessary. When manipulation of the lower cranial nerves is expected, intraoperative electrophysiological monitoring can be of significant assistance. Identifying the neurovascular structures distally, as well as proximally and monitoring their function in real time will allow the surgeon to minimize the risk of inadvertent injury.

Transcondylar Approach

Extending the retrosigmoid approach below the foramen magnum provides unimpeded access to the cervicomedullary junction, the vertebral-basilar junction and the posterior inferior cerebellar artery (PICA) origin, hypoglossal canal, and the superior cervical spine. This approach is utilized for lesions located ventrolateral to the cervicomedullary junction either intradurally (ie, meningiomas) or extradurally (Figure 1–16). The hallmark of the procedure is the subtotal removal of the occipital condyle. As the occipital condyle provides the stability for the craniocervical articulation, the greatest risk in this procedure is instability requiring an occipital-cervical fusion. To that extent, care should be taken to remove the least amount of the condyle necessary to achieve adequate visualization. As discussed with all of the posterolateral skull base approaches, intraoperative electrophysiological monitoring is generally utilized specifically monitoring CN IX to XII and somatosensory evoked potentials (SSEP).

Positioning the patient correctly is essential for this approach. Flexing the neck and extending the head away from the side of the approach without

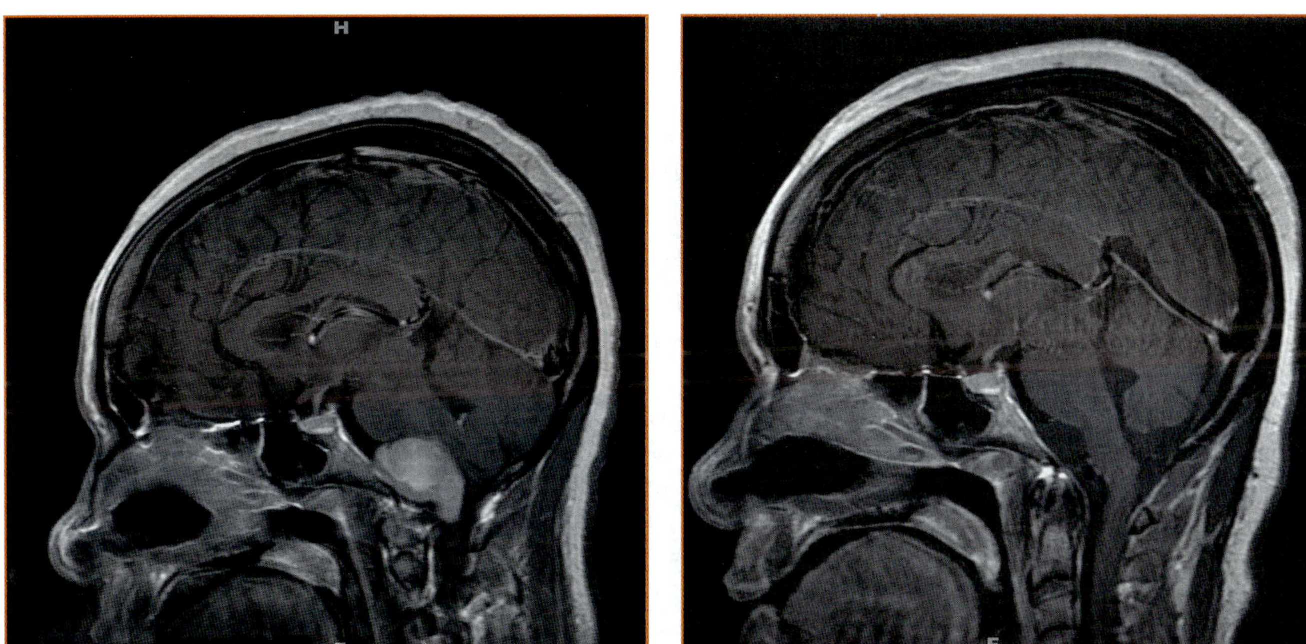

A B

Figure 1–16. Indication of the transcondylar approach. **A.** The tumor is extending through the foramen magnum resulting in significant brainstem compression. **B.** Postoperatively, the tumor has been totally removed resulting in decompression of the cervicomedullary junction.

rotation the head will provide ease of access to this region. Avoiding any rotation of the head is important as this allows the vertebral artery to maintain its neutral position. A variety of incisions have been described for this procedure. Typically, a C-shaped postauricular incision from the top of the pinna superiorly and extending inferiorly below the mastoid tip and anteriorly to the anterior border of the sternocleidomastoid muscle is utilized. In cases where an occipital fusion is expected, a hockey-stick incision can be utilized to provide access to the midline of the cervical spine posteriorly for the planned instrumentation. After the sternocleidomastoid muscle has been incised at its insertion site form the skull, the lateral aspect of the C1 lamina should be identified approximately one finger breadth below the tip of the mastoid. Once the C1 lamina is identified, the vertebral artery (VA) can more easily be located. Identifying the VA is crucial before initiating the condylectomy. Another structure to be identified prior to the condylectomy is the mastoid vein. This vein can be quite large in some case and identification and control or coagulation prior to the condylectomy will minimize unnecessary blood loss. As with the presigmoid approaches described above, obtaining a watertight dural closure is not always possible and a substantial amount of dead space can be encountered. Preparation needs to be made for autologous fat, fascia graft, or vascularized flaps for complex closures.

CONCLUSION

There are wide arrays of approaches available to access the skull base. Unfortunately, there is little uniformity in nomenclature. Additionally, for the surgeon in training poor understanding of the anatomic principles of the varied approaches can lead to an inappropriate procedure choice creating a less than optimal surgical exposure and/or outcome. Although there is no substitute for familiarity of the anatomy and comfort with the technical aspects of any surgical approach, understanding the indications and even more importantly, the limitations of each of the major approaches to the skull base will provide a foundation for the skull base surgeon.

REFERENCES

1. Rhoton AL. The anterior and middle cranial base. *Neurosurgery*. 2002;51(suppl 1):273.
2. Ammirati M, Bernardo A. Analytical evaluation of complex anterior approaches to the cranial base: an anatomic study. *Neurosurgery*. 1998;43:1398.
3. Jackson IT, Marsh WR, Bite U, Hide TAH. Craniofacial osteotomies to facilitate skull base tumor resection. *Br J Plast Surg*. 1986;39:153.
4. Biller HF, Lawson W, Sachdev VP. Estesioneuroplastoma: surgical treatment without radiation. *Laryngoscope*. 1990;100:1199.
5. Wood BG, Sadar ES, Levine HL. Surgical problems of the base of the skull. *Arch Otolaryngol*. 1980;106:1.
6. Jackson IT. Craniofacial approach to tumors of the head and neck. *Clin Plast Surg*. 1985;12:375.
7. Jackson IT, Hide TAH. A systemic approach to tumors of the base of the skull. *J Maxillofac Surg*. 1982;10:92.
8. James D, Crockard HA. Surgical access to the base of the skull and upper cervical spine by extended maxillotomy. *Neurosurgery*. 1991;29:411.
9. Eisig SB, Goodrich JT. Transfacial approaches to the cranial base. *Atlas Oral Maxillofac Surg Clin North Am*. 2002;10:73.
10. Shah JP. Surgery of the anterior skull base for malignant tumors. *Acta Otorhinolaryngol Belg*. 1999;53:1.
11. Osguthorpe JD, Patel S. Craniofacial approaches to tumors pf the anterior skull base. *Otolaryngol Clin North Am*. 2001;34:1123.
12. Lello G, Statham P, Steere J, McGurk M. Craniofacial access to the anterior and middle cranial fossae and skull base. *J Craniomaxillofac Surg*. 1997;25:285.
13. Tzortzidis F, Bejjani G, Papadas T, et al. Craniofacial osteotomies to facilitate resection of large tumors of the anterior skull base. *J Craniomaxillofac Surg*. 1996;24:224.
14. Rhoton AL. The sellar region. *Neurosurgery*. 2002;51(suppl):335.
15. Ammirati M, Ma J, Cheatham ML, Mei ZT, Bloch J, Becker DP. The mandibular swing-transcervical approach to the skull base: anatomical study. *J Neurosurg*. 1993;78:673.
16. Pieper DR, LaRouere M, Jackson, IT. Operative management of skull base malignancies: choosing the appropriate approach. *Neurosurg Focus*. 2002;12:1.
17. Moreira-Gonzalez A, Pieper DR, Balaguer CJ, Nikolis A, Jackson IT. Skull base tumors: a comprehensive review of the transfacial swing osteotomy approaches. *Plast Reconstr Surg*. 2005;115:711.
18. Jackson IT, Pieper DR. The palatal overlap flap: a modification of the maxillary swing procedure to prevent ascending infection. *Skull Base*. In press.
19. Henderson W. The pituitary adenomata: a follow-up study of the surgical results in 338 cases (Dr. Cushing's series). *Br J Surg*. 1939;26:811.

20. Cushing H. Transsphenoidal methods of access. In: Cushing H, ed. *The Pituitary Body and Its Disorders*. Philadelphia, PA: JB Lippincott; 1912:296–303.
21. Spiro RH, Gerold FP, Strong EW. Mandibular osteotomy in the surgical approach to the oral cavity. *Head Neck Surg*. 1981;3:371.
22. McArthur LL. An aseptic surgical access to the pituitary body and its neighborhood. *JAMA*. 1912;58:2009.
23. Frazier CH. An approach to the hypophysis through the anterior cranial fossa. *Ann Surg*. 1913;57:145.
24. Alaywan M, Sindou M: Fronto-temporal approach with orbito-zygomatic removal. Surgical anatomy. *Acta Neurochir*. 1990;104:79–83.
25. Al-Mefty O. The supraorbital-pterional approach to skull base lesions. *Neurosurgery*. 1987;21:474–477.
26. Blacklock JB, Weber RS, Lee YY, Goepfert H. Transcranial resection of tumors of the paranasal sinuses and nasal cavity. *J Neurosurg*. 1989;71:10–15.
27. Delfini R, Ianetti G, Belli E, Santoro A, Ciapetta P, Cantore G. Cranio-facial approaches for tumors involving the anterior half of the skull base. *Acta Neurochir*. 1993; 124:53–60.
28. Derome P. Les tumeeurs Spheno-ethmoidales. Possibilites d'exerese et de reparation chirurgicales. *Neurochirurgie*. 1972(suppl 1);18:1–164.
29. Donald PJ. Craniofacial surgery for head and neck cancer. In: Johnson JT, Blitzer A, Ossoff RH, et al, eds. *American Academy of Otolaryngology-Head and Neck Surgery: Instructional Courses. Vol 2*. St. Louis, MO: Mosby; 1989:225–253.
30. Hakuba A, Lui SS, Nishimura S. The orbitozygomatic infratemporal approach: a new surgical technique. *Surg Neurol*. 1986;26:271–276.
31. Jackson IT. Craniofacial osteotomies to facilitate resection of tumors of the skull base. In: Wilkins RH, Reganchary SS, eds. *Neurosurgery Update I*. New York, NY: McGraw-Hill; 1990: 277–291.
32. Jane JA, Park TS, Poberskin LH, Winn HR, Butler AB. The supraorbital approach: technical note. *Neurosurgery*. 1982;11:537–542.
33. Kaplan MJ, Jane JA, Park TS, Cantrell RW. Supraorbital rim approach to the anterior skull base. *Laryngoscope*. 1984;94:1137–1139.
34. Ketcham AS, Hoye RC, Van Buren JM, Johnson RH, Smith RR. Complications of intracranial facial resection for tumors of the paranasal sinuses. *Am J Surg*. 1966;112: 591–596.
35. Naumann HH. Chirurgie der Nasennebenhohle. In: Naumann HH, ed. *Kopf- und Halschirurgie. Vol. 2*. Stuttgart: Thieme; 1974: 409–530.
36. Pinsolle J, San-Galli F, Siberchicot F, Caix P, Emparanza A, Michelet FX. Modified approach for ethmoid and anterior skull base surgery. *Arch Otolaryngol Head Neck Surg*. 1991;117:779–782.
37. Raveh J. Das eintzeitige Vorgehan bei der Widerherstellung von Frontobasal-Mittelgesichtsfrakturen. Modifikationen und Behandlungsmodalitaten. *Chirurgie*. 1983; 54:677–686.
38. Raveh J. Neue Aspekte der kraniofazialen Chirurgie. *Schweiz Monatsschr Zahnmed*. 1986;96:406–424.
39. Raveh J, Laedrach K, Speiser M, et al. The subcranial approach for fronto-orbital and anteroposterior skull-base tumors. *Arch Otolaryngol Head Neck Surg*. 1993;119:385–393.
40. Raveh J, Laedrich K, Vuillemin T, Zingg M. Management of combined frontonaso-orbital/skull base fractures and telecanthus in 355 cases. *Arch Otolaryngol Head Neck Surg*. 1992;118:605–614.
41. Raveh J, Neiger M. Die Wiederherstellung bei schweren Gesichtsschadelverletzungen. *Schweiz Monatsschr Zahnheilkd*. 1981;91:206–217.
42. Raveh J, Redli M, Markwalder TM. Operative management of 194 cases of combined maxillofacial-frontobasal fractures: principles and modifications. *J Oral Maxillofac Surg*. 1984;42:555–564.
43. Raveh J, Vuillemin T. Advantages of an additional subcranial approach in correction of craniofacial deformities. *J Craniomaxillofac Surg*. 1988;16:350–358.
44. Raveh J, Vuillemin T. Subcranial management of 395 combined frontobasal-midface fractures. *Arch Otolaryngol Head Neck Surg*. 1988;114:1114–1122.
45. Raveh J, Vuillemin T. The subcranial-supraorbital temporal approach for tumor resection. *J Craniofacial Surg*. 1990;1:53–59.
46. Raveh J, Vuillemin T. The surgical one-stage management of combined cranio-maxillo-facial and frontobasal fractures. Advantages of the subcranial approach in 374 cases. *J Craniomaxillofac Surg*. 1988;16:160–178.
47. Rinehart GC, Jackson IT, Potparic Z, Tan RG, Chambers PA. Management of locally aggressive sinus disease using craniofacial exposure and the galeal frontalis fascia-muscle flap. *Plast Reconstr Surg*. 1993;92:1219–1225.
48. Schramm VL Jr, Myers EN, Maroon JC. Anterior skull base surgery for benign and malignant disease. *Laryngoscope*. 1979;89:1077–1091.
49. Sekhar LN, Janecka IP, Jones NF. Subtemporal-infratemporal and basal subfrontal approach to extensive cranial bese tumors. *Acta Neurochir*. 1988;92:83–92.
50. Sekhar LN, Nanda A, Sen CN, Snyderman CN, Janecka IP. The extended frontal approach to tumors of the anterior, middle and posterior skull base. *J Neurosurg*. 1992;76: 198–206.
51. Smith RR, Klopp CT, Williams JM. Surgical treatment of cancer of the frontal sinus and adjacent areas. *Cancer*. 1954;7:991–994.
52. Tessier P, Guiot G, Rougerie J. Osteotomies cranio-naso-orbito-faciales. Hypertelorisme. *Ann Chir Plast*. 1967;12: 103–118.
53. Van Buren JM, Ommaya AK, Ketcham AS: Ten years' experience with radical combined craniofacial resection of malignant tumors of the paranasal sinuses. *J Neurosurg*. 1969;28:341–350.

54. Raveh J, Turk JB, Ladrach K, Seiler R, et al. Extended anterior subcranial approach for skull base tumors: long-term results. *J Neurosurg*. 995;82:1002–1010.
55. Lesoin F, Pellerin P, Villete L, Jomin M. Interet de la mobilisation du volet orbito-zygomatic-malaire. *Neurochirurgie*. 1986;32:90–93.
56. Persing JA, Jane JA, Levine PA, Cantrell RW. The versatile frontal sinus approach to the floor of the anterior cranial fossa. Technical note. *J Neurosurg*. 1990;72:513–516.
57. Ray BS, McLean JM. Combined intracranial and orbital operation for retinoblastoma. *Arch Ophthalmol.* 1943;30: 437–445.
58. Sekhar LN, Sen CN, Jho HD, Janecka IP. Surgical treatment of intracavernous neoplasms: a four-year experience. *Neurosurgery*. 1989;24:18–30.
59. Sundaresan N, Shah JP. Craniofacial resection for anterior skull base tumors. *Head Neck Surg*. 1988;10:219–224.
60. Hanna E, Linskey M, Pieper D. Surgical approaches to malignant tumors of the skull base. In: Sekhar LN, ed. *Atlas of Neurosurgical Techniques*. New York, NY: Thieme Medical Publishers, Inc; 2005.
61. Pieper DR, Al-Mefty O, Hanada Y, Buechner D. Hyperostosis associated with meningiomas of the skull base: secondary changes or tumor invasion. *Neurosurg*. 1999; 44:742.
62. Pieper DR, Al-Mefty O. Management of intracranial meningiomas secondarily involving the infratemporal fossa: radiographic characteristics, pattern of tumor invasion and surgical implications. *Neurosurgery*. 1999;45:231.
63. Al-Mefty O, Anand VK. Zygomatic approach to skull base lesions. *J Neurosurg*. 1990;73:668.
64. Pieper DR, Al-Mefty O. Cranio-orbitozygomatic approach. In: Spetzler RF, ed. *Operative Techniques in Neurosurgery*. Philadelphia, PA: WB Saunders, 1999;2(1):1–6.
65. Pieper DR, Al-Mefty O. The surgical management of petroclival meningiomas. In: Black PM, Kaye A, eds. *Operative Neurosurgery*. London, UK: Harcourt Brace; 2000.
66. Pieper DR, Al-Mefty O. Petroclival/sphenopetroclival meningiomas. In: Robertson J, Robertson J, Coakham H, eds. *Cranial Base Surgery: Management, Complications and Outcome*. London, UK: Churchill Livingston/WB Saunders; 2000.
67. Al-Mefty O, Fox JL, Smith RR. Petrosal approach for petroclival meningiomas. *Neurosurgery*. 1988;22:510.
68. House WF. Acoustic neuroma (Monograph). *Arch Otolaryngol Head Neck Surg*. 1964;80:598.
69. House WF. Translabrynthine approach. In: House WF, Luetje CM, eds. *Acoustic Tumors, Vol 2: Management*. Baltimore, MD: University Park Press; 1979:43–87.
70. House WF, De La Cruz A. Transcochlear approach to the petros apex and clivus. *Trans Am Acad Ophthalmol Otolaryngol*. 1977;84:927.
71. House WF, Hitselberger WE. The transcochlear approach to the skull base. *Arch Otolaryngol Head Neck Surg*. 1976; 102:334.
72. Pieper DR, Al-Mefty O. Total petrosectomy approach. In: Spetzler RF, ed. *Operative Techniques in Neurosurgery*. Philadelphia, PA: WB Saunders; 1999.2(1):1–6.

CHAPTER 2

Surgical Approaches to the Skull Base

Rodney C. Diaz and Seilesh Babu

INTRODUCTION

The neurotology/neurosurgery team has at its disposal numerous approaches for traversing the lateral skull base and accessing the intracranial vault.[1] The discussion of approaches is divided, somewhat arbitrarily, into three general categories: transtemporal approaches, suboccipital approaches, and subtemporal approaches.

The transtemporal approaches are grouped to encompass techniques in which the temporal bone is the primary target through which dissection and intracranial access are achieved. The suboccipital approaches group those procedures where variations in suboccipital craniotomies provide access to the posterior fossa. The subtemporal approaches are those procedures where access to varying regions of the middle or posterior fossae is achieved caudal to the temporal lobe.

Finally, combined middle fossa–posterior fossa approaches is discussed. As to be demonstrated, many approaches combine elements of subtemporal, suboccipital, and transtemporal vectors and can be considered in multiple ways.

TRANSTEMPORAL APPROACHES

Lateral Temporal Bone Resection

The lateral temporal bone resection is performed when the tumor involves the external auditory canal and extends to, but not beyond, the tympanic membrane (Figure 2–1). In cases where the tumor has extended beyond the bony confines of the external auditory canal or through the tympanic membrane and involving the mesotympanum or mastoid air cells, a subtotal or total temporal bone resection is indicated (Figures 2–2 and 2–3).

These surgical approaches are described in detail in Chapter 3.

Translabyrinthine Approach

The translabyrinthine approach to the lateral skull base is considered the workhorse of surgical approaches to the cerebellopontine angle used by neurotologists. It provides excellent visualization of the facial nerve along its entire course, shortened depth of tumor dissection from the outer cortex, complete visualization of the internal auditory canal, wide access to the cerebellopontine angle, and minimal cerebellar retraction. The anatomy of the mastoid and posterior otic capsule is familiar, and the approach is a natural extension of the commonly dissected anatomic spaces within the temporal bone (Figure 2–4).

Surgical Technique

In preparation for a translabyrinthine approach, the patient is positioned supine and rotated 180 degrees away from anesthesia. The head is turned and secured with approximately 60 degrees rotation away from the side of tumor and with maximal flexion of the chin onto the shoulder.

Preoperative preparation of the surgical wound site begins with adequate shaving of scalp hair

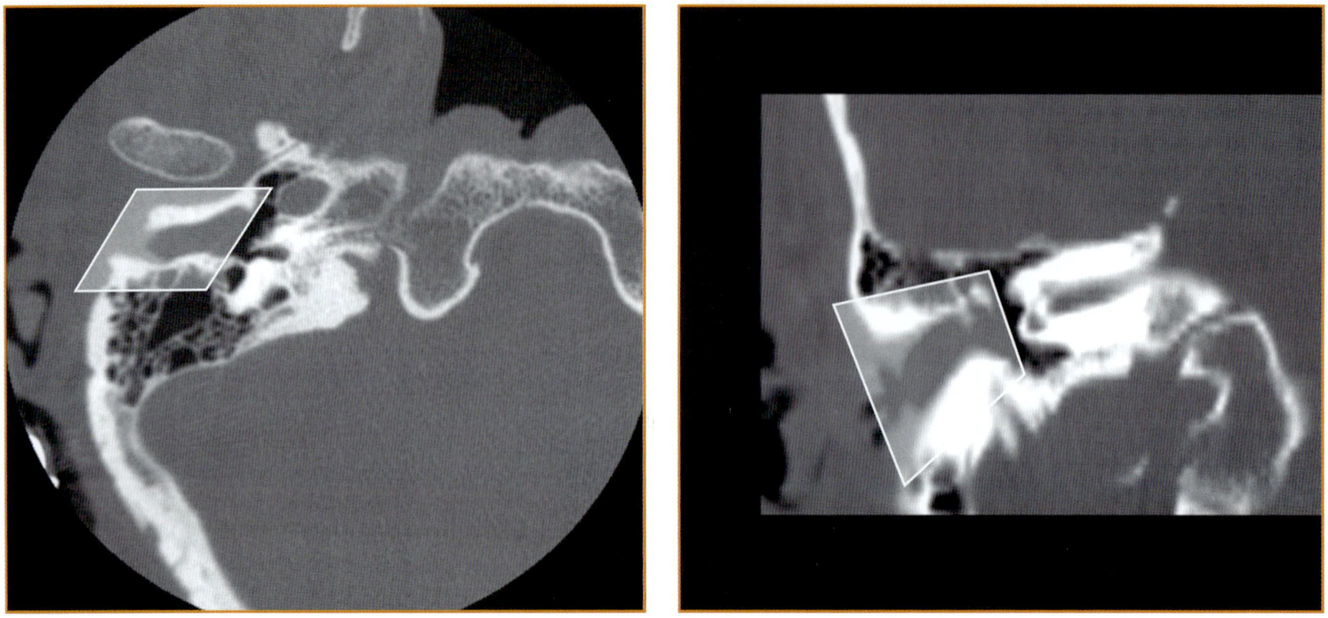

A B

Figure 2–1. Lateral temporal bone resection, schematic, axial (**A**) and coronal (**B**).

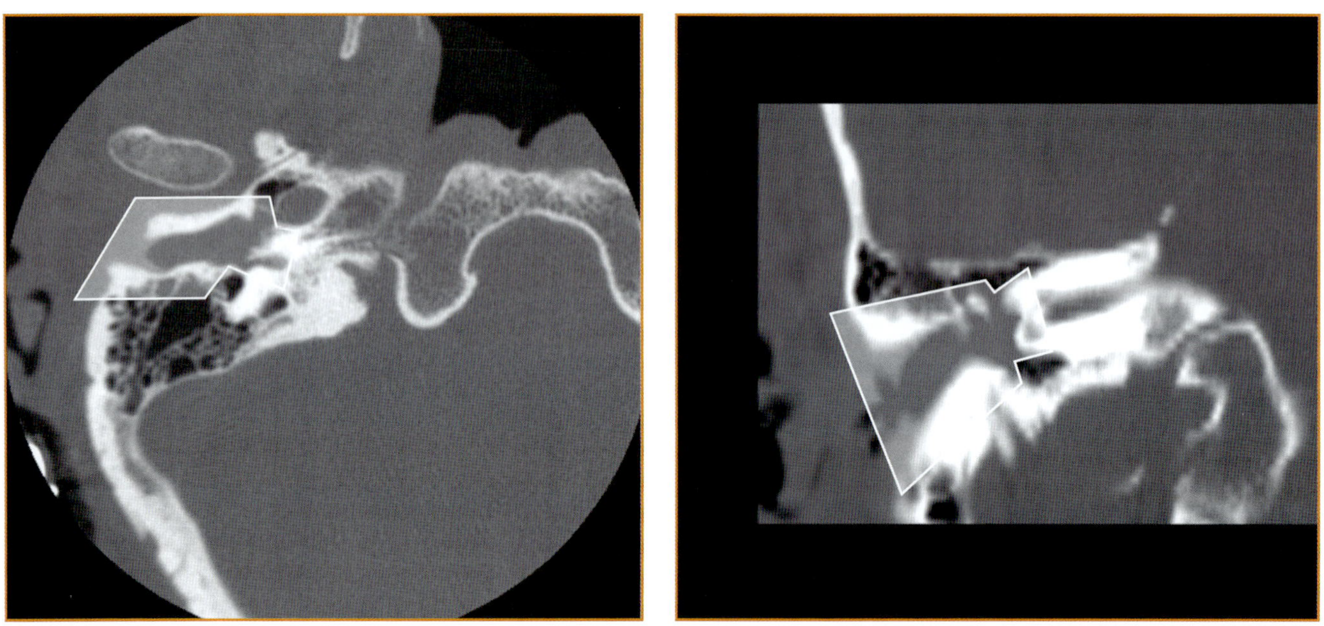

A B

Figure 2–2. Subtotal temporal bone resection, schematic, axial (**A**) and coronal (**B**).

above and behind the planned surgical wound. The skin circumferential to the auricle is thoroughly cleansed with alcohol to ensure removal of loose keratin debris and skin oils, and a layer of mastisol or benzoin ointment is applied to the cleansed skin. After the antibiotic adhesive is completely dried,

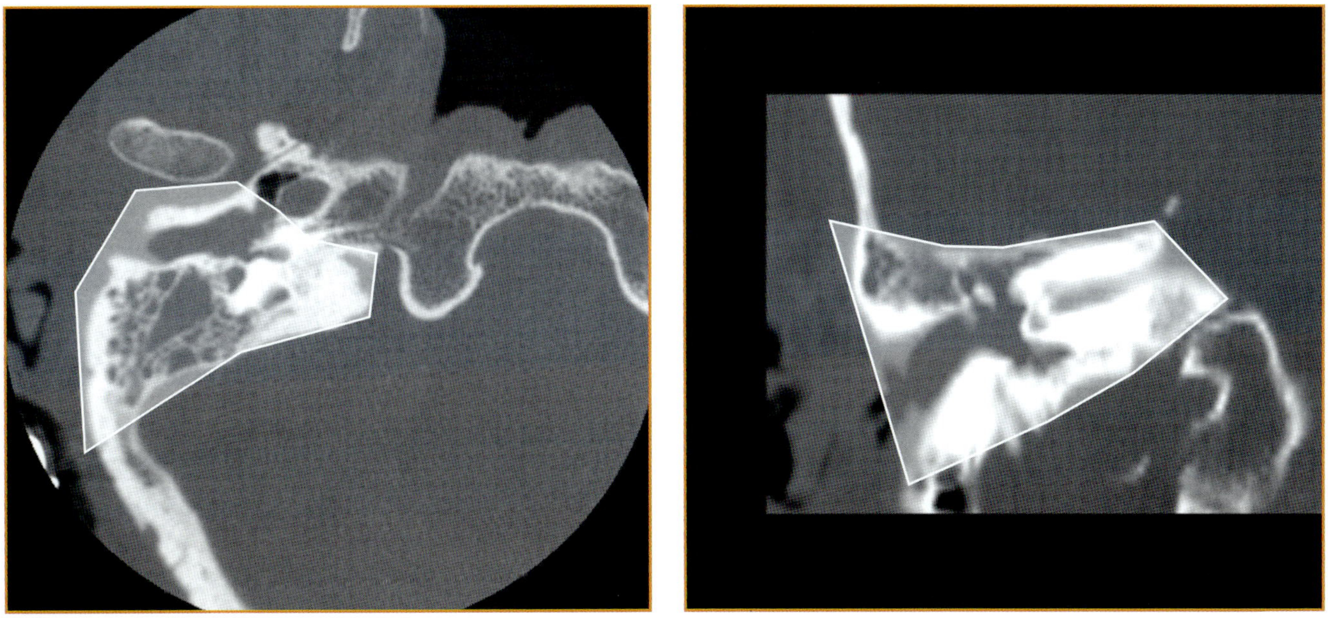

A B

Figure 2–3. Total temporal bone resection, schematic, axial (**A**) and coronal (**B**).

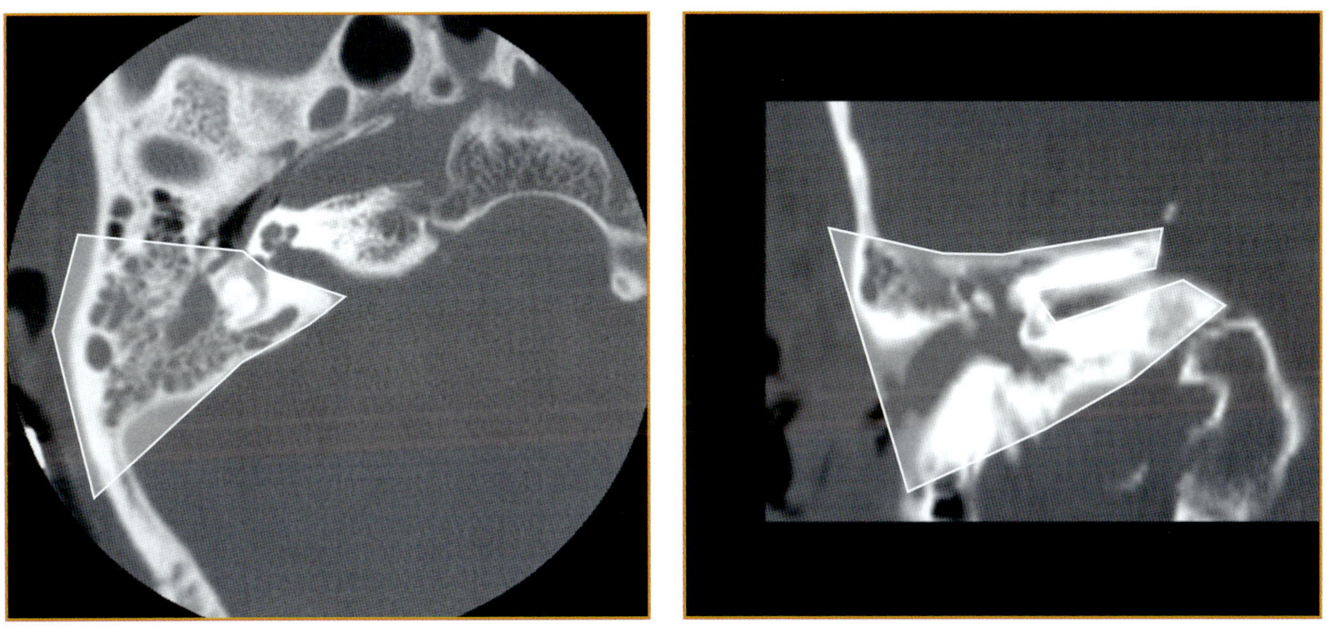

A B

Figure 2–4. Translabyrinthine approach, schematic, axial (**A**) and coronal (**B**).

quartered sheets of 3M 1000 drape or other adhesive drape are applied circumferentially around the auricle to delineate the region to be prepared.

Betadine or chlorhexidine is used to sterilely prepare the delineated periauricular skin as well as the surrounding clear drapes. Although the external auditory canal is not routinely entered in translabyrinthine surgery, Betadine is generously applied to fill the external auditory canal and is left in place. The Betadine serves not only as an antiseptic but as a dissection marker: during mastoid drilling and skeletonization of the posterior canal wall, any sign of Betadine in the mastoid cavity implies fistulization of the posterior canal wall and injury of the canal skin or tympanic membrane, necessitating a canal wall down procedure and overclosure of the ear canal to avoid CSF otorrhea and minimize the risk of postoperative meningitis.

Abdominal or other adipose fat is required for adequate watertight closure of the translabyrinthine defect following tumor removal. Therefore, the abdomen must be sterilely prepared in addition to the primary surgical site. Abdominal subcutaneous fat is typically harvested most easily from a midline low abdominal or bikini line incision. A periumbilical incision is more cosmetically favorable, but harvesting an adequate amount of fat is often more challenging. The chosen donor site is shaved and similarly delineated with 1000 drapes in a rectangular fashion. The delineated site is sterilely prepared with a Betadine or chlorhexidine solution.

The translabyrinthine approach begins with a large C-shaped postauricular incision positioned more posteriorly than a standard otological postauricular incision. This is often three to four fingerbreadths behind the postauricular crease and two to three fingerbreadths above the superior helical root and below the lobule, as the bony dissection is much more extensive posteriorly, superiorly, and inferiorly compared to that in a standard mastoidectomy for chronic ear disease. However, in cases in which there is limited tumor extension posterolaterally into the cerebellum and hence limited need for posterior intracranial dissection, a postauricular incision close to the auricle can be used with good results.

Soft tissue dissection is carried down to the temporalis muscle fascia superiorly, the mastoid periosteum mid-level, and the lateral sternocleidomastoid muscle inferiorly. A slip of occipitofrontalis muscle and fascia is harvested and partitioned into small segments for later use in packing off the eustachian tube, mesotympanum, and epitympanum. Superiorly, a large temporalis muscle fascia graft is harvested for later use in obstructing the aditus ad antrum during closure. Mid-level, a thick, healthy layer of mastoid periosteum must be maintained to provide adequate strength in the periosteal reapproximation over fat packing during closure. Inferiorly, the superior fringe of platysma is encountered just deep to the subcutaneous fat; this platysma is raised in continuity with the skin flap, keeping the skin flap adequately thick. The sternocleidomastoid muscle belly is kept down, maintaining dissection at a safe distance from the facial nerve. The skin and muscle flap is raised anteriorly to the external canal without violating it.

Mastoid periosteum is incised and elevated to widely expose the mastoid cortex, squamosal cortex, and anterior occipital cortex. The asterion posterosuperiorly, mastoid tip inferiorly, and bony external canal anteriorly should all be fully visible. The surgical field is irrigated copiously with a Bacitracin saline solution prior to and intermittently throughout bony dissection.

A cortical mastoidectomy is performed in the usual fashion and dissections carried down and through Koerner's septum to widely open the antrum. The mastoid cavity laterally is widely expanded to completely skeletonize the tegmen mastoideum superiorly, with further removal of squamosal bone up to 2 cm superior to the level of the tegmen. Posteriorly, the lateral sinus is identified and skeletonized, and the cortex is resected up to 2 cm posterior to the lateral sinus from Citelli's angle superiorly down to the mastoid tip inferiorly. This degree of resection often includes the anterior border of the occipital bone and exposes the retrosigmoid posterior fossa dura. The mastoid tip is fully resected, with identification of the digastric ridge pointing to the stylomastoid foramen along the anterior border of the tip. The posterior external auditory canal wall is thoroughly skeletonized.

The tegmen mastoideum and superior squamosal bone are skeletonized until eggshell thin, then gently elevated and resected off of the underlying dura of the middle fossa convexity and floor. The exposed middle fossa dura is contracted by tangential application of bipolar electrocautery under irrigation. Contraction of this dura can be quite significant and beneficial for exposure of the cerebellopontine angle, particularly for larger tumors.

The sigmoid sinus is often decompressed by development of a bony island overlying the most anterior aspect of the sigmoid portion of the lateral sinus, the so-called "Bill's Island." This technique is useful in modestly displacing the sigmoid sinus posteriorly. However, a more aggressive and much more effective technique is, as with the tegmen above, to completely dissect and remove all the bone overlying the sigmoid sinus and lateral to it to the mastoid cortex, up to 2 cm posterior to the interface of the sigmoid sinus and posterior fossa dura. The bone overlying the sigmoid sinus is similarly thinned and resected, with additional care taken as the sigmoid sinus dura is generally more attenuated and fragile than the middle fossa dura. Mastoid emissary veins should be identified exiting the sigmoid sinus posteriorly and appropriately transected, electrocauterized, or ligated. After fully unroofing the sigmoid sinus, it too is contracted by tangential application of bipolar electrocautery under irrigation. Posterior contraction of the sigmoid sinus and occipital convexity dura can increase posterior exposure by up to 2 to 3 cm.

Following decompression of the sigmoid sinus, the leading edge of posterior fossa dura distally is gently elevated and decompressed out from under the bone of Trautmann's triangle, that is, the bony plate separating the posterior fossa from the mastoid cavity, between the sigmoid sinus, otic capsule, and jugular bulb. With the posterior fossa dura compressed and retracted away from this bone, the bone of Trautmann's triangle can be drilled away with cutting burs or drilled down toward the otic capsule with diamond burs. Again, extreme care is taken in bony removal near the superior petrosal sinus along Citelli's angle superiorly and near the jugular bulb inferiorly. Sinus bleeding from either region can be extremely time consuming to control, and it is often wise to leave intact adherent small islands of bone overlying the major sinuses in these regions rather than completely resect all bone on principle.

With the majority of the lateral bone now completely resected and with underlying posterior and middle fossa dura maximally contracted, the posterior petrous apex now comes into excellent view and can be systematically resected. All overlying spiculated bone is first drilled fully away in order to define the contours of the semicircular canals. The off-white color of the overlying spiculated mastoid bone is often easily contrasted to the more yellow or cream colored appearance of the dense, endochondral bone of the underlying otic capsule.

Although not essential to the translabyrinthine approach, a technique favored by the author is to find the lateral facial nerve and delineate its vertical course. Prior to labyrinthectomy, the bone between the otic capsule and facial recess is carefully drilled under copious irrigation until the second genu and vertical facial nerve are identified. The lateral fallopian canal is then skeletonized but kept intact distally to the stylomastoid foramen. By delineating the course of the vertical facial nerve, the labyrinthectomy can proceed efficiently with close approximation to the facial nerve.

The standard method for performing labyrinthectomy involves first blue-lining each semicircular canal: the body of the canal is gradually drilled down along the long axis of the canal until the gray or blue coloration of the lumen comes into contrast or is "blue-lined" juxtaposed against the surrounding dense yellow bone of the canal. The horizontal canal is blue-lined first as it lies most lateral, followed by the posterior semicircular canal, whose arc is bisected by the long axis of the horizontal canal, that is, Donaldson's line. The superior semicircular canal is blue-lined last, with its posterior limb discovered by following the superior limb of the posterior semicircular canal up to the crus communis. The superior canal is followed and blue-lined forward to its ampulla, which lies directly suprajacent to the ampulla of the horizontal semicircular canal. Each canal lumen is then fully opened, and the otic capsule bone central to all the canals is resected, thereby exposing the vestibule.

The condensed bone that lies between the ampullae of the horizontal and posterior semicircular canals is then removed. Removal of this bone essentially resects the lateral wall of the vestibule, and thorough removal enhances the view of the vestibule and, hence, the fundus of the internal auditory canal after deeper dissection. However, this otic capsule bone lies in very close proximity to the second genu of the facial nerve, and careful removal with copious irrigation is warranted to avoid injury.

In addition, undercutting the bone in this region is strictly prohibited, as the vestibular cavity extends medial to the facial nerve; premature removal of bone from the undersurface of this ledge can lead to facial nerve injury along its medial face.

An alternative conception of executing the labyrinthectomy involves the development and gradual expansion of a cavity of dissection, or "Malcolm's cup" as it has become known, from the solid angle. After removal of overlying mastoid air cells and bony spiculations, the "solid angle" or "hard angle" of dense otic capsule bone that lies posterosuperior to the horizontal and posterior semicircular canals is identified. A cavity of dissection is then developed within this solid angle and gradually expanded in all directions. The posterior and middle fossa dural plates and sinodural angle denote the limits of dissection posterosuperiorly. Malcolm's cup is expanded anteroinferiorly to follow the lumina of the posterior and horizontal canals, and it is expanded deep to outline the superior semicircular canal lumen. The ampullae of each semicircular canal mark the anterior and inferior ends of dissection, as the facial nerve lies in very close proximity to each ampulla. The lateral wall of the vestibule is again taken down until the fallopian canal is skeletonized, just shy of the lateral facial nerve. During labyrinthectomy, usage of cutting burs instead of diamond burs prevents bone dust from plugging canal lumina and aids in positive identification of the canal lumina out to the vestibule and ampullae. Maintaining dissection within the confines of a recessed cup or cavity also enhances safety of cutting bur usage at this stage.

With the vertical facial nerve previously outlined, the retrofacial air cell tract is then exenterated. This tract may be expansive or contracted in nature, but the limits of dissection are constant: facial nerve anteriorly, jugular bulb inferiorly, and posterior fossa dura and endolymphatic sac posteriorly. Superior dissection is brought in continuity with the labyrinthectomy dissection. As the posterior fossa dural plate and operculum are outlined, the endolymphatic duct is brought into view and transected.

The internal auditory canal is embedded within the remaining dense bone of the posterior petrous apex. Skeletonization of the internal auditory canal begins with exenteration of "pillars," or more precisely wells, inferior and superior to its estimated position. The inferior pillar is developed until the jugular bulb is skeletonized inferiorly and the lower border of the internal auditory canal skeletonized superiorly. The dissection is carried medially until the cochlear aqueduct is identified, sometimes with egress of CSF. The superior pillar is developed until the superior border of the internal auditory canal is skeletonized inferiorly, while maintaining thin bone over the superior petrosal sinus. Because of the tangential inclination of the internal auditory canal from the translabyrinthine perspective, the pillars are naturally developed more deeply medially around the porus acousticus and more superficially laterally around the fundus.

Final exenteration of the superior pillar laterally is performed carefully, as the labyrinthine segment of the facial nerve curves upward superior to the level of the internal auditory canal. Medial facial nerve decompression of the labyrinthine segment is advocated and routinely performed to reduce the incidence of postoperative inflammatory facial paresis or paralysis.[2]

The porus acousticus is skeletonized along the medial-most aspect of the internal auditory canal. This area often must be drilled out using sequentially smaller diamond burs to effect complete removal of the bony collar without damaging the underlying dura. Any remaining bone of the posterior fossa dural plate is removed as well, allowing full exposure of the posterior fossa dura from the sigmoid sinus laterally to the porus acousticus medially and from the sinodural angle superiorly to the jugular bulb inferiorly.

The dense bone overlying the lateral face of the internal auditory canal is drilled down until eggshell thin similarly to the inferior and superior faces of the internal auditory canal. This amount of dissection now provides 270 degrees of exposure of the internal auditory canal. The eggshell-thin bone of the internal auditory canal is then elevated and removed from the underlying internal auditory canal dura, which is well developed at the porus but significantly attenuates laterally and is absent at the fundus.

Bony removal is carried further laterally to the elliptical recess of the vestibule until the macula cribrosa superioris is identified. The macula cribrosa superioris, or Mike's dot, localizes the bony perforation along the medial wall of the elliptical recess through which pass the fibers of the superior vestibular nerve supplying the utricular macula. Lateral dissection to the level of Mike's dot verifies the location of the medial wall of the vestibule and assures the surgeon of ample lateral dissection of the internal auditory canal to fully expose the fundus. In conjunction with the remaining eggshell-thin posterior wall of the internal auditory canal, Mike's dot is then unroofed, beneath which lies the superior vestibular nerve and internal auditory canal fundus. Just inferior to Mike's dot is the crista falciformis, or horizontal crest, further confirming dissection to the fundus.

Prior to opening the dura, an osmotic diuretic such as mannitol is administered to lower CSF production and minimize intracranial pressure. This is usually administered during dissection of the mastoid or labyrinth, timed to maximize efficacy prior to dural opening. Hyperventilation to achieve a pCO_2 of 25 to 28 mm Hg can also aid in this regard.

Before incising the dura, the entire surgical field is copiously irrigated and evacuated of all residual bone dust. The posterior fossa dura is first opened, incising just anterior to the sigmoid sinus. The dural incision is carried to the porus acousticus. A triangle of posterior fossa dura is often excised to aid in exposure of particularly large tumors. The dural incision is extended onto the intracanalicular dura from the porus to the fundus, along the inferior aspect of the canal to minimize risk to the facial nerve.

Complete exposure of the fundus, via dissection of Mike's dot, is advantageous in that within the lateral most extent of the internal auditory canal, the superior vestibular nerve lies separated from the facial nerve by a vertical bony crest, or Bill's bar. Gentle palpation and dissection of the superficially located superior vestibular nerve allows for a natural dissection plane to be formed between the superior vestibular nerve and the facial nerve, which lies deep to Bill's bar. This dissection plane can then be developed in a lateral to medial direction, enabling efficient and safe dissection of the superior vestibular nerve and associated acoustic tumor off of the underlying facial nerve down to the porus.

The acoustic tumor is now completely exposed within its cerebellopontine angle and internal auditory canal compartments through the translabyrinthine cavity. The facial nerve should first be localized both visually and electrically within the internal auditory canal. As stated, this is easiest accomplished at the fundus, where a natural plane of dissection can be developed from Bill's bar separating the superior vestibular nerve superficially from the deeper facial nerve. The superior vestibular nerve is transected or shelled out from its lateral bony canal and gently peeled away from the internal auditory canal in a lateral to medial dissection. The inferior vestibular nerve is also identified, transected, and elevated similarly. With elevation of both vestibular branches, the lateral border of the acoustic tumor is elevated in continuity and can often be easily elevated off of the underlying facial nerve nearly to the porus. The facial nerve can now be directly tested at lowest stimulator setting (0.01 to 0.05 mA) to verify electrical and functional integrity from the porus distally.

The tumor bulk within the cerebellopontine angle is removed next. Prior to tumor dissection, the tumor envelope is thoroughly mapped with the facial nerve stimulator at moderate setting (0.1 to 0.3 mA) to ensure that no functional branches of the facial nerve have been displaced posteriorly onto the superficial face of the tumor. Following this, the posterior envelope of tumor is cauterized and resected. The interior mass of tumor is then debulked, taking care to electrically stimulate when dissecting near or just underneath the tumor envelope. The displaced facial nerve is most commonly compressed onto the tumor envelope anteriorly, but attenuated nerve fascicles may be present along any or all sides of the tumor envelope. After adequate dissection of the tumor centrally, the tumor envelope can be collapsed inward along all sides to gently dissect the tumor off of the surrounding cerebellum. As the tumor envelope is reduced from cerebellar tissue, it is sequentially resected after confirmation of clearance of the facial nerve with electrical stimulation. With significant clearance of tumor volume, the brainstem comes into view, and the root entry zone of the facial nerve, and if possible the cochleovestibular nerve, should be positively identified. The facial nerve stimulator is set to its lowest current setting (0.01 to 0.02 mA), and the root entry zone of the facial nerve should be stimulated to confirm electrical functional integrity of the nerve prior to continuation and completion of the tumor dissection.

The tumor is gently dissected off of the brainstem, taking care to identify and preserve the facial nerve at the root entry zone. During brainstem dissection, communication between the surgeon and anesthesiology team is critical, as compression of the brainstem from tumor dissection can lead to dangerous bradycardia and hypotension and must be countered quickly with atropine.

The remaining tumor is now dissected off of the facial nerve within the cerebellopontine angle in a medial to lateral direction. The tumor is often most adherent to the facial nerve near the porus acousticus, and it is this region that demonstrates the most tumor compression and nerve attenuation. As a result, it is in this final region where a decision must be made whether to attempt total tumor removal and place the structural integrity and function of the facial nerve in jeopardy versus leave a microscopic residual of tumor on the nerve with the benefit of minimizing trauma and risk of injury to the facial nerve. Near total tumor resection, where a microscopic tumor residuum is left on the facial nerve, results in postoperative tumor control rates comparable to total tumor removal, provides better rates of postoperative facial nerve function, and is generally accepted as a reasonable and oncologically sound compromise for this benign disease.[3] In contrast, subtotal tumor resection, where a macroscopic amount of tumor bulk is left behind, does not benefit the patient and is not generally accepted as an adequate solitary treatment.

Following completion of tumor dissection, the facial nerve is checked electrically for functional integrity. Bleeding is checked and controlled with thrombin, surgicel, and occasionally bipolar electrocautery. Verification that all bleeding vessels have been secured can be accomplished by having anesthesia perform Valsalva maneuvers to 20 and 40 cm H_2O and checking for active bleeders within the dissection cavity, with the patient supine or in slight Trendelenburg. After hemostasis is confirmed, excess CSF is evacuated and the patient is placed into reverse Trendelenburg. The translabyrinthine cavity is now ready for closure.

Access to the epitympanum and eustachian tube is improved by removal of the incus. The malleus head may also be drilled or nipped away if desired, although this is not requisite and risks injury to the tympanic membrane. The previously harvested muscle and fascial segments are gently inserted through the aditus ad antrum and securely packed into the bony eustachian tube. This process is done blindly, and the orientation of the eustachian tube must be verified by gentle palpation with extended blunt instrumentation prior to packing. As the eustachian tube is filled, the mesotympanum and epitympanum are also gently packed as well. The aditus ad antrum is then sealed off with the large sheet of temporalis muscle fascia.

Abdominal fat graft harvest is fairly straightforward; however, a few important details must be considered. Ideally no subcutaneous anesthetic at all should be used in the abdominal incision site, or if excessive bleeding is a major concern, an epinephrine-only infiltrate should be used. If local anesthetic is used, this should be infiltrated in a subdermal fashion only with care taken to avoid any infiltration of anesthetic deeper into the subcutaneous fat. This fat will eventually be harvested and used to pack the translabyrinthine defect, and any local anesthetic within this fat graft can leach into the wound cavity and cause a temporary anesthesia of the facial nerve anywhere along its course from internal auditory canal to stylomastoid foramen. The cause of an immediate postoperative facial paralysis cannot be determined a priori, and therefore immediate return to the operating room is often warranted. Avoidance of local anesthetic in the fat graft can prevent such an inadvertent if temporary chemical facial paralysis as well as prevent the attendant but ultimately unnecessary immediate re-exploration.

Harvested fat is prepared into tear-drop shapes and held in sterile saline until ready for use. After packing of the eustachian tube and epitympanum and closure of the aditus ad antrum, strips of fat are gently inserted into the translabyrinthine cavity with the medial ends extending slightly beyond the posterior fossa dural defect. As fat strips are inserted, attention is paid to the location of the facial nerve to avoid impingement. The facial nerve monitor is also utilized to monitor for compression or other stimulation to the facial nerve during packing. After secure packing of the dural defect and deep cavity, the remaining superficial cavity is overfilled with additional fat packing.

The mastoid periosteum is reapproximated and closed securely over the packed fat. High-density porous polyethylene sheeting or other cranioplasty material can assist closure by placement over the overfilled fat and under the reapproximated periosteum. The skin is closed in layers to form a secure, watertight repair.

The external auditory canal is thoroughly cleansed of all residual betadine and closely inspected to ensure the tympanic membrane is intact. A defect in the tympanic membrane must be repaired in a watertight fashion, or the canal must be taken down and overclosed to prevent postoperative CSF otorrhea.

The wound is cleansed and dressed with a mastoid pressure dressing. The dressing is changed once on postoperative day three and kept in place for a total of one week. The wound is checked daily for any sign of CSF otorrhea, CSF wound leak, or CSF fluid collection.

Modified Translabyrinthine Approach

The advantages of the translabyrinthine approach are tempered by the singular disadvantage of postoperative anacusis. In order to avoid this outcome, the labyrinth can be resected in a modified fashion in an attempt to preserve hearing.[4,5]

The standard translabyrinthine approach is performed laterally, with wide excision of the mastoid air cells and resection of the tegmen mastoideum, tegmen tympani, and posterior bony skeleton overlying the sigmoid sinus and posterior fossa dura. Mastoid air cells and bony spiculations overlying the otic capsule bone are removed to delineate the contour of the posterior otic capsule.

The labyrinthectomy is then performed in an abbreviated fashion to avoid injury to the membranous labyrinth. The semicircular canals are bluelined as far anteriorly, posteriorly, and inferiorly as possible without entering the lumina. Using diamond burs, each limb of each semicircular canal is transected and then plugged immediately with bone wax. The horizontal semicircular canal is used as a starting point, with its anterior and posterior limbs transected and plugged. The posterior semicircular canal is followed inferiorly to the ampullated end and transected, followed by transection and plugging of the crus communis. Finally, the ampullated end of the superior semicircular canal is transected and plugged.

The central otic capsule bone overlying the vestibule is gradually thinned until attenuated to near eggshell thickness. Previous reports of translabyrinthine modification described opening and then plugging the vestibule with bone wax.[4] However, the rate of success in hearing preservation appears to be greater when the vestibule is not violated at all.[6]

The remaining otic capsule bone posterior to the vestibule is resected posteriorly down to the posterior fossa plate and medially to the porus acousticus (Figure 2–5). The internal auditory canal is skeletonized as laterally as possible, without violating the vestibule. The posterior fossa and medial internal auditory canal dura are opened, and the exposed tumor is resected in the usual fashion.

The modified translabyrinthine technique can be considered in a similar light as the posterior semicircular canal occlusion procedure for intractable benign paroxysmal positional vertigo, but involving occlusion of all three semicircular canals instead of just one. Occlusion of the posterior semicircular canal for intractable vertigo allows for excellent postoperative hearing outcomes, with the vast majority of surgical recipients maintaining normal hearing.[7] In contrast, occlusion of all three canals and skeletonization of the vestibule, in conjunction with intracanalicular tumor dissection performed in the modified translabyrinthine approach, yields postoperative preservation of serviceable hearing in at best 40 to 50% of patients.[6,8]

Because of the limitation in anatomic dissection by preservation of the vestibule, only the medial half of the internal auditory canal is directly visible via this approach. In addition, resection of the entire otic capsule bone posterior to the vestibule necessarily transects the vestibular aqueduct and endolymphatic duct, placing the patient at risk for latent endolymphatic hydrops, especially in the "fortunate" case of those patients whose endolymphatic function and hearing are preserved following surgery.

Retrolabyrinthine Approach

Occasionally, a small tumor of the cerebellopontine angle has little or no extension into the internal auditory canal, or a tumor of the mastoid has extended through the posterior fossa dural plate into the

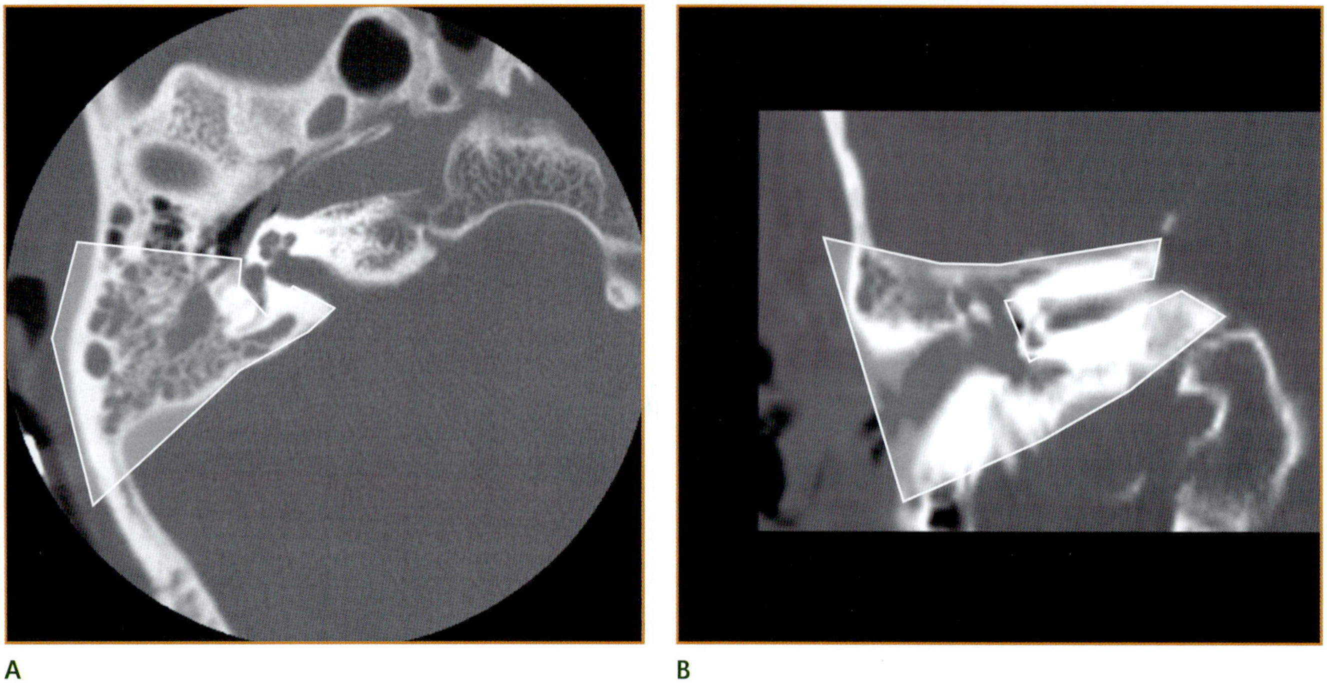

Figure 2–5. Modified translabyrinthine approach, schematic, axial (**A**) and coronal (**B**).

cerebellopontine angle. In such cases in which transmastoid access to the cerebellopontine angle can be significantly restricted without impeding tumor removal, a strictly retrolabyrinthine dissection can be performed.

The retrolabyrinthine approach is a restricted version of the translabyrinthine approach in which the entire posterior otic capsule is functionally preserved. Limits of dissection continue to be the middle fossa dura and tentorium cerebelli superiorly, the jugular bulb inferiorly, and the posterior fossa dura and sigmoid sinus posteriorly (Figure 2–6). Anteriorly, rather than traverse the posterior otic capsule, the semicircular canals are blue-lined posteriorly to maximize anterior exposure without opening the lumina. Trautmann's triangle of bone overlying the posterior fossa dura is fully resected between the sigmoid and otic capsule, and the sigmoid itself can be completely decompressed to effect additional retraction and exposure posteriorly.

Despite the potential to preserve hearing, the retrolabyrinthine approach has limited application due to its extremely narrow window of intracranial exposure.

Transotic Approach

On the opposite end of the spectrum, the transotic and transcochlear approaches expand rather than restrict the limits of dissection.[9] In cases in which the tumor being accessed has significant anterior petrous apex or cerebellopontine angle extension, the translabyrinthine approach may be extended anteriorly.

The transotic approach follows in similar fashion to the translabyrinthine approach, with wide and complete mastoidectomy and skeletonization of the middle and posterior fossa petrous dura. Departing from the standard translabyrinthine technique, the external auditory meatus is transected and overclosed, the canal wall is taken down, and the external auditory canal, tympanic membrane, and lateral ossicles resected (Figure 2–7). This lateral temporal bone resection is described in greater detail at the beginning of the section.

There is now direct access to the anterior mesotympanum. The cochlea is then fully resected to expose the anterior petrous apex, and a variable amount of resection of the anterior apex can be performed depending on the size and location of tumor.

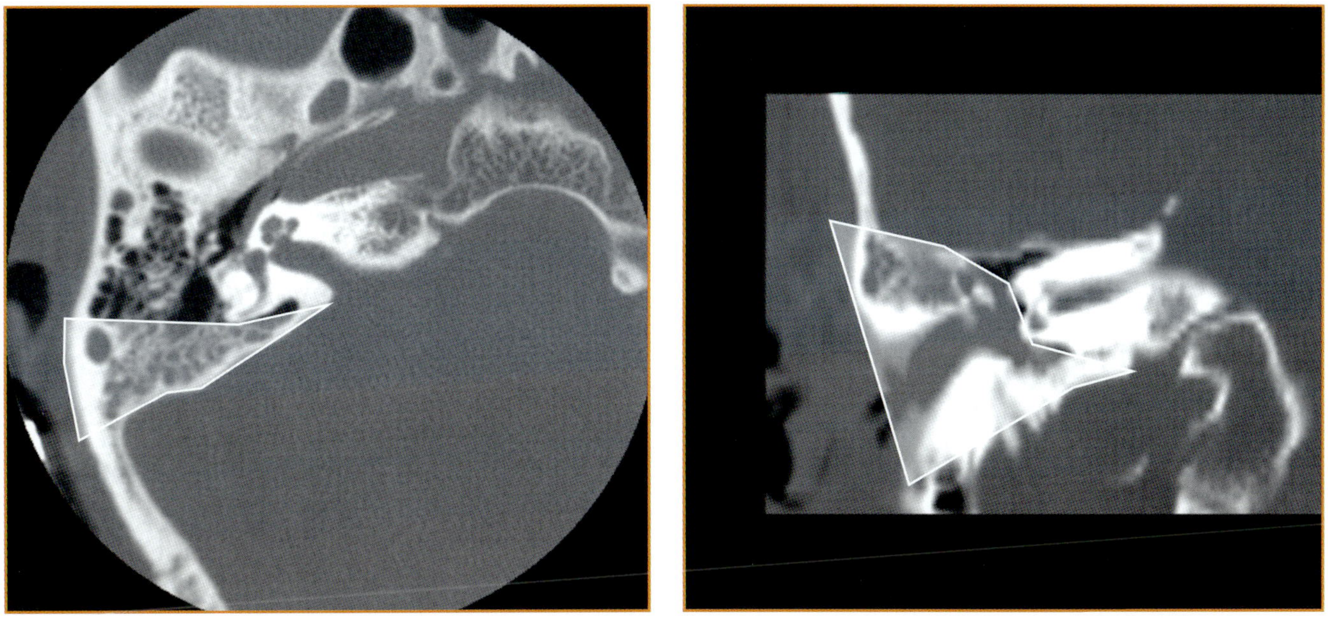

A B

Figure 2–6. Retrolabyrinthine approach, schematic, axial (**A**) and coronal (**B**).

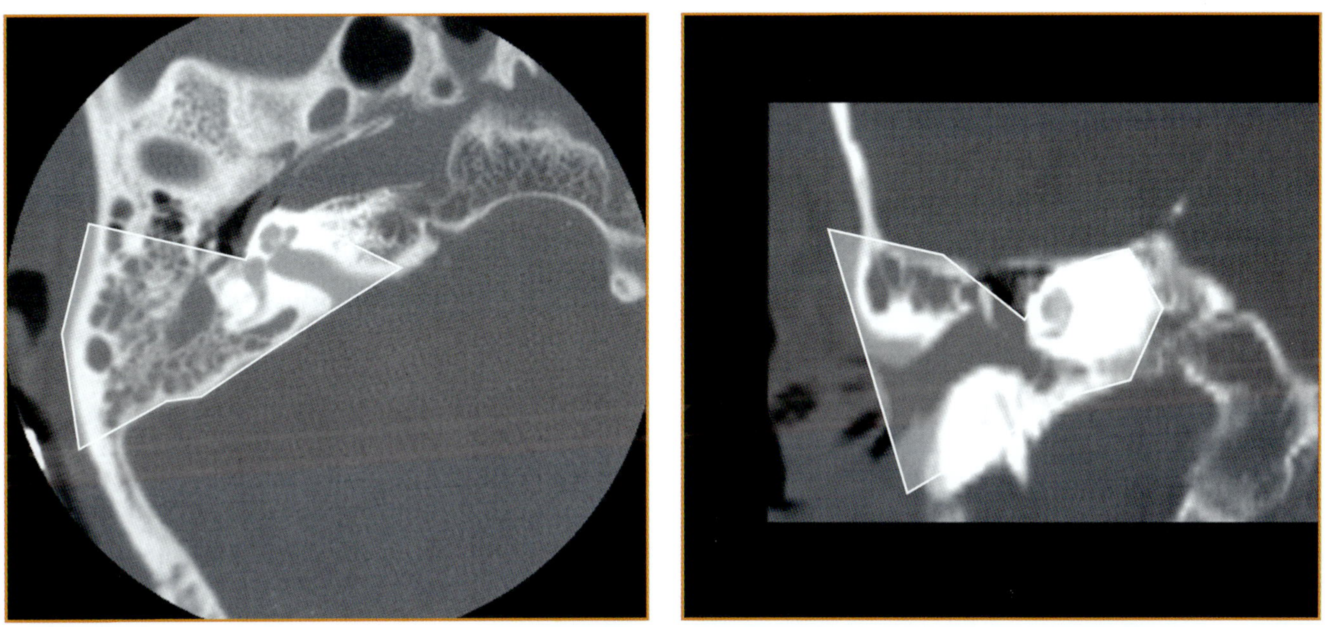

A B

Figure 2–7. Transotic approach, schematic, axial (**A**) and coronal (**B**).

The anterior face of the internal auditory canal is skeletonized, and the intracranial vault is accessed through the dura overlying the petrous apex to expose the prepontine cistern. If a posterior labyrinthectomy is performed also, the entire internal auditory canal can be skeletonized and exposed.

The transotic approach makes use of lateral anterior exposure by means of external auditory canal resection and overclosure to provide access to the anterior petrous apex medially. The facial nerve is left in situ throughout its course, from within the internal auditory canal, through the temporal bone, and out the stylomastoid foramen. If additional exposure is necessary, a transcochlear approach is used.

Transcochlear Approach

When wide anterior petrous apex exposure is necessary, the facial nerve can be removed from its entire course within the bony fallopian canal and transposed posteriorly. This anterior petrous apex exposure is termed the transcochlear approach.

The transotic approach is performed as described above. Following labyrinthectomy, the fallopian canal is skeletonized, and the facial nerve is unroofed from the meatal foramen to the stylomastoid foramen. The internal auditory canal is opened from fundus to porus, and the posterior fossa dura is opened to expose the cerebellum and brainstem. The facial nerve is elevated completely out of the bony fallopian canal, fully mobilized from the brainstem to the stylomastoid foramen, and transposed posteriorly to rest on the cerebellum.

With the facial nerve completely transposed posteriorly, the remaining cochlea can be resected, if not already done so. The anterior petrous apex to the clivus can be resected, and the anterior limit of dissection becomes the petrosal internal carotid artery. Through this approach, the entire lateral and ventral aspects of the brainstem, the clivus, and the prepontine cistern are directly visible with minimal or no cerebellar retraction (Figure 2–8).

Infratemporal Fossa Type A Approach

When wide exposure along the posterior petrous apex and jugular bulb are required, the infratemporal fossa type A approach is used. This approach is commonly used when resecting tumors of the jugular bulb, such as glomus jugulare tumors (Figure 2–9).

A wide mastoidectomy is performed. The posterior wall of the external auditory canal is skeleton-

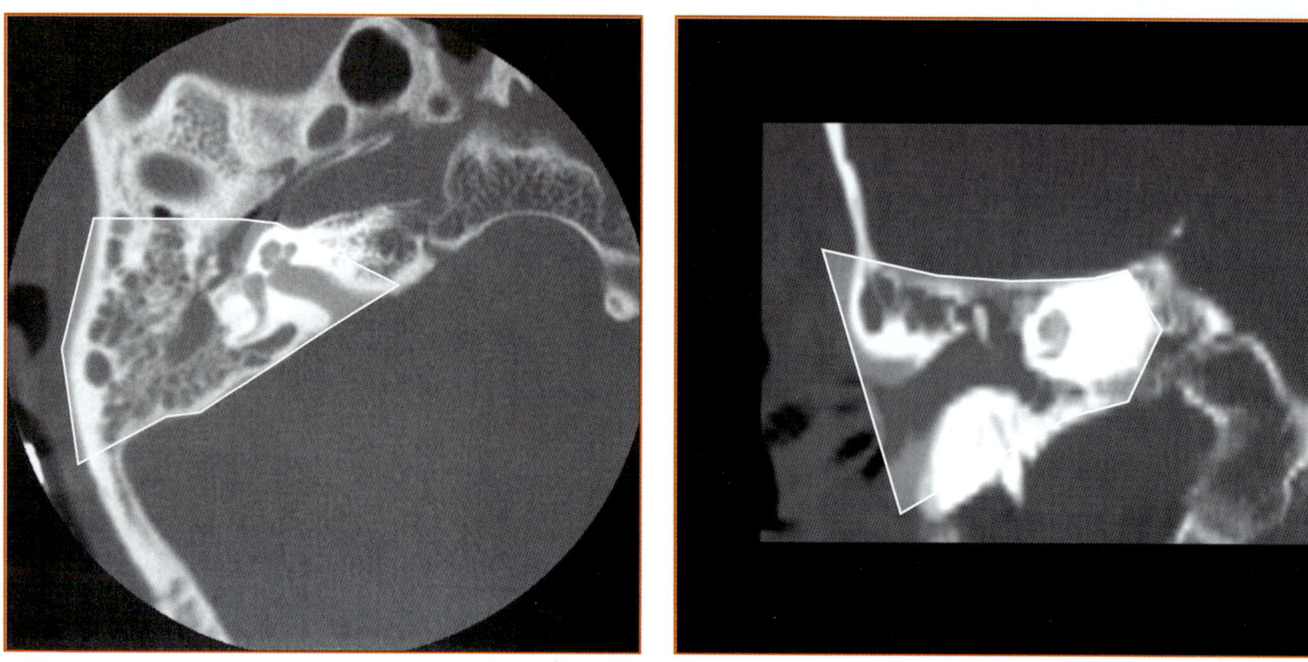

A **B**

Figure 2–8. Transcochlear approach, schematic, axial (**A**) and coronal (**B**).

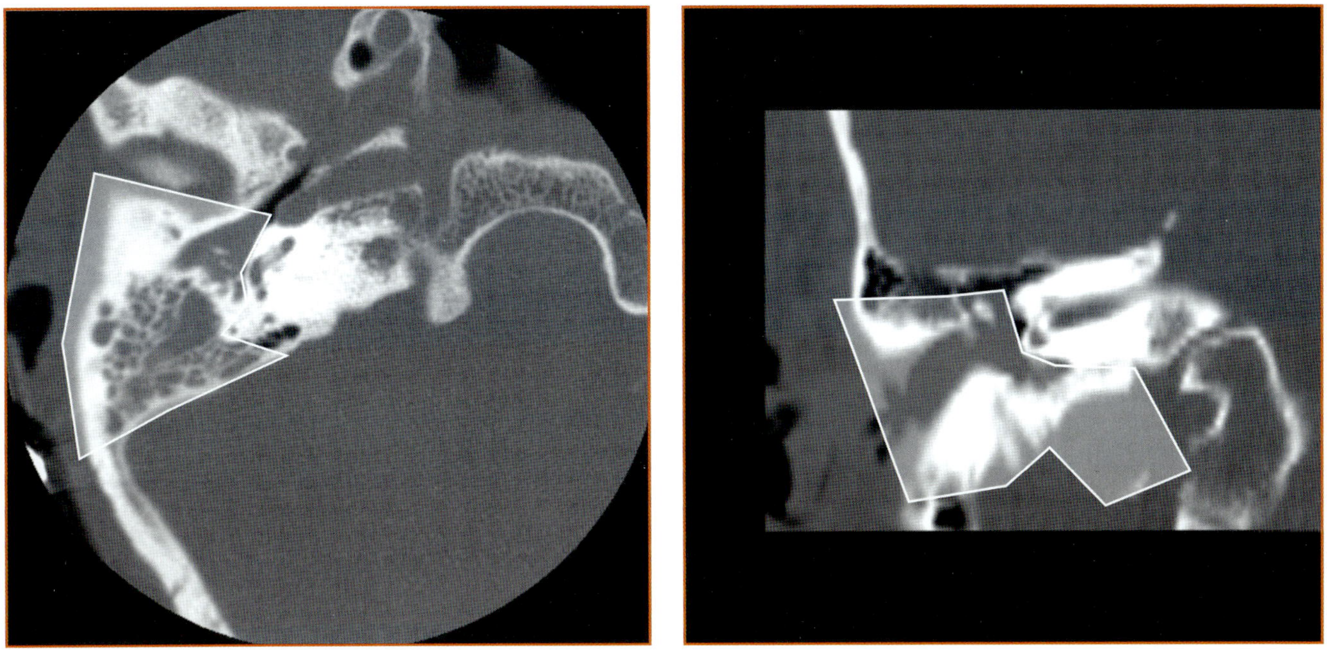

A B

Figure 2–9. Infratemporal fossa type A approach, schematic, axial (**A**) and coronal (**B**).

ized in preparation for later resection. The lateral sinus is skeletonized from its transition from the transverse sinus superiorly to the jugular bulb inferiorly. This requires complete resection of the mastoid tip in order to expose the jugular vein's exit out the skull base inferiorly. The exit of the facial nerve through the stylomastoid foramen is in close proximity; therefore the facial nerve must be identified and preserved prior to skeletonization of the jugular bulb and foramen.

The inferior facial nerve can be easily localized by two means. The facial nerve can be skeletonized along its vertical or transmastoid course from the second genu superiorly down to the stylomastoid foramen inferiorly. Alternatively, the digastric ridge can be identified within the mastoid tip laterally and followed medially to the stylomastoid foramen.

The facial nerve is skeletonized from the second genu to the stylomastoid foramen, and an extended facial recess is performed. The lateral temporal bone is described as in a lateral temporal bone resection.

Following removal of the lateral temporal bone, the entire course of the fallopian canal is now visible, from the tympanic segment to the stylomastoid foramen. The entire bony fallopian canal is skeletonized and then gently dissected away from the facial nerve. The facial nerve is then lifted away from the remaining trough of the fallopian canal and transposed anteriorly, taking as its points of rotation the geniculate ganglion and the stylomastoid foramen. The infratemporal facial nerve can be dissected further along the main trunk to provide additional mobility anteriorly.

The postauricular incision is carried inferiorly into the upper neck, which is dissected to expose and provide control of the carotid artery and jugular vein. With the facial nerve out of the way, the jugular bulb can be dissected completely of its bony skeleton within the temporal bone. The lateral sinus is either extraluminally packed or suture ligated above the level of the jugular bulb tumor, and the jugular vein is suture ligated and transected in the upper neck. The tumor is then resected between the two ligated ends.

The tumor residual within the jugular bulb itself is resected last, as removal at this site will cause brisk bleeding from the inferior petrosal sinus, which, because of its medial location within the cranial base, cannot be controlled prior to tumor resection. Control of the inferior petrosal sinus is only accomplished following complete tumor resection within the jugular bulb, when the lumen of the inferior petrosal sinus can be identified and packed off with oxidized cellulose polymer or other hemostatic packing agent.

Considerable care must be taking during tumor dissection and packing of the jugular bulb and foramen, as the lower cranial nerves exit the medial wall of the jugular foramen. Excessive pressure on the lower nerves, even if they are maintained anatomically intact, can easily lead to dysphagia, dysphonia, vocal cord paralysis, and shoulder weakness.

If the tumor extends intracranially, the posterior fossa dura can be incised and resected in continuity with the jugular bulb, and the intracranial portion of the tumor can be removed through this dural opening.

Following completion of tumor resection, the external auditory meatus is overclosed as in the procedure for lateral temporal bone resection. The facial nerve is replaced to a neutral, anatomic position, and the bony defect can be filled with a temporalis muscle flap or other local rotation flap.

Fallopian Bridge Technique

A significant morbidity to the infratemporal fossa A approach is the necessity for facial nerve transposition. Facial nerve transposition causes a complete facial paralysis acutely. Long-term facial function rarely exceeds a House-Brackmann grade 3, as there is almost always long-term facial synkinesis as a result of bulk movement of the nerve.

An alternative approach to achieving lateral exposure of the jugular bulb is to perform the so-called "fallopian bridge" technique. The fallopian canal is completely skeletonized along its vertical or mastoid component. Rather than remove the bone and transpose the facial nerve, the nerve is kept intact within the canal and wide dissection is performed anteriorly within the tympanic ring and posteriorly within the retrofacial air cell tract (Figure 2–10).

The vertical facial nerve is kept in situ, and tumor dissection medial to the fallopian bridge is carried out

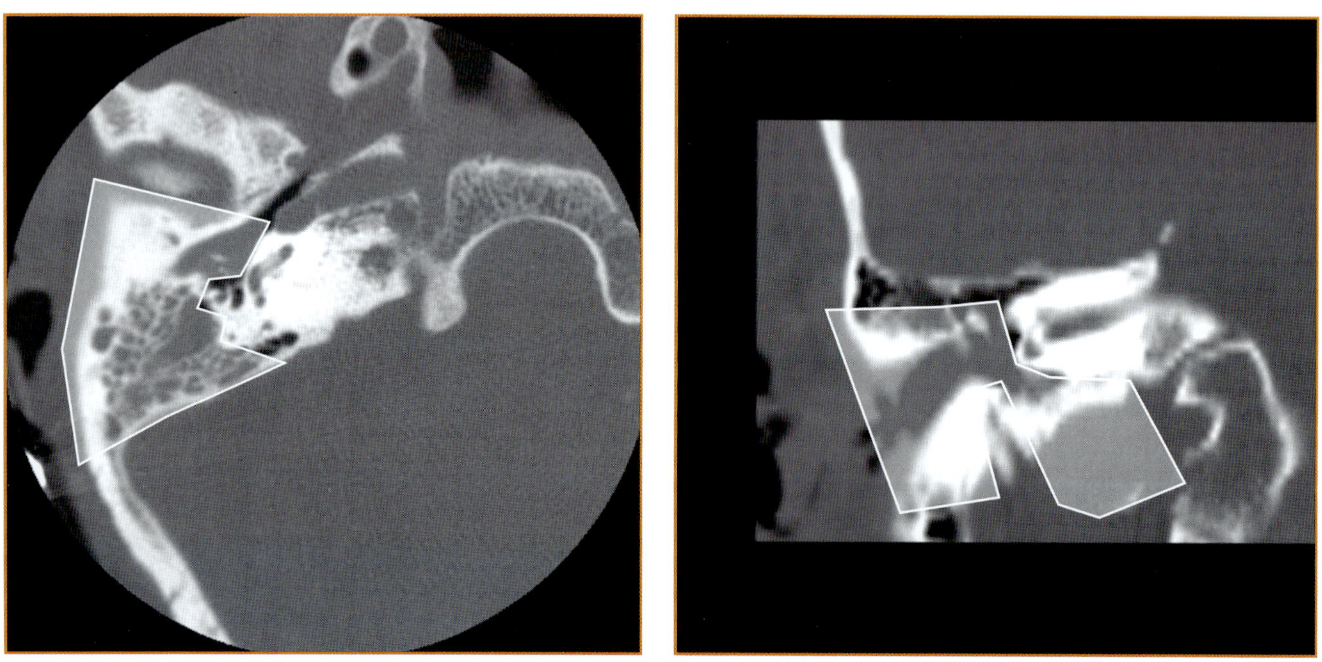

A B

Figure 2–10. Fallopian bridge technique, schematic, axial (**A**) and coronal (**B**).

in piecemeal fashion, accessing the tumor anterior and posterior to the bridge. This technique is most effective for small glomus jugulare tumors and in temporal bones with very well developed air cell tracts.

Transjugular Approach

The transjugular approach is used to expose the jugular bulb, jugular foramen, and cerebellopontine angle for resection of combined extracranial-intracranial jugular foramen tumors.[10]

The transjugular approach begins with a wide mastoidectomy and complete skeletonization of the lateral sinus from the transverse: sigmoid junction superiorly to the jugular bulb inferiorly. Trautmann's triangle of bone is removed to fully expose the presigmoid posterior fossa dura. The posterior mastoid is widely resected to expose the retrosigmoid posterior fossa dura. The mastoid tip is resected, and the jugular foramen is exposed. The vertical facial nerve is delineated and skeletonized to the stylomastoid foramen. The retrofacial air cell tract is extirpated, as is the inferior tympanic ring, with the facial nerve left in place to form the fallopian bridge.

The upper neck is dissected to identify and control the carotid artery and jugular vein and locate and preserve the lower cranial nerves. The jugular vein is ligated, divided, and dissected superiorly to the jugular foramen. The lateral sinus is then ligated and transected in continuity with the surrounding posterior fossa dura anteriorly and posteriorly.

The transected section of lateral sinus and jugular bulb is then resected in similar fashion to the infratemporal fossa A approach, but with more posterior retraction, dural resection, and wider exposure of the intracranial vault. As this is a presigmoid-postsigmoid approach, access to the jugular bulb, jugular foramen, and intracranial vault can be achieved from a more posterior vector, and the facial nerve does not need to be mobilized and transposed anteriorly as is done in the infratemporal fossa A approach. In addition, the external auditory canal does not need to be resected; thereby preserving the native middle ear mechanics and conductive hearing normally lost in the infratemporal fossa A approach (Figure 2–11).

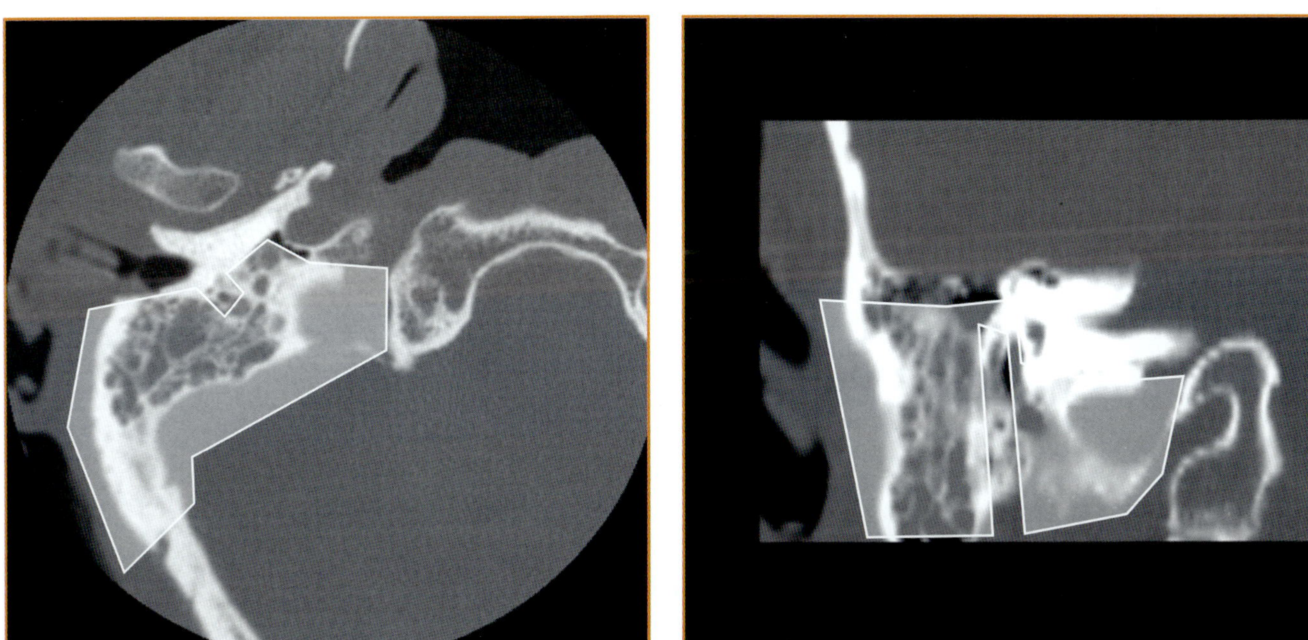

A B

Figure 2–11. Transjugular approach, schematic, axial (**A**) and coronal (**B**).

SUBOCCIPITAL APPROACHES

Retrosigmoid Approach

The retrosigmoid approach as utilized by neurotologists places a suboccipital craniotomy as far anteriorly and laterally as possible, minimizing cerebellar retraction and minimizing the depth of the surgical dissection from the craniotomy to the cerebellopontine angle. Its great strength lies in the ability to fully visualize the entire posterior fossa from tentorium to foramen magnum (Figure 2–12). This approach is useful for large tumors over 3 to 4 cm or with significant inferior or superior extension, and tumors in which the jugular bulb is high, constricting inferior access to the cerebellopontine angle through a translabyrinthine craniotomy. The retrosigmoid approach is also employed when a hearing conservation approach to tumor removal is desired, particularly in tumors with significant cisternal extension not amenable to middle fossa approach. The retrosigmoid approach is described in detail in Chapter 4 with description of vestibular schwannoma management.

Far Lateral Approach/Transcondylar Approach

The far lateral approach, also called the transcondylar approach when modified in such a manner, is an extension of the retrosigmoid approach caudally to the foramen magnum. The standard retrosigmoid approach exposes the posterior fossa at its superior and lateral limits, along the transverse and lateral sinuses, respectively.

The far lateral approach extends this craniotomy inferiorly to encompass the foramen magnum (Figure 2–13). The occipital bone alone can be removed, but if inadequate for tumor exposure, the condyle can be partially resected in continuity with this craniotomy to extend exposure anteriorly.[11]

A C-shaped or S-shaped incision is made approximately midway between the postauricular crease and the occipital midline. The occipital attachments of the sternocleidomastoid and posterior occipital musculature are released. The C1 lamina is palpated, adjacent to which is the vertebral artery. The vertebral artery is found with assistance of Doppler if necessary. A suboccipital craniotomy is performed and extended to the foramen magnum and

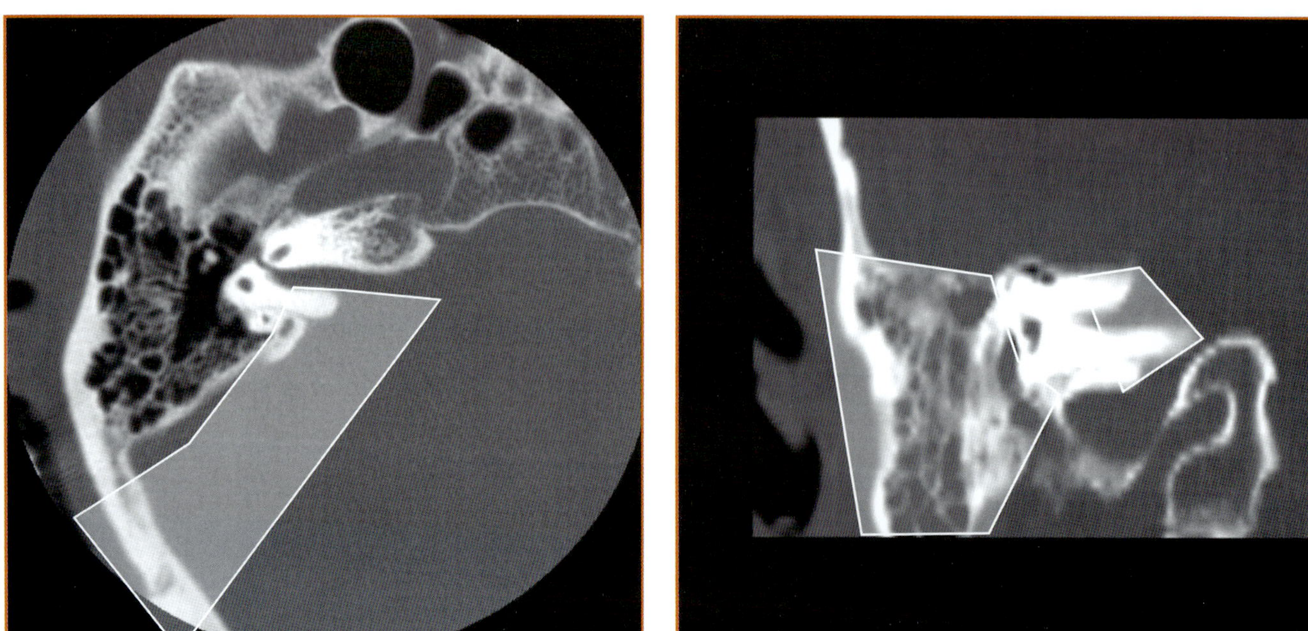

A B

Figure 2–12. Retrosigmoid approach, schematic, axial (**A**) and coronal (**B**).

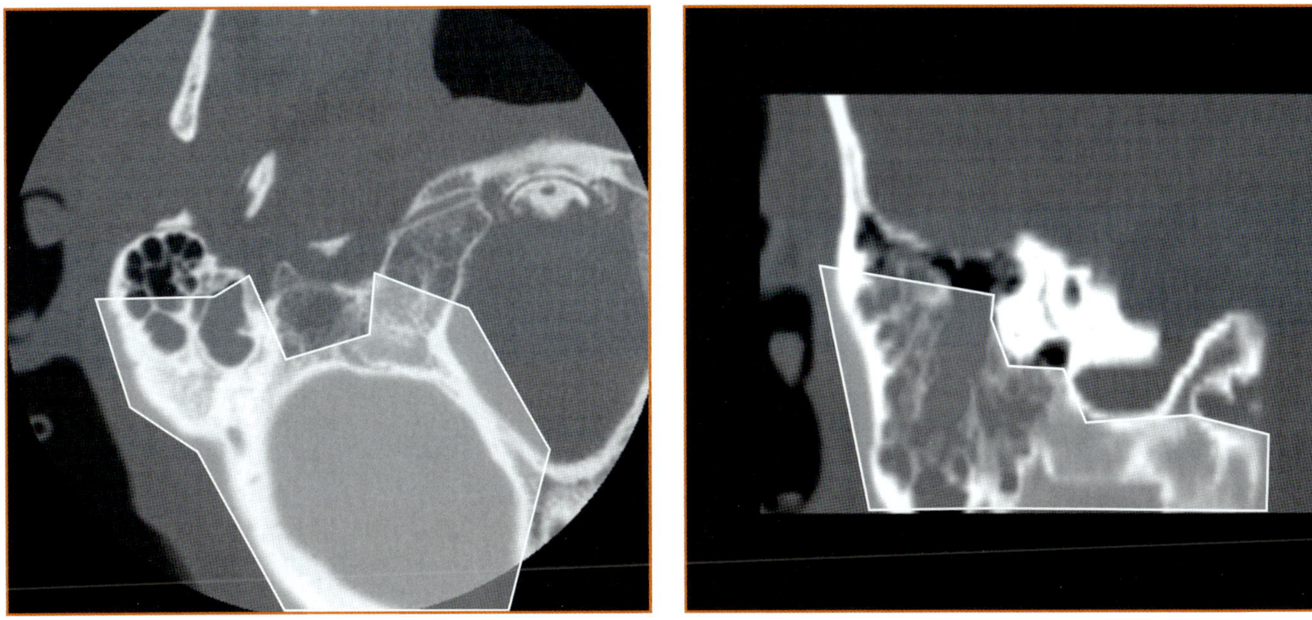

A B

Figure 2–13. Transcondylar approach (far lateral), schematic, axial (**A**) and coronal (**B**).

to partially resect the posterior third to half of the occipital condyle, with care taken around the vertebral artery. If more than half of the occipital condyle is resected, an occipitocervical fusion must be performed to avoid the risk of craniocervical instability.

The transcondylar approach offers extended access to the posterior fossa from the tentorium to the cervicomedullary junction.

Extreme Lateral Approach

The transcondylar approach can be extended to encompass the lateral sinus, jugular bulb, and jugular foramen. This lateral extension provides access to the ventral cervicomedullary junction, or to the jugular foramen itself.[12] The approach is often combined with a retrolabyrinthine extension superiorly into the mastoid cavity, which is employed when the target of dissection is the jugular bulb and jugular foramen as opposed to the ventral cervicomedullary junction (Figure 2–14). This approach is termed the extreme lateral approach.

The extreme lateral approach can be thought of as an extension of the transcondylar approach laterally, that is, traversing the lateral sinus, which denotes the lateral limit of dissection in the transcondylar approach. It can also be thought of as an extension of the transjugular approach inferiorly, with resection of the lower lateral sinus superiorly and extension of intracranial access through the foramen magnum and as low as C1 or C2 inferiorly.[13]

SUBTEMPORAL APPROACHES

Postauricular Subtemporal Approach/Posterior Petrosectomy/Middle Fossa Approach

The standard middle fossa approach used in neurotology to access the internal auditory canal via subtemporal craniotomy is often termed a posterior subtemporal approach or posterior petrosectomy in the neurosurgical literature.

The middle fossa approach is applicable for tumors which are intracanalicular. The great advantage to the middle fossa approach is the ability to visualize the entire internal auditory canal from

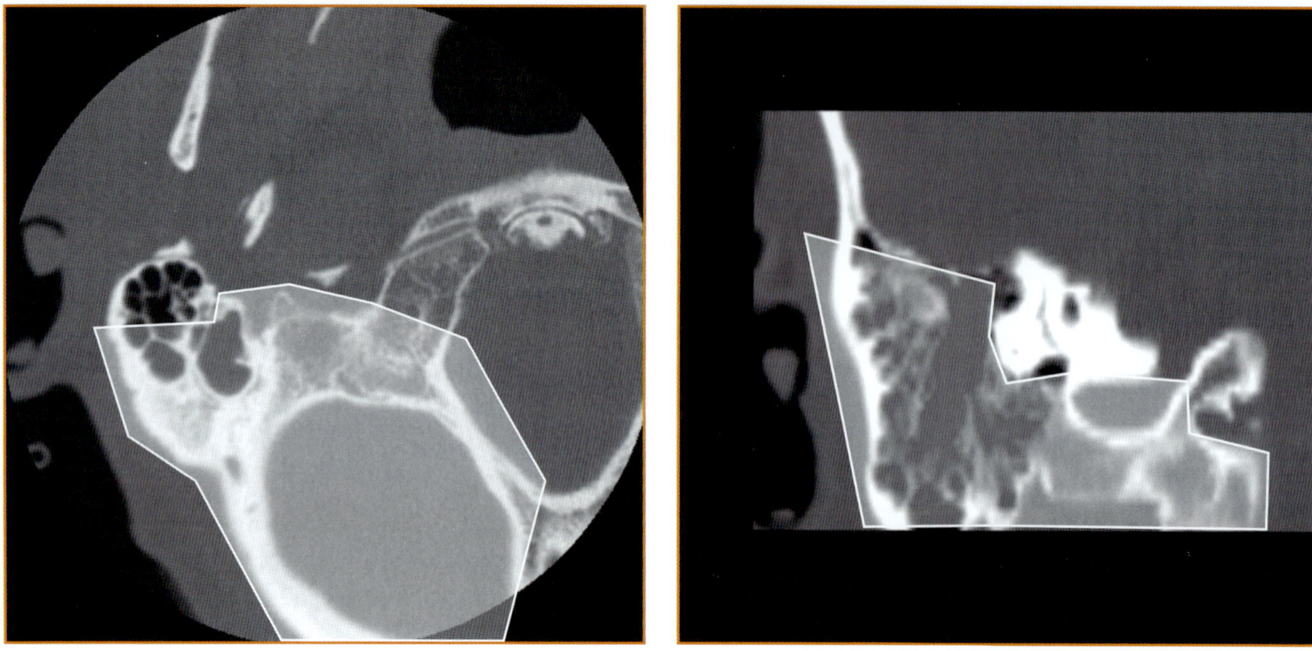

A B

Figure 2–14. Extreme lateral approach, schematic, axial (**A**) and coronal (**B**).

fundus to porus and resect tumors completely with good hope for hearing preservation (Figure 2–15). However, this approach, without modification, does not provide adequate posterior fossa exposure and hence is not appropriate for tumors extending more than 3 to 5 mm beyond the porus acousticus. The middle fossa approach is described in detail in Chapter 4 with description of vestibular schwannoma management.

Preauricular Subtemporal Approach/ Anterior Petrosectomy

The middle fossa approach is sometimes termed the posterior or postauricular subtemporal approach in the neurosurgical literature. By contrast, the preauricular subtemporal approach or anterior petrosectomy takes the internal auditory canal as its posterior limit of dissection rather than as the center of dissection.

Anterior petrosectomy is often aided first by additional lateral exposure by means of osteotomy and downward mobilization of the zygomatic arch, allowing for lower subtemporal craniotomy and wider exposure for Kawase's triangle.

The anterior petrous apex bone between Meckel's cave and the internal auditory canal is then removed. The limits of this anterior petrosectomy, dubbed Kawase's triangle, or more appropriately Kawase's quadrangle, are the gasserian ganglion and mandibular nerve anteriorly, the confluence of the superior petrosal sinus and anterior dural edge of the internal auditory canal medially and posteromedially, the cochlea posterolaterally, and the line parallel to the horizontal petrous carotid artery that passes from the geniculate ganglion to the gasserian ganglion laterally.[14] (Figure 2–16)

Removal of the bone delineated within this quadrangle exposes the posterior fossa dural lining of the anterior petrous apex, beyond which provides access to the prepontine cistern and clivus.

Infratemporal Fossa Type B Approach

If additional anterior extension is desired, the mandibular nerve (V2) is transected proximal to foramen

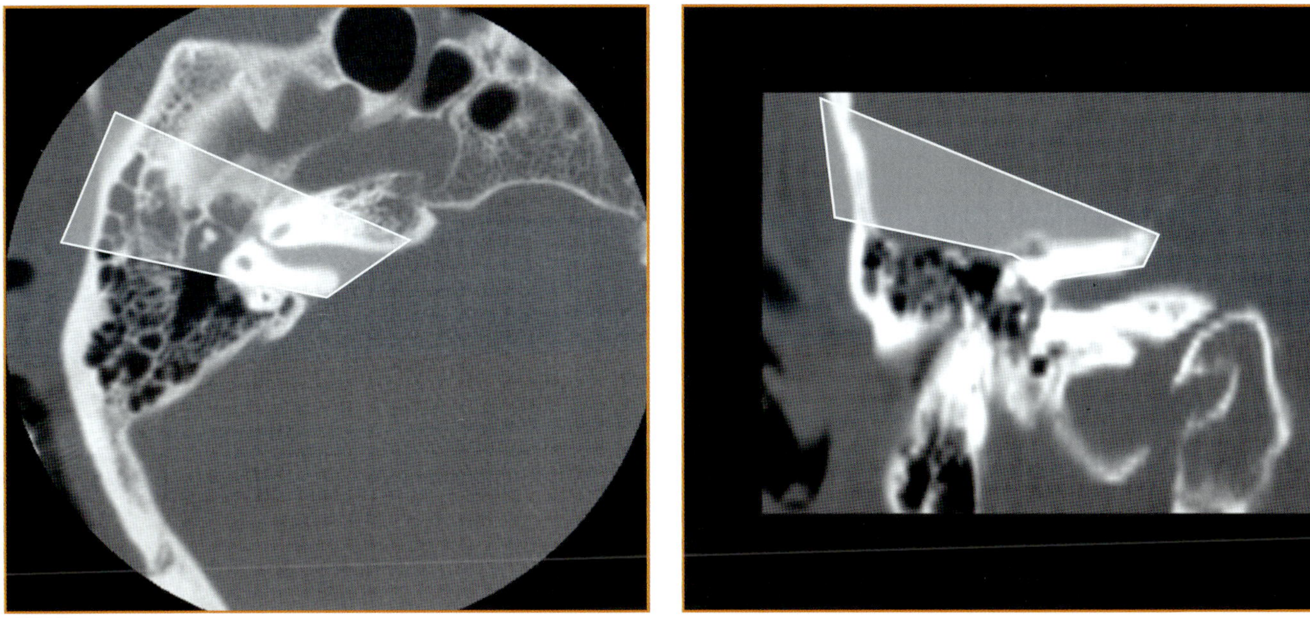

A B

Figure 2–15. Middle fossa approach (postauricular subtemporal), schematic, axial (**A**) and coronal (**B**).

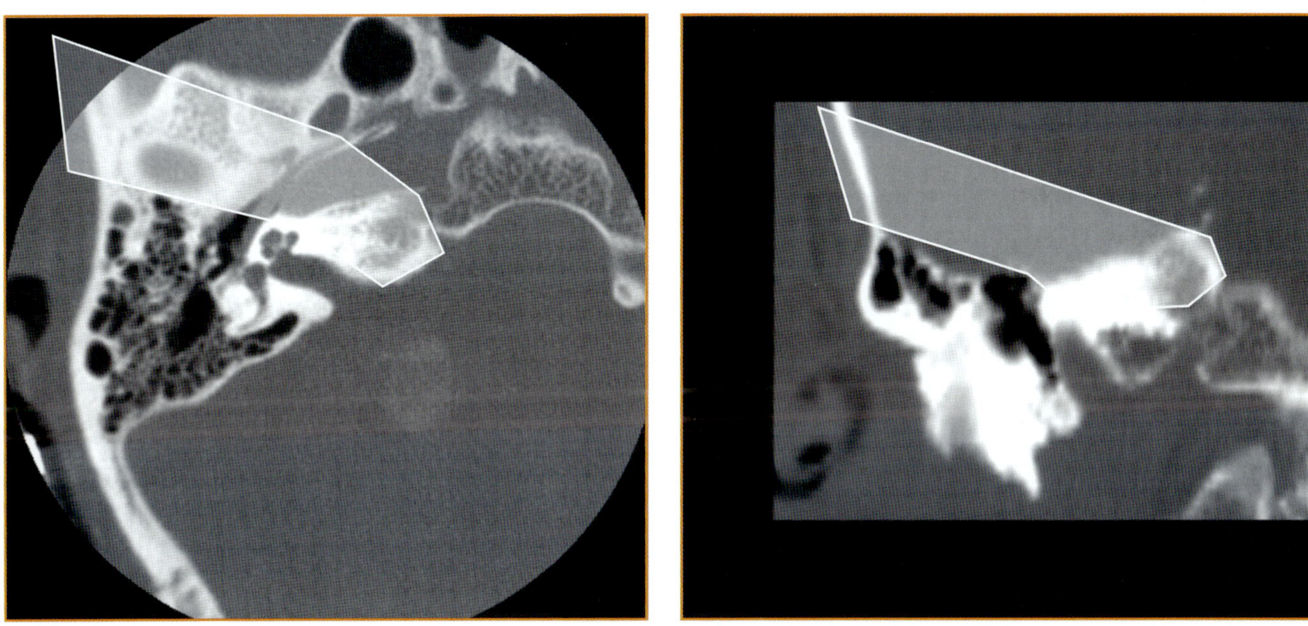

A B

Figure 2–16. Anterior petrosectomy (preauricular subtemporal), schematic, axial (**A**) and coronal (**B**).

ovale and separated from the gasserian ganglion. This provides unimpeded access to the anterolateral triangle of the middle fossa floor and the lateral sphenoid wing (Figure 2–17). For basal tumors with infratemporal fossa extension, the greater wing of the sphenoid can be resected and the infratemporal

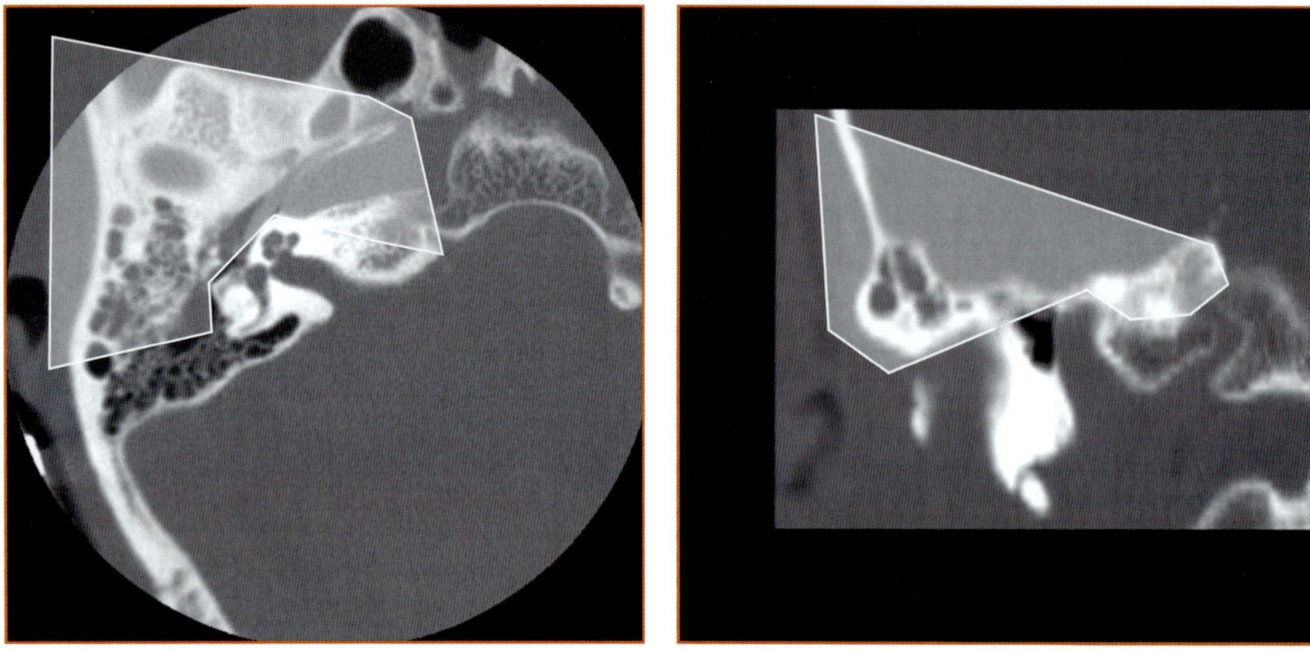

A B

Figure 2–17. Infratemporal fossa type B approach, schematic, axial (**A**) and coronal (**B**).

fossa opened. This exposure of the anterior petrous apex extending to the foramen ovale, transecting the mandibular nerve, with access to the infratemporal fossa via a subtemporal approach is termed the infratemporal fossa B approach. As originally described, the infratemporal fossa B approach utilized a postauricular incision, ear canal overclosure and lateral temporal bone resection for exposure of the eustachian tube and petrous apex in conjunction with the subtemporal craniotomy.

Infratemporal Fossa Type C Approach

The infratemporal fossa type C approach is utilized for tumors along the anterior extent of the petrous bone and clivus, but with more significant extension subcranially within the infratemporal fossa and pterygomaxillary fissure. The infratemporal fossa type C approach continues the shift of transbasal exposure anteriorly; from infratemporal fossa type A where exposure is centered along the jugular bulb, to the infratemporal fossa type B, where exposure is centered along the petrous carotid artery.

The infratemporal fossa type C approach is an extended anterior petrosectomy approach with a preauricular incision and posterior limit of dissection, thereby preserving the external auditory canal and middle ear mechanics. Anteriorly, dissection traverses the mandibular and maxillary nerves to encompass a greater degree of the sphenoid greater wing, including the anterolateral and anteromedial triangles (Figure 2–18). Zygomatic osteotomy and a down fracture are again performed to allow unimpeded access to resection of the lateral sphenoid wing and exposure of the infratemporal fossa.

Extended Middle Fossa Approach

When additional exposure is needed within the cerebellopontine angle through a subtemporal craniotomy, the middle fossa or postauricular subtemporal approach can be combined with the preauricular

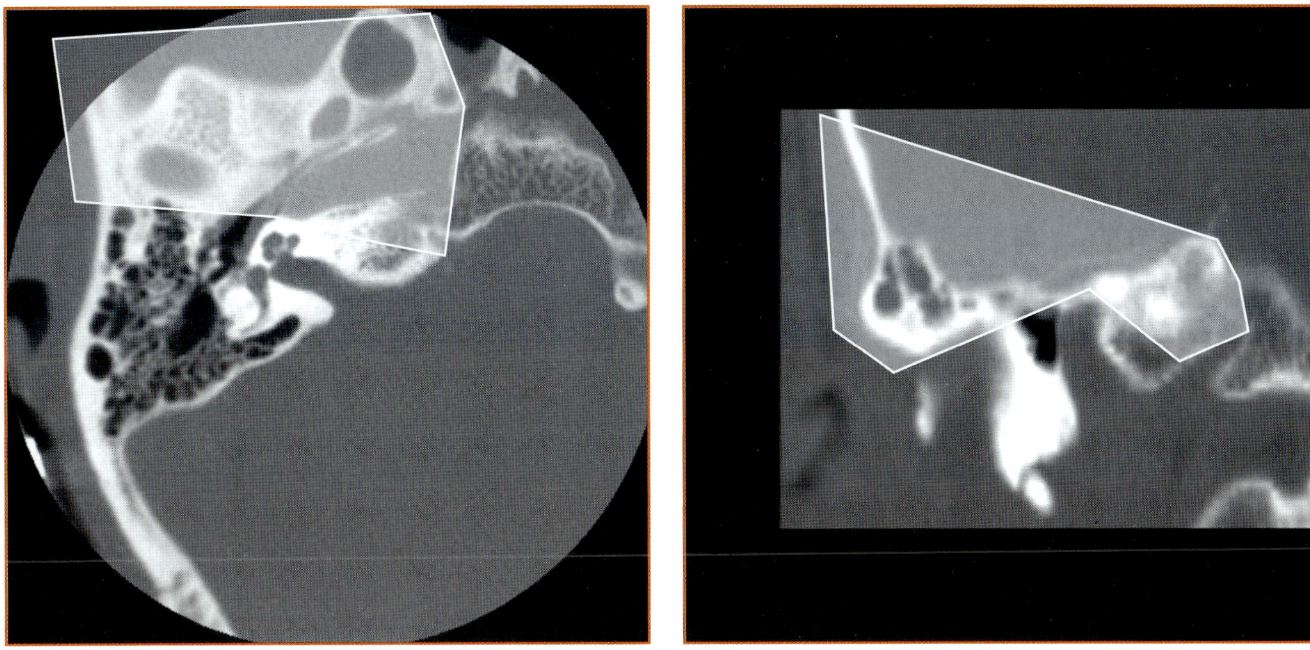

A B

Figure 2–18. Infratemporal fossa type C approach, schematic, axial (**A**) and coronal (**B**).

subtemporal approach to provide such exposure. This extended middle fossa approach provides adequate access to the cerebellopontine angle to allow for tumor removal for intracanalicular tumors with significant cisternal component.[15] This approach is of limited utility for tumors with significant brainstem compression, however.

The standard middle fossa approach is performed. Dissection is carried to the petrous ridge and superior petrosal sinus posteriorly. Anteriorly, dissection is carried beyond the middle meningeal artery, which is ligated and transected at the foramen spinosum. Anterior dissection along the middle fossa floor is extended to Meckel's cave, and the three branches of the trigeminal nerve are delineated and preserved. Anterior petrosectomy is then performed as described above, with extirpation of the bone within Kawase's triangle or quadrangle (Figure 2–19).

All bone above and behind the internal auditory canal is resected, providing a 270° dissection around the porus acousticus medially. The dural around the porus and along the face of the petrous ridge is incised and followed into the internal auditory canal, allowing access to both the internal auditory canal space as well as limited access to the cerebellopontine cistern.

If additional exposure is desired, the tentorium cerebelli can be divided superior to the middle fossa exposure, after ligation or clipping of the superior petrosal sinus. Care must be taken to avoid injury to the trochlear nerve (CN IV) as it runs along the tentorium. The limits of exposure in the extended middle fossa technique are the otic capsule laterally, the petrous carotid artery anteroinferiorly, Meckel's cave and the gasserian ganglion anteromedially, and the safe limit of temporal lobe retraction superiorly. Safe temporal lobe retraction, as with standard middle fossa approaches, is limited in part by traction on the vein of Labbé. The anastamotic vein of Labbé, which bridges the inferior surface of the temporal lobe and the transverse sinus, drains the temporal and parietal lobes. Injury to this vein may lead to speech, memory, and/or other cognitive disorders. Labbé may course in close proximity to the

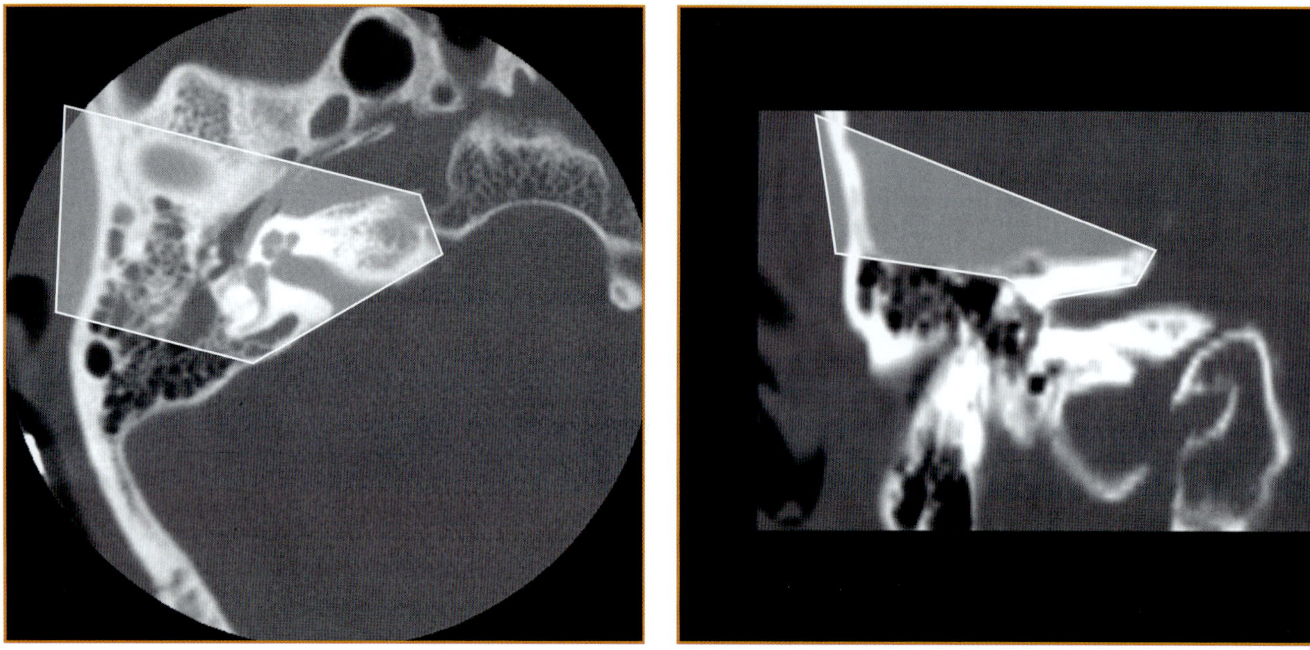

A B

Figure 2–19. Extended middle fossa approach, schematic, axial (**A**) and coronal (**B**).

upper surface of the tentorium or even travel within it for a short segment of its course en route to the transverse sinus.

COMBINED MIDDLE FOSSA-POSTERIOR FOSSA APPROACHES

Large intracranial tumors that traverse both the middle and posterior fossae often cannot be fully accessed by a subtemporal or suboccipital approach alone. Combining subtemporal and suboccipital approaches allows for wide exposure of the prepontine cistern, clivus, and petroclival junction, where such tumors present.

Subtemporal-Retrosigmoid Petrosal Approach

Combining a subtemporal with a retrosigmoid approach provides better access to the petroclival junction than either approach alone (Figure 2–20). However, a significant disadvantage lies in the integrity of the lateral sinus via this approach. This anatomic limitation forces dissection to be performed within two compartments, the presigmoid/subtemporal compartment and the retrosigmoid/suboccipital compartment. This approach has been of limited value since recognition of the greater versatility of the presigmoid varieties of the petrosal approach.

Subtemporal-Retrolabyrinthine Petrosal Approach

Combinations of a subtemporal approach with a presigmoid approach are termed petrosal or transpetrosal approaches. The subtemporal component typically involves a subtemporal craniotomy without significant additional dissection along the middle fossa floor. The presigmoid component can vary based on the amount of the petrous apex is kept intact or resected. The superior petrosal sinus is

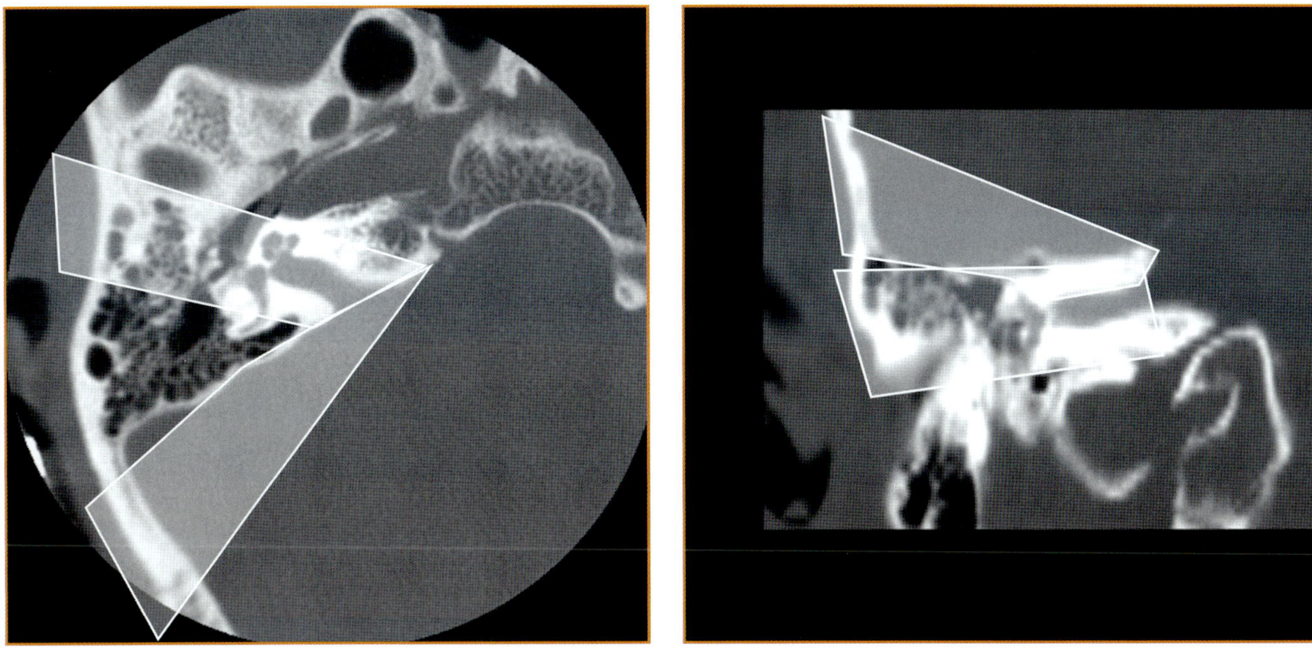

A B

Figure 2–20. Subtemporal-retrosigmoid approach, schematic, axial (**A**) and coronal (**B**).

ligated or clipped and transected, and the tentorium cerebelli is divided to bring the middle and posterior fossa spaces into continuity.

The subtemporal-retrolabyrinthine petrosal craniotomy provides good exposure to the petroclival region and some direct prepontine and clival exposure without sacrificing the otic capsule (Figure 2–21). Retrolabyrinthine dissection is carried to completely resect the posterior fossa dural plate. The semicircular canals are blue-lined but preserved.

Subtemporal-Translabyrinthine Petrosal Approach

The subtemporal-translabyrinthine petrosal craniotomy provides even greater anterior exposure not just to the petroclival region but a complete view of the internal auditory canal as well. The advantage of greater anterior exposure is tempered by the postoperative anacusis induced through this approach (Figure 2–22). A variation of this approach, the transcrusal approach, attempts to maintain neurosensory hearing function by limiting translabyrinthine resection to just the superior and posterior semicircular canals. A technique similar to posterior semicircular canal occlusion or modified translabyrinthine approach is used, with semicircular canal resection and lumen packing up to the ampullae and crus communis, hence the name transcrusal.

Subtemporal-Transcochlear Petrosal Approach

The subtemporal-transcochlear approach extends transpetrosal dissection even further anteriorly, enabling direct view of the entire clivus and prepontine cistern with no brain retraction (Figure 2–23).

Anterior Transpetrosal Approach/ Total Petrosectomy Approach

Removal of the entire petrous bone to access the clivus can be termed an anterior transpetrosal approach. This dissection is essentially equivalent

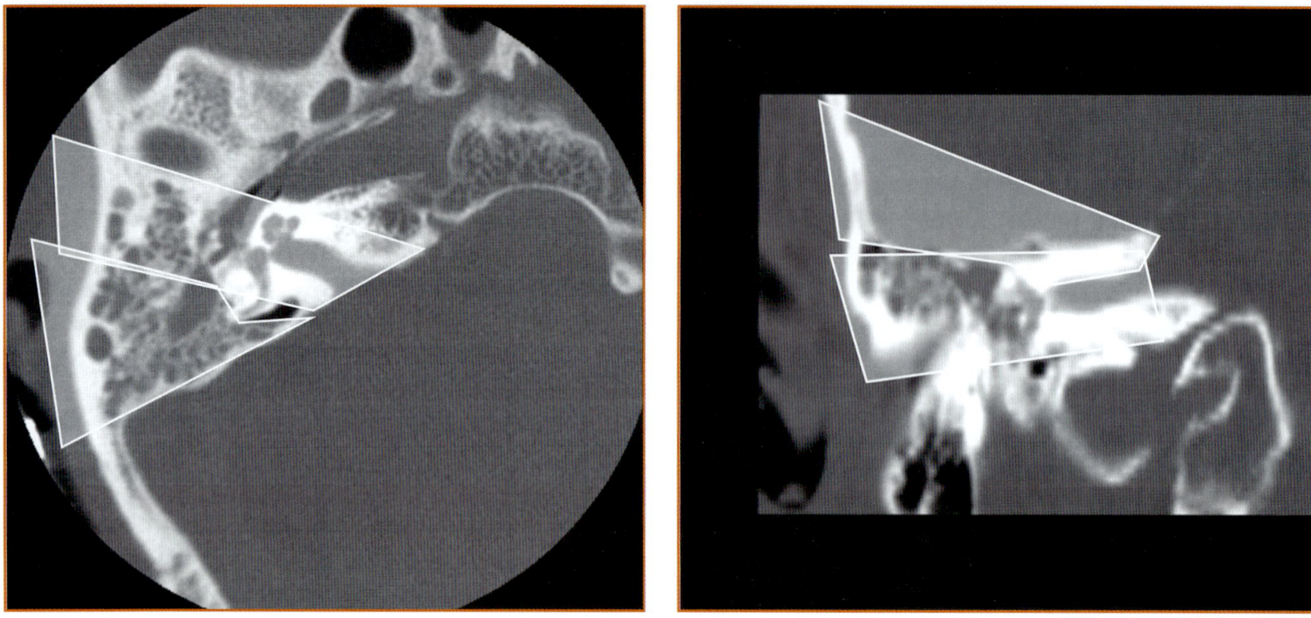

A B

Figure 2–21. Subtemporal-retrolabyrinthine approach, schematic, axial (**A**) and coronal (**B**).

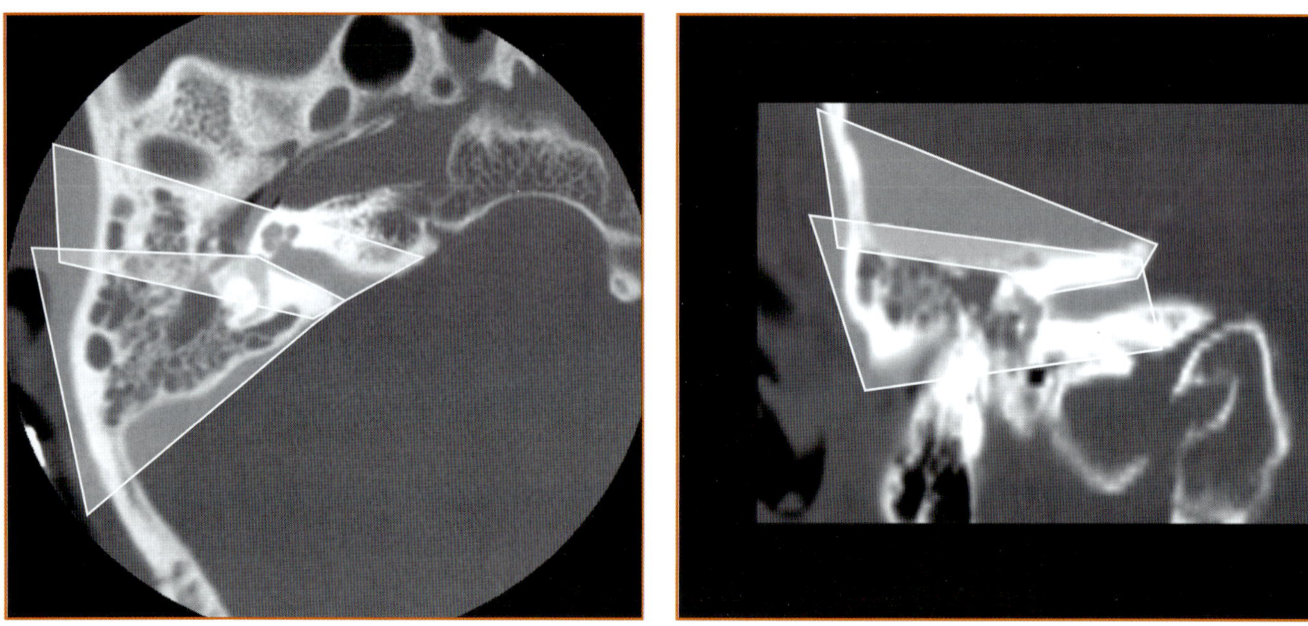

A B

Figure 2–22. Subtemporal-translabyrinthine approach, schematic, axial (**A**) and coronal (**B**).

to the total petrosectomy approach, but the two terms are used in different settings: the petrosal approaches are used to access the middle fossa/posterior fossa, whereas the total petrosectomy is performed to extirpate disease that is embedded within the petrous temporal bone proper (Figure 2–24).

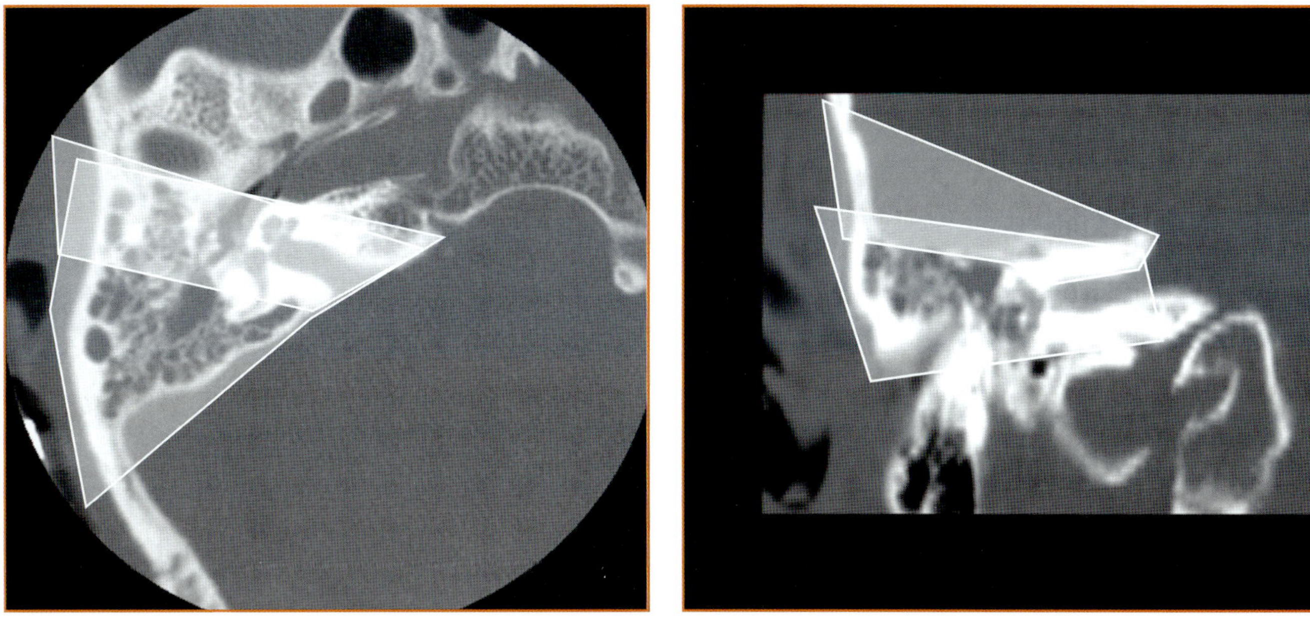

A B

Figure 2–23. Subtemporal-transcochlear approach, schematic, axial (**A**) and coronal (**B**).

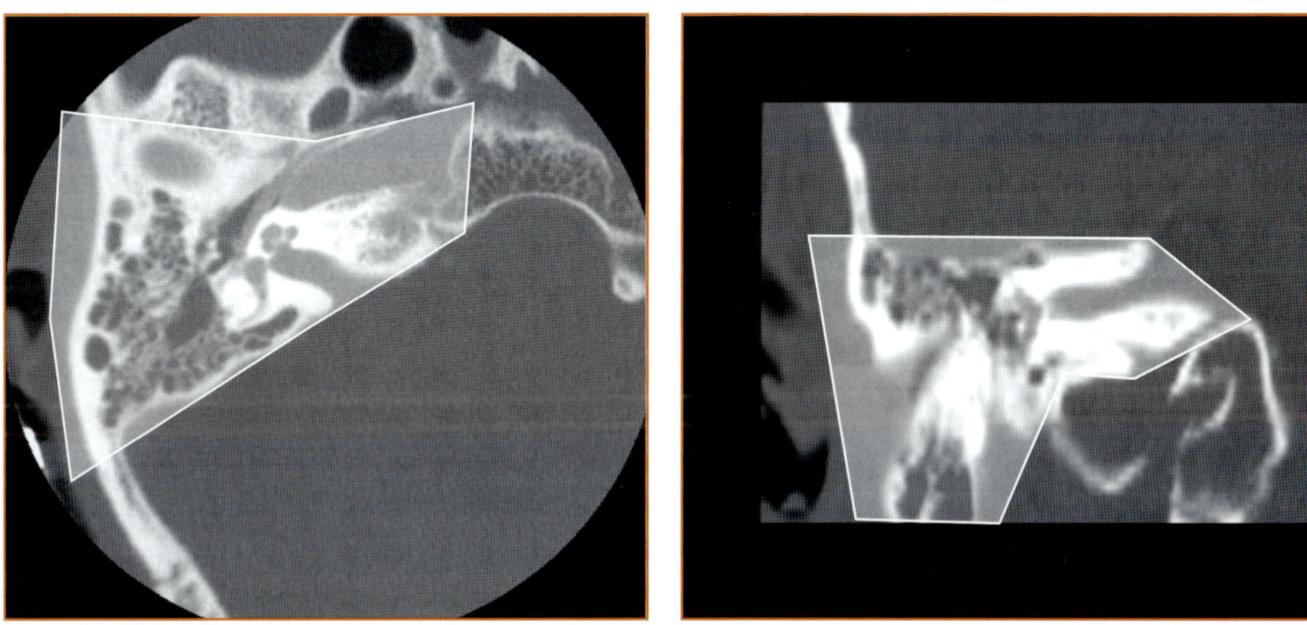

A B

Figure 2–24. Total petrosectomy, schematic, axial (**A**) and coronal (**B**).

This temporal bone dissection, under either name, is uncommonly performed. The entire anterior petrous apex does not need to be resected to visualize the clivus and prepontine cistern: this can be partially accessed with a subtemporal-retrolabyrinthine approach or completely accessed with a subtemporal-transcochlear approach without brain retraction. Total petrosectomy for advanced, invasive malignant disease will cause significant perioperative morbidity and possibly mortality yet will do little to improve prognosis.

SUMMARY

From the varied names and descriptions of the many approaches to the lateral skull base, it is clear that most named approaches share commonalities in regional dissections with other, adjacent approaches. The approach chosen for a given tumor can be tailored very specifically to the anatomic regions encompassed by that tumor, and intimate knowledge of the surrounding cranial base can ensure that proper techniques are employed. Equally importantly, if a chosen approach ends up being inadequate for management of a given tumor, knowledge of the lateral skull base allows one to modify and expand an existing approach to provide more effective exposure for successful tumor extirpation.

REFERENCES

1. Pieper DR, LaRouere M, Jackson IT. Operative management of skull base malignancies: choosing the appropriate approach. *Neurosurg Focus*. 2002;12(5):e6.
2. Sargent EW, Kartush JM, Graham MD. Meatal facial nerve decompression in acoustic neuroma resection. *Am J Otol*. 1995;16(4):457–464.
3. Bloch DC, Oghalai JS, Jackler RK, Osofsky M, Pitts LH. The fate of the tumor remnant after less-than-complete acoustic neuroma resection. *Otolaryngol Head Neck Surg*. 2004;130(1):104–112.
4. McElveen JT Jr., Wilkins RH, Molter DW, Erwin AC, Wolford RD. Hearing preservation using the modified translabyrinthine approach. *Otolaryngol Head Neck Surg*. 1993;108(6):671–679.
5. Tringali S, Bertholon P, Chelikh L, Jacquet C, Prades JM, Martin C. Hearing preservation after modified translabyrinthine approach performed to remove a vestibular schwannoma. *Ann Otol Rhinol Laryngol*. 2004;113(2):152–155.
6. Magliulo G, Stasolla A, Parrotto D, Marini M. Modified translabyrinthine approach and hearing preservation: imaging evaluation. *J Laryngol Otol*. 2007;121(8):736–741.
7. Shaia WT, Zappia JJ, Bojrab DI, LaRouere ML, Sargent EW, Diaz RC. Success of posterior semicircular canal occlusion and application of the dizziness handicap inventory. *Otolaryngol Head Neck Surg*. 2006;134(3):424–430.
8. Magliulo G, Parrotto D, Stasolla A, Marini M. Modified translabyrinthine approach and hearing preservation. *Laryngoscope*. 2004;114(6):1133–1138.
9. Jenkins HA, Fisch U. The transotic approach to resection of difficult acoustic tumors of the cerebellopontine angle. *Am J Otol*. 1980;2(2):70–76.
10. Oghalai JS, Leung MK, Jackler RK, McDermott MW. Transjugular craniotomy for the management of jugular foramen tumors with intracranial extension. *Otol Neurotol*. 2004;25(4):570–579; discussion 579.
11. Rhoton AL, Jr. The far-lateral approach and its transcondylar, supracondylar, and paracondylar extensions. *Neurosurgery*. 2000;47(3 suppl):S195–209.
12. Kumar CV, Satyanarayana S, Rao BR, Palur RS. Extreme lateral approach to ventral and ventrolaterally situated lesions of the lower brainstem and upper cervical cord. *Skull Base*. 2001;11(4):265–275.
13. Liu JK, Sameshima T, Gottfried ON, Couldwell WT, Fukushima T. The combined transmastoid retro- and infralabyrinthine transjugular transcondylar transtubercular high cervical approach for resection of glomus jugulare tumors. *Neurosurgery*. 2006;59(1 suppl 1):ONS115–125; discussion ONS115–125.
14. Naguib MB, Sanna M. Subtemporal exposure of the intrapetrous internal carotid artery. An anatomical study with surgical application. *J Laryngol Otol*. 1999;113(8):717–720.
15. Aristegui M, Cokkeser Y, Saleh E, et al. Surgical anatomy of the extended middle cranial fossa approach. *Skull Base Surg*. 1994;4(4):181–188.

CHAPTER 3

Minimally Invasive and Endoscopic Approaches to the Skull Base

Gregory Artz, Marc Rosen, James Evans, and Daniel Pieper

INTRODUCTION

Since the pioneering research and clinical experience in Austria by Messerklinger and Stamberger and the first publication in the United States by Kennedy in 1985, endoscopic sinus surgery has become one the most common procedures performed by otolaryngologists.[1] With the early work of these and many other surgeons combined with the development of improved optics, visualization, and instrumentation, endoscopic sinus surgery has become a routine part of all otolaryngology training programs. For the last decade, it has been commonly used in conjunction with digital video imagery and image-guidance technology with improved outcomes.

Only recently has this technology been introduced into the field of skull base surgery and for the past several years there has been an increase in surgeons attempting and succeeding in performing minimally-invasive endoscopic skull base surgery with acceptable outcomes, less morbidity, and improved cosmetic results when compared to the traditional open skull base approaches.

Initially, there was resistance to endoscopic approaches to the skull base by some surgeons unfamiliar with the technology, uncomfortable with the limited exposure, and unwilling to give up the traditional microscopic approaches requiring extensive soft tissue dissection and large craniotomies. However, through a younger generation of surgeons trained in endoscopic techniques, otolaryngologists and neurosurgical teams now collaborate and the field of minimally invasive skull base surgery has emerged.

This chapter will discuss minimally-invasive endoscopic skull base surgery for the anterior and posterolateral skull base with attention to indications, surgical technique complications and outcomes.

ENDOSCOPIC ANTERIOR SKULL BASE SURGERY

One of the most common endoscopic skull base surgeries performed today is the transsphenoidal hypophysectomy (TSH) for pituitary lesions. Some of the first publications to describe this technique were by Jankowski et al and Jho et al followed by several other surgeons who found success with similar techniques.[2–4] The days of the sublabial incisions, Hardy nasal speculums, septal flaps, microscopic visualization, and limited resections due to poor visualization are gone. Postoperative complications related to the sublabial approach are no longer seen and nasal complications such as septal perforations are rare.

Pituitary adenomas are the third most common intracranial tumor and can be classified as micro or macroadenoma and secreting or non-secreting tumors. Symptoms are related to hormone excesses in secreting-tumors (ie, acromegaly from growth hormone or hyperprolactinemia) or due to compression of surrounding structures in the cases of macroadenomas. Commonly presenting symptoms include visual disturbances, field defects, and headaches. Options include medications for prolactinomas, observation with serial MRI for small asymptomatic lesions, or surgical resection for those symptomatic or progressive tumors. Recurrent lesions have been traditionally treated with radiotherapy, stereotactic radiosurgery, and medical therapy; however, with the success of the endoscopic approach along with a signifivcant reduction in morbidity even with recurrent tumors, revision surgery is now being argued by many surgeons as an equally viable option. Access to the pituitary and area of the sella turcica in revision surgery is often quite easy and the success of resection depends only on the amount of residual scarring in the adenoma. A publication by Barker et al[5] reviewed complication rates in traditional open, microscopic pituitary surgery. Major complications such as patient mortality and intracranial hemorrhage were low and outcomes were significantly better at high-volume centers. White et al[6] published data on the endoscopic approach showing similar complication rates with improvement in minor complications such as numbness, septal perforation, and other nasal complaints. The endoscopic approach decreases the need for nasal packing, reduces hospital stays, and may result in fewer patients requiring revision surgery.

In addition to pituitary surgery, the endoscopic approach is also being applied to other pathologies that were traditionally approached via large open craniotomies. CSF leaks, suprasellar lesions, esthesioneuroblastomas, clival chordomas, epidermoids, petrous apex lesions, and even anterior fossa meningiomas have been successfully treated with endoscopic approaches.

Prior to surgery for any skull base lesion, a patient should be thoroughly evaluated by a neurosurgeon and an otolaryngologist who specializes in endoscopic skull base surgery. The work-up should include endoscopic evaluation of the sinonasal cavity to assess for septal deviation, perforation, infection, polyps, or other anatomic abnormalities. In addition, MRI and CT imaging of the brain, skull base, and sinuses are essential for proper planning of the surgical procedure. Large tumors, aberrant carotid anatomy precluding an approach through the posterior wall of the sphenoid sinus, poorly aerated sinuses, and active sinusitis are the few contraindications to the endoscopic approach.

Instrumentation

Surgical instrumentation continues to be a work in progress for many high volume centers as tools specifically designed for endoscopic skull base surgery are being designed and developed. Standard endoscopic sinus surgery instrumentation are often used, however they are limited by length, as they are not designed for the depth of field often required for skull base surgery. Bayoneted neurosurgical instruments used for microsurgery to keep the surgeon's fingers out of line-of-sight are not needed for endoscopic surgery and their shape can be counterproductive. Straight, "pistol-grip" retractable/guarded blades and dual functioning suction currettes are better suited for endoscopic procedures.[7]

Endoscopic Transphenoidal Hypophysectomy Surgical Technique

There has been an evolution of transnasal endoscopic surgery from an endoscopic-assisted version through the sublabial/transseptal approach to a purely transnasal technique that is used today. Sinonasal anatomy should be preserved when possible, while allowing the operating surgeon the adequate exposure to comfortably perform two-handed surgery. A septoplasty is performed when indicated to improve the nasal airway. A posterior ethmoidectomy can be helpful for access to the sella floor and planum sphenoidale and a partial middle turbinate resection is done when needed. The middle turbinate is an important sinonasal landmark, and helps protect the posterior septectomy and skull base defect.

Once the patient is intubated the bed is turned 180 degrees from the anesthesiologist. The bed is lowered and the head/back of the table raised 20 degrees with the head and neck in neutral position. The navigation system is then set up and calibrated.

The nasal cavity is then prepared for surgery by decongesting the nasal mucosa with Cottonoids soaked in 4% cocaine solution. Ten cc of 1% lidocaine with 1:100,000 epinephrine is used to inject the inferior turbinate, middle turbinate, posterior septum, and sphenoid face. If needed, a septoplasty and a partial resection of the middle turbinate are performed. For most portions of our procedures, a 0-degree rigid endoscope equipped with an irrigating system (Xomed Endoscrub, Jacksonville, FL) fitted with a high-definition digital camera is used.

The sphenoid os on one side of the nasal cavity is identified and is enlarged with cutting forceps and 2 and 3-mm rotating Kerrison punches. Access to the sphenoid sinus is enlarged by performing a posterior septectomy with straight cutting forceps and backbiters. The contralateral sphenoid sinus in enlarged using Kerrison punches straight cutting forceps. Jansen-Middleton forceps or even high-speed drills are occasionally required to remove the thick bone of the sphenoid rostrum. Once the sphenoid has been entered one must cautiously remove the intersphenoid septum as it is often eccentrically located and can insert onto the carotid canal. Depending on the access required, the sphenoidotomy can be extended superiorly to the planum, laterally to the carotids, and inferiorly to the clivus. Access to the planum can be further facilitated by removal of posterior ethmoid air cells. This "access" portion of the procedure is usually performed with a two-handed technique: one hand holding the camera and the other using instrumentation. The foot pedals for a monopolar, bipolar, and the endoscope irrigating system all should be arranged on the floor for easy access by the surgeon.

Once access has been created to the skull base, the minimally invasive approach is performed through both nares with the camera usually positioned in the left nare either held by an assistant or by a polyarticulated pneumatic camera holder that is attached to the bed frame. Adequate sinonasal exposure is critical so the operating surgeon can use a two-handed technique either from the right nare or using both nares to triangulate and be able to freely dissect both medially and laterally. A right-handed operating surgeon will stand at the patient's right side with an image guidance suction-tip in the left hand and instrumentation in the right.

When the sella has been exposed, bipolar cautery is used to cauterize the mucosa and the thin bone can usually be fractured and easily removed using Kerrison punches. If the bone of the sella is thick, straight cutting forceps, small chisels, or even diamond and cutting high-speed drills, specifically designed for endoscopic skull base surgery, can be used to expose dura. A cruciate dural incision is made using a retractable blade and tumor dissection is performed. To facilitate maximal tumor removal, a 30-degree scope can be used as well as image-guidance instrumentation and a carotid doppler.

At the completion of tumor resection, a Valsalva maneuver is performed to identify any occult CSF leak. Hemostasis is achieved using surgifoam and specially designed "Flo-balls," which are small spheres of Floseal™ wrapped with Surgicel. The dural incision in the sella is repaired using a few sheets of Surgicel in an overlay pattern. If there is an indentified CSF leak, dura repair material and Dura Seal™ are also used to create a "watertight" seal. Sphenoid packing is not routinely performed. The middle turbinates are medialized and Gelfilm sheeting is placed along the septum and in the middle meatus bilaterally to prevent synechiae.

Technical Notes

1. Occasionally, a large, posteriorly pedicled mucosal flap is used for reconstruction in extended skull base surgeries. In these instances, a posterior septectomy of both mucosal septal surfaces is not performed; instead, on the contralateral side of the intended mucosal flap, a small vertical incision in made in the posterior septal mucosa and raised off the sphenoid os. The exposed bone of the sphenoid, rostrum, and posterior septum is them removed while preserving the entire septal mucosa on the contralateral side. This pedicled septal flap can also be used for reconstruction of large cribriform plate defects.
2. For large dural defects, a reconstructive technique has been developed called the "facial-button." A large homograft of fascia lata is harvested and cut into two pieces that are approximated 30 to 40% larger than the dural defect. One or 2 stitches are placed in the middle of each piece to secure them together. The pieces are then

placed in the defect in an underlay or overlay technique and then either a mucosalized flap or Dura Seal™ is used to secure and cover the graft.

3. For planum or cribriform plate defects, preserving the middle turbinate is important as it can be used as a rotational osteoplastic flap ("MTOP"—middle turbinated osteoplastic flap). The medial surface of the middle turbinate is denuded of mucosa and it is up fractured to fill in the bony defect. This technique is successfully used, as well as a "STOP" (superior turbinate osteoplastic flap) for smaller skull base reconstruction (ie, spontaneous CSF leak of the cribriform plate).

Image Guidance

An image-guidance navigation system is essential in performing safe endoscopic skull base surgery. It allows the operating surgeon to accurately locate the midline and establish and confirm the skull base anatomy. For pituitary surgery, it is important to accurately identify the location of the carotid arteries to ensure a safe craniotomy and dural incisions. If there is any question of accuracy, doppler signals are used to confirm carotid artery location as image guidance accuracy can be limited by an error range of 1 to 3 mm.[8] A frameless navigation system can be used that is set up in minutes and uses a CT/MRI fusion image that gives both bony skull base anatomy as well soft tissue detail. Despite not giving real-time information we do feel it helps us decrease operating time and allows for a more complete resection. Future technology such as intraoperative MRI and CT imaging is currently becoming available to further help with tumor removal; however, it seems to prolong surgical time and is not being widely used due to its high cost.

Complications

Major complications related to open pituitary surgery include cerebrospinal fluid leak (1 to 3%), diabetes insipidus (0.4 to 3%), ophthalmoplegia, and rarely intracranial hemorrhage.[9] The endoscopic approach appears to have similar or better rates of these complications when compared to the microscopic approach.[6] Minor complications such as post-op epistaxis, lip anesthesia, septal deviation, or septal perforation have been significantly reduced or eliminated by the endoscopic approach. At our institution, there has been a decrease in length of stay, cerebrospinal fluid leaks, and more complete tumor resection. This has resulted in a decrease in the number of revision TSH procedures being performed. At high-volume centers, with experienced surgeons, the endoscopic approach is a safe procedure that has reduced complication rates and improved outcomes.[10]

ADVANTAGES/ DISADVANTAGES

The endoscopic skull base approach, particularly for pituitary surgery offers several key advantages. Endoscopy allows for dramatically better visualization of the surgical area than the microscopic view. The depth of field and the straight field of view required for illumination has always made the microscopic approach challenging. With straight and angled endoscopes, one is able to visualize around corners, inspect the carotid arteries, access the suprasellar space and lateral recesses that were never able to be seen with the microscopic approach. There is less need for a transseptal or sublabial approach. Nasal packing is rarely required, improving postoperative patient comfort. The wide sphenoidotomy and posterior septectomy provide the ability to survey the surgical site in the outpatient setting. In patients who require revision surgery, access to the sella region has already been established, making the approach easy. Preserving all or part of the middle turbinate is important, as it serves as a key sinonasal landmark for orientation and it aids in nasal airflow, olfaction, and humidification. The middle turbinate can be protective, as it will often re-direct nasogastric tubing downward that potentially could enter a skull base defect when introduced blindly. It is recommended that endoscopic guidance of any nasogastric tubing be performed in all patients having had previous surgery on the anterior skull base.

A disadvantage of the endoscopic approach is the monoptical two-dimensional image that it provides. While the microscopic does offer a stereoscopic view that more closely replicates a three-dimensional view, the modern optics, image guidance technology and the freedom of visualization at the surgical site, all make the endoscope superior, despite the two-dimensional view.

There has been some concern regarding the exposed dura in the sinonasal cavity and the potential for meningitis. While this is a theoretical risk, it does not seem to translate into much of a risk. We have observed that our skull base repairs form a thick, tough scar that becomes a well-mucosalized barrier. Re-ossification of the surgical access site has also been observed.

ENDOSCOPIC POSTEROLATERAL SKULL BASE SURGERY

Endoscopic surgery for the anterior skull base is becoming a well-accepted approach for skull base lesions, while endoscopic surgery for the posterolateral skull base is a relatively new frontier. Posterior fossa endoscopy is being performed at only a few centers for vascular compression disorders (trigeminal neuralgia and hemifacial spasm) and for small meningiomas or schwannomas, and those that do, use it as an adjunct to the microscope. Very few centers are using the endoscope exclusively. When used without the microscope, endoscopy of the posterior fossa has the ability to limit craniotomy size, procedure-time, and hospital length of stay while maintaining or improving the outcomes seen in microscopic surgery.

Microvascular decompression (MVD) is a well-accepted, highly successful surgical procedure for the treatment of trigeminal neuralgia (TGN) and hemifacial spasm (HFS). It also has been shown to be successful in the treatment of patients with less common vascular compressive syndromes such as glossopharyngeal neuralgia (GPN) and cochleovestibular nerve compressive syndrome (CNCS). MVD is well accepted and remains the most successful intervention for immediate and long-term relief of symptoms in patients with TGN and HFS.[10,11] Alternative interventions that are well tolerated, but less successful than MVD for the treatment of TGN include percutaneous radiofrequency rhizotomy, glycerol rhizotomy, ballon-compression, and stereotactic radiosurgery. Endoscopic assisted microvascular decompression (EAMVD) is a recent variation on the traditional procedure that has been reported to provide better intraoperative visualization with the potential for better results. Many articles on this topic detail the endoscopic anatomy of the cerebellopontine angle (CPA) and use the endoscopic technique only after traditional craniotomy and vascular decompression has been performed using the operating microscope.[12–14] Only a few articles discuss a fully endoscopic technique without the aid of an operating microscope, performed through a more limited incision and craniotomy.[15–17]

The benefits of EVD include a smaller incision with less soft tissue mobilization, smaller craniotomy, less cerebellar retraction, and panoramic visualization of the intracranial space from lower cranial nerves to the tentorium (Figure 3–1). Straight and angled endoscopes improve the ability to visualize areas of vascular compression not seen with the microscope, leading to a higher rate of successful outcomes.[14,18] Potential additional benefits of EVD include lower complication rates, shorter hospitals stays, and less postoperative pain resulting in quicker recoveries.[15] Patients may be able to more quickly return to work and resume normal daily activities.

Despite its success, EVD does present technical challenges. Finding the exact position of the transverse-sigmoid sinus junction based on surface landmarks can be challenging and is a critical

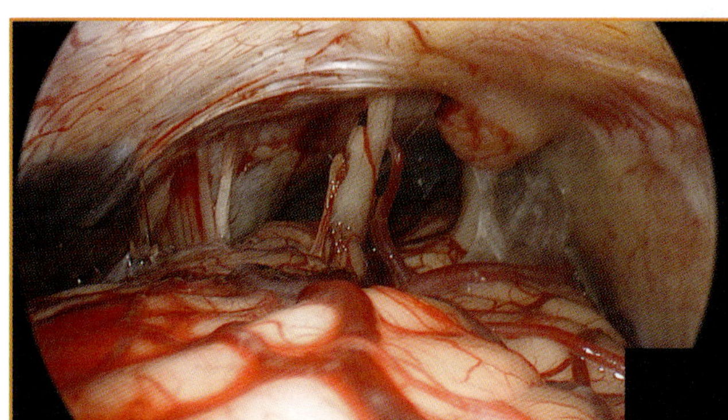

Figure 3–1. Endoscopic view of posterior skull base, left. Tentorium is to the right with VII/VIII in middle of view.

step to minimize both the size of the incision and craniotomy. Another problem is the lack of depth perception and stereoscopic visualization that the microscope can provide. This creates a steep-learning curve that can significantly increase operative time until a certain level of experience is obtained. There is also additional equipment, which can increase the operating room setup, turnover time, and the capital expense required to perform the procedure.

Endoscopic Vascular Decompression Technique

A retrosigmoid craniotomy approach is used for all of posterior fossa endoscopic cases, including the EVD. Facial nerve monitoring with The NIM-response (Medtronic USA, Inc, Minneapolis, MN) and auditory brainstem response (ABR) monitoring with the Cascade system (Cadwell Laboratories, Inc, Kennewick, WA) are used. The patient is placed in a supine position and the head is immobilized in a Mayfield head clamp to avoid any unforeseen movement of the head while the endoscope is within the cerebellopontine angle. The intracranial pressure is reduced by elevating the head to 30°, administering 1 gm/kg of mannitol (not exceeding 75 gm) followed by 20 mg of furosemide intravenously and reducing the arterial pCO_2 to 28 to 30 mm Hg. Lumbar drain is not utilized. Prior to the skin incision, the craniotomy site is estimated by the intersection of two anatomical lines. The first line approximates the inferior border of the transverse sinus by drawing a line from the zygomatic root to the inion, also called the superior nuchal line. The second line is along the posterior mastoid groove, which approximates the occipitomastoid suture line. The intersection of these two lines is an accurate estimation of the transverse-sigmoid sinus junction and will be the anteriosuperior limit of our 1.5-cm craniotomy once the calvarium has been exposed. A 3 to 4 cm oblique incision along the hairline is marked and centered over the estimated craniotomy site (Figure 3–2).

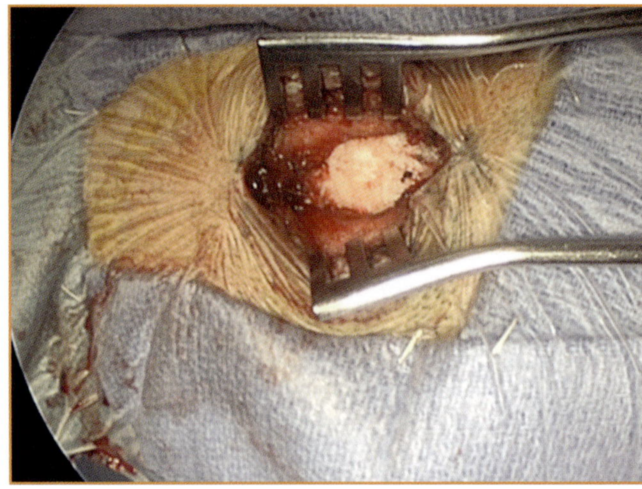

Figure 3–2. Right posterior skin incision is made and the muscles have been transected with cranium visible. Incision is 3 cm.

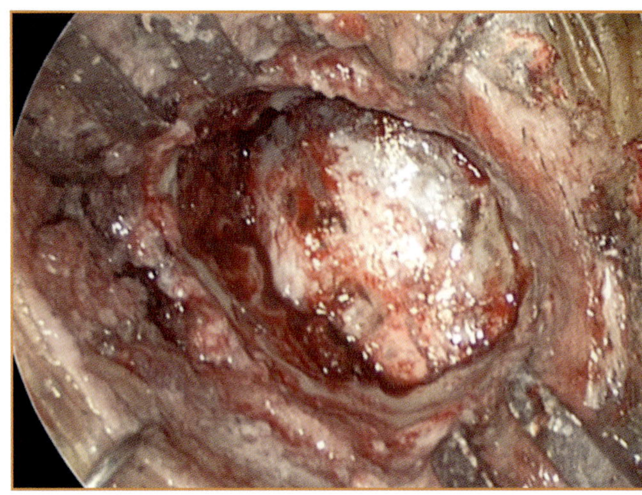

Figure 3–3. Right retrosigmoid craniotomy is performed and the junction of the tranverse and sigmoid sinus veins is identified. The dura is exposed. Craniotomy is 2 by 2 cm.

The craniotomy may be performed in two ways, either with a high-speed drill with cutting and diamond burs or with a 14-mm perforator (Figure 3–3). The transverse-sigmoid sinus junction is identified and the dura posterior to this is carefully exposed. A dural incision is made in the retrosigmoid dura paralleling the transverse and sigmoid sinuses regardless of the cranial nerve of interest as this provides access from the interpeduncular cistern and cranial nerve III through the foramen magnum and cranial nerve XII. A 0-degree, 4-mm endoscope is used as the working endoscope, whereas the 30-degree endoscope is used for supplemental visualization. Once the dura has been entered and the endoscope secured in the pneumatic arm, it is advanced along

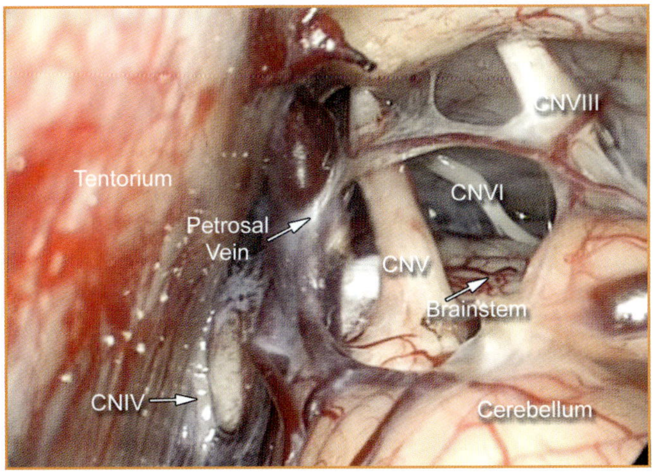

A

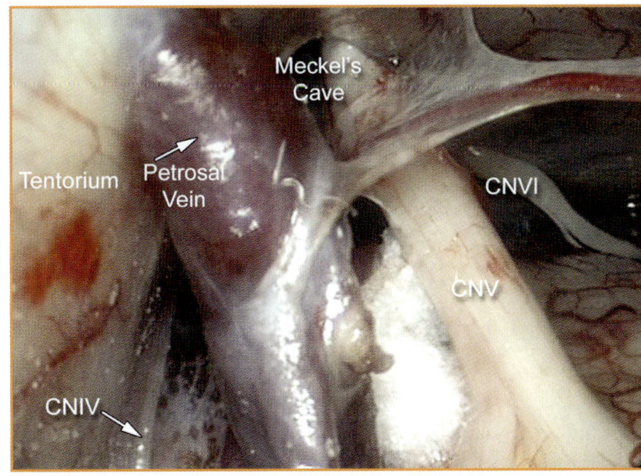

B

Figure 3–4. Endoscopic view of posterior skull base, right. **A.** CN V can be seen entering Meckel's cave. Note CN IV along tentorium. **B.** Zoomed-in view of superior portion.

the tentorium to the prepontine and interpeduncular cisterns. The arachnoid is then released from these cisterns and CSF is evacuated to provide maximal cerebellar relaxation. It is important to take time to evacuate the CSF to allow maximal exposure and avoid the need for any retractors. The endoscope is then positioned over the cranial nerve of interest for the critical portion of the procedure (Figure 3–4). The Endoscrub™ irrigation system (Medtronic, Minneapolis, MN) is used to maintain clear visualization as well as continuously cool the heat emitted from the xenon light source. The vascular decompression is performed by placing a small piece of PTFE felt between the offending vessel and nerve at the root entry zone (Figure 3–5). Prior to closure, any exposed mastoid air cells are obliterated with bone wax. The dura is closed in a watertight fashion and the craniotomy site can be reconstructed with hydroxyapatite bone cement, Medpore implant, or titanium mesh. All have been used with equal success. A head dressing is used to apply pressure to the surgical site.

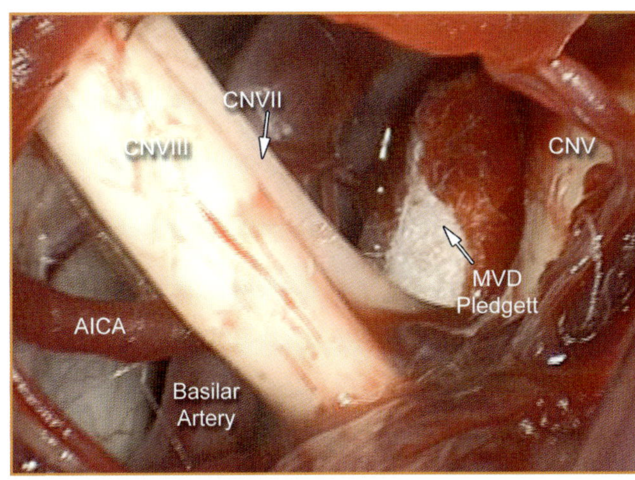

Figure 3–5. Endoscopic view of posterior skull base, left. Pledget placed between vessel and CN V for trigeminal neuralgia.

Technical Notes

1. There are skull base surgeons who perform retrosigmoid approaches and advocate slight modifications of craniotomy position and size based on which cranial nerve(s) are to be approached. With the endoscopic approach this is not necessary. The 1.5 to 2.0-cm craniotomy posteroinferior to the transverse-sigmoid sinus junction is versatile and allows access to cranial nerves III to XII.
2. Unlike anterior cranial base surgery, where an assistant surgeon may be necessary; the polyarticulated pneumatic arm is used to stabilize

the camera. This is due to patient positioning and the lower margin of error that can be tolerated when performing intradural endoscopy.

3. Intraoperative navigation for posterior fossa endoscopy is not done routinely. When in the posterior fossa, the intradural, subarachnoid space provides a panoramic view and navigation is usually not required. This is in contrast to anterior skull base surgery where visualization can be limited due to bony anatomy, and image guidance can help confirm the location of critical structures such as the carotid arteries and optic nerves prior to the craniotomy and dura incisions.

RESULTS/COMPLICATIONS

Trigeminal Neuralgia: Outcomes

For the traditional MVD procedure, several large series reporting on TGN patients have shown an 82 to 100% rate for complete relief of symptoms with a slight decline in these results as patient are followed over time.[18–20] Barker[10] published a landmark article of 1,185 patients undergoing MVD for TGN. Their initial success rate was 94 to 97%, which decreased to 70% in those patients that were followed for 10 years.[10]

In 2008, Artz et al[21] published a paper on EVD in TGN and HFS patients. They reported an 86% success rate in 14 TGN patients and 80% in 5 patients with HFS. Kabil[15] performed the EVD in 255 patients with TGN with 95% having complete resolution of their symptoms in the immediate postoperative period. Those results remained relatively stable with 93% of patients still symptom-free at three years. Currently, these are the only 2 series reporting the EVD procedure and their results compare favorably with the results of the traditional MVD procedure.

Hemifacial Spasm: Outcomes

For HFS patients undergoing MVD, Moffat reviewed several major studies that reported success rates varying from 79 to 97%.[11] There is evidence that with long-term follow-up, these successful outcomes decline slowly over time as some patients have a recurrence of symptoms, similar to the reported studies on trigeminal neuralgia patients. Long-term follow-up studies show HFS recurrence rates ranging from 1 to 13%.[12,14,22] Artz et al[21] reported their EVD results in HFS patients. Their data are limited with 5 patients, 4 of whom had complete resolution of their symptoms (80%). There are other isolated case reports describing success with this procedure.[23]

The incidence of complications from the MVD and EVD are low. The major complications are those related to the cranial nerve being decompressed or those nerves that are in close approximation. For trigeminal neuralgia patients undergoing decompression, the most common complication is facial numbness that is usually temporary. Other complications include facial weakness (0.8 to 9.5%), hearing loss (1.2 to 5.5%), and rare reports of cerebrospinal fluid leaks.[15,21]

For patients undergoing MVD or EVD for HFS, the risk of facial weakness (3 to 20%) and hearing loss (5 to 20%) is greater than for TGN patients.[12,14,20,21,23] Dizziness and vertigo can be a common postoperative complaint due the proximity of the vestibular nerve to the area of decompression and it usually resolved in hours to days.[21]

Advantages/Disadvantages

Endoscopic approaches to the posterior fossa offer several advantages to the traditional microscopic approach. Endoscopic surgery does not require the access or exposure required by the operating microscope resulting in smaller incisions, less soft tissue dissection, and smaller craniotomies. The lack of cerebellar retraction potentially increases the accuracy of identifying the offending compressive vessel(s) due to preservation of neurovascular relationships.[24] Smaller craniotomies result in less skull base reconstruction and faster recovery. Patients usually have decreased postoperative pain and studies have shown a decrease in hospital length of stay.[15,21] Improved visualization is another advantage of the endoscope. Using both the straight and angled endoscopes, the surgeons can visualize around corners and see anterior to neurovascular bundles not accessible by the microscopic view. In vascular decompression surgery, a negative exploration can mean either a misdiagnosis or failure to locate the compressive vessel. Teo et al[25] reported that 8% of their cases of arterial compression in MVD surgery were missed by the operating microscope and then correctly identified later when using the endoscope. Endoscopic surgery seems to provide surgeons the ability to more often identify the offending vessel(s) and therefore improve surgical outcomes.[25]

There are a few reported limitations of endoscopic surgery that need to be addressed to safely perform posterior fossa surgery. Most endoscopic-assisted MVD procedures have been performed by the surgeon holding the endoscope in one hand, thereby, preventing bimanual dexterity. The positioning of the patient and equipment for these procedures does not comfortably allow an assistant to safely hold the camera. The introduction of a polyarticulated pneumatic arm with the ability to hold the endoscope securely in the CPA has made EVD possible. Poor visualization can be a problem with all endoscopic surgeries due to blood, CSF, or condensation affecting the distal end of the endoscope. With the use of an irrigator (Endoscrub™) that cleans the distal end of the endoscope, visualization and heat are not issues.

Endoscopic Approach for Other Indications

The endoscopic approach may also be used for other indications, such as vestibular neurectomy, resection of meningiomas, and acoustic neuromas (Figures 3–6 and 3–7). This may become more common as comfort and expertise develops in this field.

CONCLUSIONS

The field of endoscopic skull base surgery is maturing and becoming a well-accepted option to the traditional open skull base approaches with comparable disease related outcomes, decreased patient morbidity, and dramatically improved cosmetic results. Improved equipment, instrumentation, surgical expertise, real-time intraoperative imaging, and the advancement of robotic surgery will continue to advance endoscopic skull base surgery and keep it the forefront of surgical achievements for many years to come.

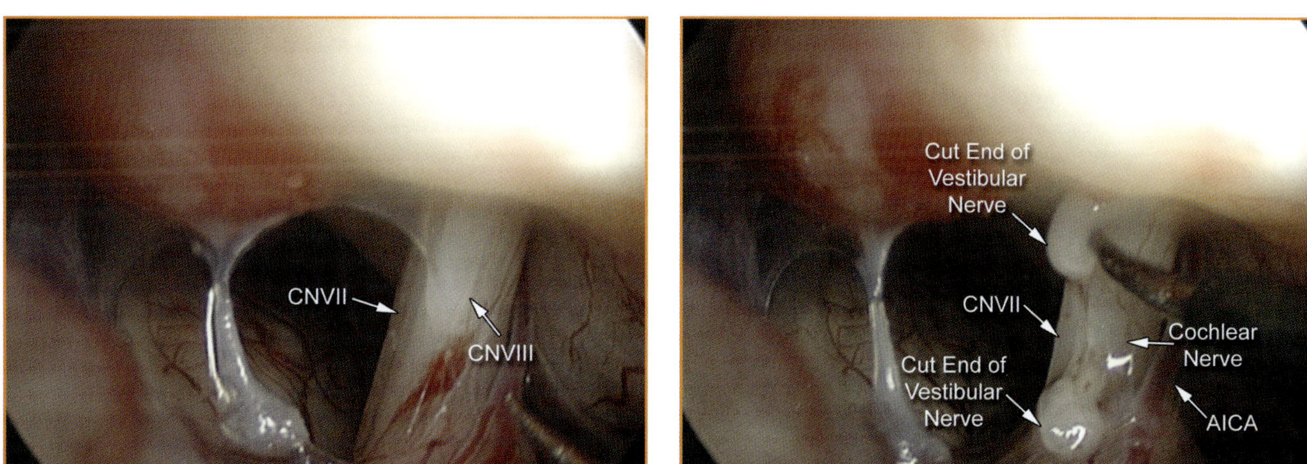

A B

Figure 3–6. A. Endoscopic view of posterior skull base, left with view of VII/VIII nerve complex. **B.** Vestibular neurectomy performed for Ménière's disease.

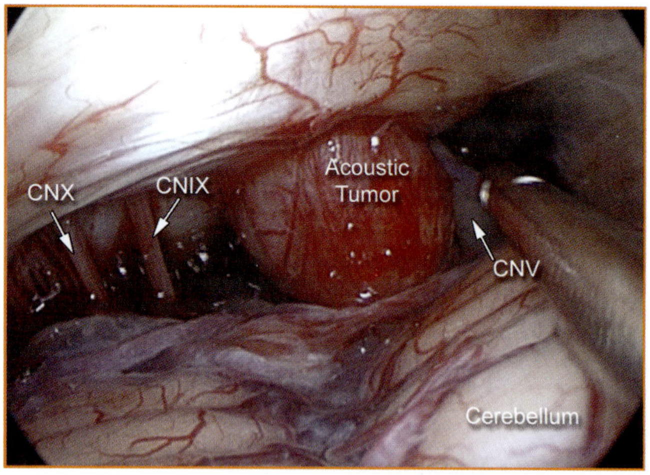

A

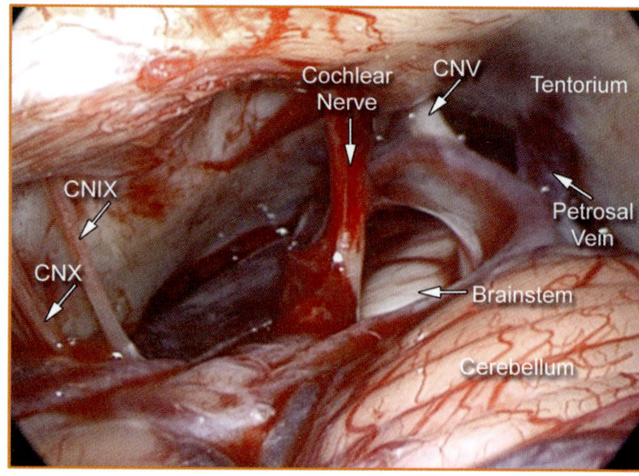

B

Figure 3–7. A. Endoscopic view of posterior skull base, left with acoustic neuroma easily visualized. **B.** View after resection with preservation of cochlear nerve.

REFERENCES

1. Kennedy DW. Functional endoscopic sinus surgery technique. *Arch Otolaryngol*. 1985;111(10): 643–649.
2. Jankowski R, Auque J, Simon C. Endoscopic pituitary tumor surgery. *Laryngoscope*. 1992;102:198–202.
3. Jho,HD, Carrau RL, Ko Y. Endoscopic pituitary surgery. In: Wilkins RH, Rengarchary SS, eds. *Neurosurgical Operative Atlas*. 1996:1–12.
4. Ghopal HV. Endoscopic transnasal pituitary surgery. *Curr Opin Oto Head Neck Surg*. 2000;91:43–48.
5. Barker FG, Klibanski A, Swearingen B. Transsphenoidal surgery for pituitary tumors in the United States, 1996–2000: mortality, morbidity, and the effects of hospital and surgeon volume. *J Clin Endocrinol Metab*. 2003;88(10):4709–4719.
6. White DR, Sonnenburg RE. Safety of minimally invasive pituitary surgery (MIPS) compared with a traditional approach. *Laryngoscope*. 2004;114:1945–1948.
7. Cappabianca P, Cavallo LM, DeDivitiis E. Endoscopic endonasal transphenoidal surgery. *Neurosurgery*. 2004;55: 933–941.
8. McCutcheon IE, Kitagawa RS, et al. Frameless stereotactic navigation in transsphenoidal surgery: comparison with fluoroscopy. *Stereotactic Funct Neurosurg*. 2004;82:43–48.
9. Ciric I, Ragin A, Baumgartner C. Complications of transphenoidal surgery: results of a national survey, review of literature, and personal experience. *Neurosurgery*. 2005; 40:225–236.
10. Barker FG, Jannetta PJ, Bissonette DJ, et al. Microvascular decompression for hemifacial spasm. *J Neurosurg*. 1995;82:201–210.
11. Moffat DA, Durvasula VSP, Stevens King A, Hardy DG. Outcome following retrosigmoid microvascular decompression of the facial nerve for hemifacial spasm. *J Laryngol Otol*. 2005;119:779–783
12. Miyazaki H, Deveze A, Magnan J. Neuro-otologic surgery through minimally invasive retrosigmoid approach: endoscope assisted microvascular decompression, vestibular neurotomy and tumor removal. *Laryngoscope*. 2005;115:1612–1617.
13. Rak R, Sekhar LN, Stimac D, Hechl P. Endoscope-assisted microsurgery for microvascular compression syndromes. *Neurosurgery*. 2004;54(4):876–883.
14. Magnan J, Chays A, Lepetre C, Pencroffi E, Locatelli P. Surgical perspective of endoscopy of the cerebellopontine angle. *Am J Otol*. 1994;15(3):366–370.
15. Kabil MS, Eby JB, Shahinian HK. Endoscopic vascular decompression versus microvascular decompression of the trigeminal nerve. *Minim Invas Neurosurg*. 2005;48: 207–212.
16. Jarrahy R, Eby JB, Cha ST, Shahinian HK. Fully endoscopic vascular decompression of the trigeminal nerve. *Minim Invas Neurosurg*. 2002;45:32–35.
17. Eby JB, Cha ST, Shahinian HK. Fully endoscopic vascular decompression of the facial nerve for hemifacial spasm. *Skull Base*. 2001;11(3):189–197.
18. Kondo A. Follow-up results of microvascular decompression in trigeminal neuralgia and hemifacial spasm. *Neurosurgery*. 1997;40:46–51; discussion 51–52.
19. Broggi G, Ferroli P, Franzini A, Servello D, Dones I. Microvascular decompression for trigeminal neuralgia: comments on a series of 250 cases, including 10 patients with multiple sclerosis. *J Neurol Neurosurg Psychiatry*. 2000;68:59–64.

20. Kolluri S, Heros RC. Microvascular decompression for trigeminal neuralgia. A five-year follow-up study. *Surg Neurol.* 1984;22:235–240.
21. Artz G, Hux F, LaRoucre M, Bojrab D, Babu S, Pieper D. Endoscopic vascular decompression. *Otol Neurotol.* 2008;29:995–1000.
22. Samii M, Gunther T, Iaconetta G, Muehling M, Vorkapic P, Samii A. Microvascular decompression to treat hemifacial spasm: long-term results for a consecutive series of 143 patients. *Neurosurgery.* 2002;50(4):712–717.
23. Payner TD, Tew JM Jr. Recurrence of hemifacial spasm after microvascular decompression. *Neurosurgery.* 1996; 38:686–690.
24. O'Donoghue G, O'Flynn P. Endoscopic anatomy of the cerebellopontine angle. *Am J Otol.* 1993;14(2):122–125.
25. Teo C, Nakaji P, Mobbs R. Endoscope-assisted microvascular decompression for trigeminal neuralgia: technical case note. *Neurosurgery.* 2006;59(4 suppl 2):489–490.

CHAPTER 4

Vestibular Schwannoma

Rodney C. Diaz

INTRODUCTION

Acoustic neuromas are the most common benign tumor of the cerebellopontine angle (CPA) and are the most common intracranial tumor treated by neurotologists. The term "acoustic neuroma" is technically incorrect, as the tumor neither arises from the acoustic nerve nor does it arise from neuronal cells. "Vestibular schwannoma" or "vestibular neurilemmoma" is more commonly accepted and more accurate. However, the otolaryngological, neurotological, and neurosurgical communities still often frequently use the term "acoustic neuroma" in daily parlance.

HISTORICAL PERSPECTIVE

The first reputed case of an acoustic neuroma reported in the medical literature was in 1777 by Sandifort. Bell gave the first accurate description of an acoustic neuroma in 1830, and the first successful surgical removal of an acoustic neuroma was by Ballance in 1894.

Surgery for removal of acoustic neuromas was routinely accomplished first in the early 1900s by neurosurgeons approaching the tumor via a unilateral or bilateral suboccipital craniotomy. Finger dissection was commonly employed when possible. Tumors were diagnosed based on purely clinical findings and thus, unsurprisingly, were often huge when discovered. Bioccipital craniotomy and partial cerebellar resection were employed to access such large tumors. Despite the extremely wide access, such tumors were still often incompletely resected.

Dandy advocated the use of a smaller, unilateral suboccipital craniotomy and stressed the importance of total tumor resection. Quix reported the first translabyrinthine approach to the cerebellopontine angle in 1912, but this approach did not gain wide support from either the neurosurgical or otological communities until several decades later. Otologists did not become involved in the surgical treatment of acoustic neuromas and other cerebellopontine angle and posterior fossa tumors until the techniques of microscopic dissection, microsurgical drilling, and otological-neurosurgical cooperation were popularized by House and Hitselberger in the 1960s.

Management of acoustic neuromas in the modern age is typically handled in a team fashion between neurotologists and neurosurgeons. Cranial base approaches are performed by the neurotologist, whereas definitive resection of the tumor is the responsibility of the neurosurgeon. However, there are a number of academic medical centers, neurotological practices, and neurosurgical practices where one surgeon, whether neurotologist or neurosurgeon, routinely handle the entire surgical management of the acoustic neuroma, as many neurotologists are dually trained in tumor dissection and removal, and many neurosurgeons have training in temporal bone dissection and skull base drillouts. Gigantic tumors, on the other hand, with significant brainstem compression, obstructive hydrocephalus, and need for maximization of skull base dissection for optimizing transtemporal exposure, are best managed by exploiting the best training qualities of both the neurosurgeon and neurotologist.

The team approach to acoustic neuroma management also extends to nonsurgical therapy. Gamma Knife and other stereotactic radiotherapy modalities commonly employ a team of treating physicians including neurotologist or neurosurgeon, radiation oncologist, and radiation physicist. The treatment team collaborates to determine candidate suitability, treatment protocol, and prescription dosing for specific tumors.

EPIDEMIOLOGY

Acoustic neuromas comprise approximately 80 to 90% of all cerebellopontine angle tumors and approximately 6 to 8% of all intracranial tumors. Acoustic neuromas have an incidence of approximately 1 in 100,000 to 2 in 100,000 per year. They have a mean age of presentation in the 50- to 60-year age range but can have a wide range of presentation, from the teens to the 80s. Men and women are equally affected.

Approximately 1 in every 10 to 20 patients with acoustic neuroma has neurofibromatosis type II. Approximately 50% of cases of neurofibromatosis type II are of familial autosomal dominant inheritance, the remaining equivalent being of de novo genetic mutations. The birth incidence of neurofibromatosis type II is 1 in 25,000 to 1 in 50,000.

PATHOPHYSIOLOGY

Acoustic neuromas are benign tumors of the vestibular nerve, thought to arise lateral to the junction between the peripheral nervous system and central nervous system. This region, the so-called Obersteiner-Redlich zone, defines the location where the peripheral Schwann cell neural sheathing transitions to the central oligodendrocyte sheathing. This narrow zone is typically located near the porus acousticus.

Occasionally, an acoustic neuroma may be identified in a completely intralabyrinthine or intracochlear location (in the latter case, truly being an acoustic tumor or cochlear schwannoma). Intracochlear or intralabyrinthine enhancement is possible in inflammatory or infectious processes within the inner ear; however, if stable contrast enhancement is noted over a prolonged imaging period, such localized enhancement may represent such an intralabyrinthine tumor. While such tumors may be resected, the vast majority are simply observed, as tumor growth and periotic expansion are not observed, and surgical resection would result in anacusis (Figure 4–1).

Macroscopically, these tumors tend to appear encapsulated and, historically, were often removed by finger dissection. However, acoustic neuromas do not have a histologically defined capsule. Viable tumor cells are only a few microns separated from the outer fibrous layers of the tumor.

Centrally, acoustic neuromas display histologic characteristics typical of peripheral schwannomas. The solid tumor bulk consists of an arrangement of compact spindle cells, termed Antoni A areas, or a loose, hypocellular, disorderly cellular arrangement, myxoid stroma, and chronic inflammatory

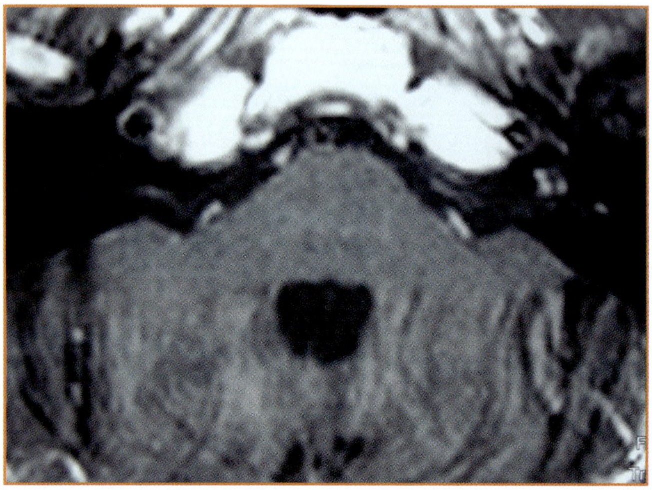

Figure 4–1. Intracochlear schwannoma, left. MRI, T1 weighted with gadolinium contrast, axial. This patient exhibited mild asymmetric SNHL and underwent MR imaging, demonstrating enhancement along the basal turn and modiolus of the cochlea. Serologic testing was normal. Subsequent imaging at 6 and 12 months was unchanged. The patient was managed by continued observation and serial imaging.

cellular infiltrate, termed Antoni B areas. Both types of cellular arrangement in fact often coexist within different regions of the same tumor. Antoni A areas contain regions where fusiform cell bodies arrange in short interlacing fascicles with whirling or palisading nuclei, called Verocay bodies. Sparse mitoses are present, consistent with the benign nature of the tumor. There is, however, cellular pleomorphism with hypochromasia.

Occasionally, tumors can display retrogressive changes including cystic degeneration, central tumor necrosis, hyalinization, calcification, and intratumor hemorrhage. Intratumor calcification can lead to suspicion of meningioma preoperatively; as such intratumor calcifications mimic the CT and MR radiographic appearance of meningiomas (Figure 4–2).

Tumor immunohistochemistry of acoustic neuromas displays diffuse positive affinity for the neural crest marker S-100, thereby differentiating them from the more focal S-100 staining of malignant neural lesions and the variable S-100 staining of meningiomas. Acoustics stain negatively for cytokeratin, an epithelial marker, and chromogranin and synaptophysin, both neuroendocrine cell markers, helping to differentiate them from glomus jugulare tumors.

Acoustic neuromas can have variable growth in relation to the vestibular nerve of origin. Some tumors display a biased or more pedunculated growth off to the side of the nerve cable, whereas other tumors appear densely integrated into the nerve cable itself.

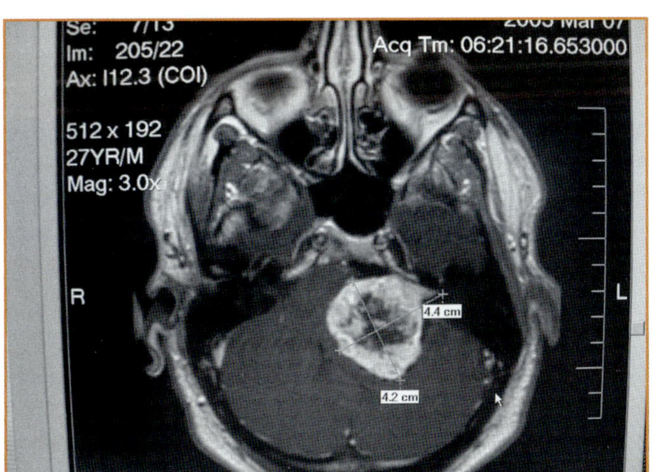

Figure 4–2. Large acoustic neuroma, left, with central tumor necrosis. MRI, T1 weighted with gadolinium contrast, axial.

Histologic studies show that acoustic neuromas invariably demonstrate cochlear nerve invasion, thereby challenging the concept of performing hearing conservation surgery in an oncologically sound fashion.[1] That is, one cannot claim total tumor resection if one has conserved hearing, as there will invariably be microscopic tumor residual embedded within the density of the preserved cochlear nerve. Despite this assertion, such tumor residual seems to have minimal clinical significance, as hearing conservation surgery has been successfully performed for small and medium acoustic neuromas for many decades.

GENETICS

Biallelic mutations of the NF2 gene are responsible for the generation of both the sporadic form of acoustic neuromas as well as the familial form of bilateral acoustic neuromas seen in neurofibromatosis type II, from which the gene receives its name.[2,3] The NF2 gene is a tumor suppressor gene localized on the long arm of chromosome 22, 22q12. The NF2 gene product is termed schwannomin or more commonly merlin, after its relative homology to the moesin, ezrin, and radixin proteins. Like these proteins, merlin localizes to the cell membrane and appears to manage cellular proliferation by inhibiting multiple cell signaling pathways controlling regulation of growth factors, cell cycle proteins, apoptosis cascades, Schwann cell-axonal interaction, and cell-cell adhesion during tissue fusion.[4] The NF2 tumor suppressor gene is highly expressed in Schwann cells, neurons, meninges, and lens, explaining the propensity for neoplastic disease in these tissues in neurofibromatosis type II.

Genetic defects in neurofibromatosis type I, or von Recklinghausen's disease, are localized to chromosome 17. The discrete NF1 gene product neurofibromin is involved in modulation of distinctly different signal transduction pathways from those of merlin, thereby confirming on a genetic basis the clinical differentiation between neurofibromatosis type I and neurofibromatosis type II.

SIZE

Categorization of acoustic neuromas is typically performed based on general size. A useful categorization follows: small tumors <1 cm in diameter (Figures 4–3A and 4–3B), medium tumors 1 to 2.5 cm in diameter (Figures 4–4A and 4–4B), large tumors 2.5 to 4 cm in diameter (Figures 4–5A and 4–5B), and giant tumors >4 cm in diameter (Figures 4–6A and 4–6B). This general categorization in size can be thought to correlate roughly to a designation based on anatomical location: intracanalicular, cisternal, brainstem compressive, and hydrocephalic. In this sense, a completely intracanalicular tumor is typically 1 cm or less in maximal dimension, a tumor that extends into the cerebellopontine angle is typically 2.5 cm or less in diameter, a tumor with obvious brainstem contact is typically over 2.5 cm in diameter, and a tumor that is 4 cm or larger in diameter likely is compressing the brainstem and 4th ventricle to the point of causing an obstructive hydrocephalus.

A different way of classifying acoustic neuroma size classification is based on candidacy for different therapeutic criteria: small tumors <1.5 cm in diameter can be accessed by a middle fossa approach; medium-sized tumors >1.5 cm have cerebellopontine angle components large enough to necessitate a posterior fossa craniotomy of some kind, whether it be translabyrinthine or retrosigmoid; and those large tumors >3 cm in diameter, because of their intimate proximity to the brainstem and possible ventricular compression, are not amenable to stereotactic radiotherapy and must be surgically resected as the primary modality of treatment. In addition, some authors suggest consideration for two-stage resection of acoustic neuroma for tumors larger than 3 cm in diameter.

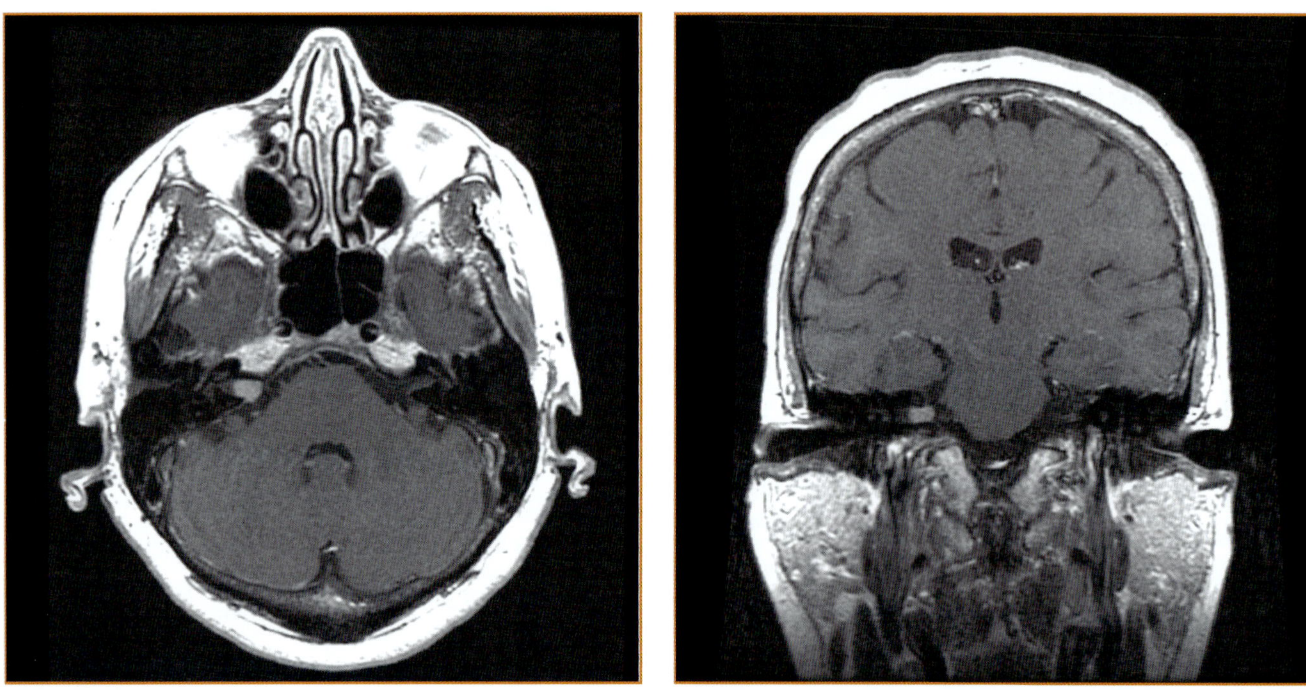

A B

Figure 4–3. Small acoustic neuroma, right. MRI, T1 weighted with gadolinium contrast, axial **(A)** and coronal **(B)**. This intracanalicular tumor extended from the fundus laterally to the porus acousticus medially, without significant extension into the cerebellopontine angle.

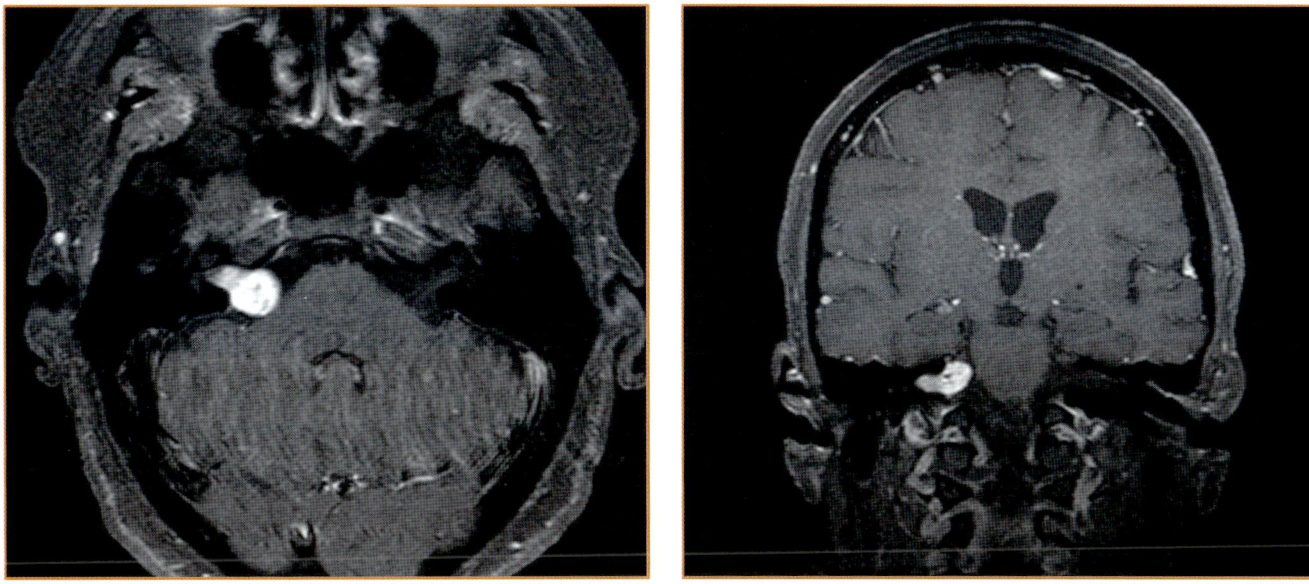

A B

Figure 4–4. Medium acoustic neuroma, right. MRI, T1 weighted with gadolinium contrast, axial (**A**) and coronal (**B**). This cisternal tumor extended from the fundus laterally to the cerebellopontine angle medially, with minimal brainstem contact.

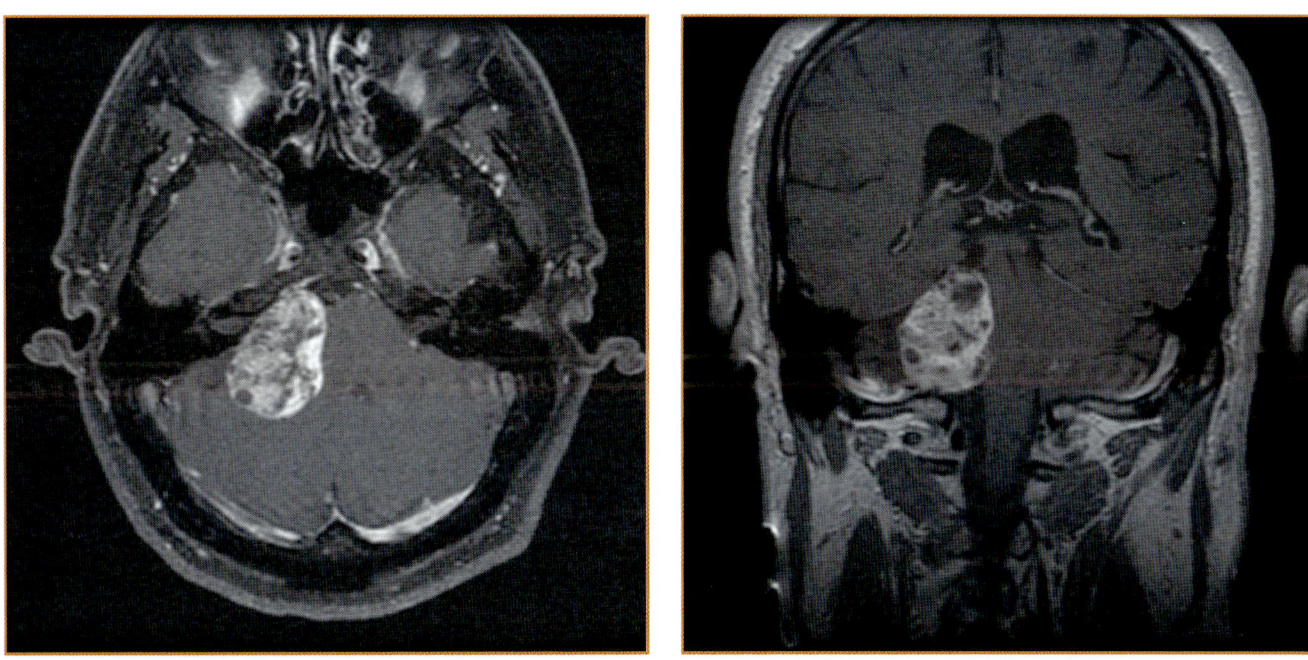

A B

Figure 4–5. Large acoustic neuroma, right. MRI, T1 weighted with gadolinium contrast, axial (**A**) and coronal (**B**). This brainstem compressive tumor extended from the midportion of the internal auditory canal laterally to highly compress and displace the brainstem medially and cerebellum posteriorly. The tumor exhibited cystic degeneration and scattered tumor necrosis with large intratumor vessels, seen in both views. On the coronal image, the lateral ventricles demonstrate mild dilation but are not yet convex.

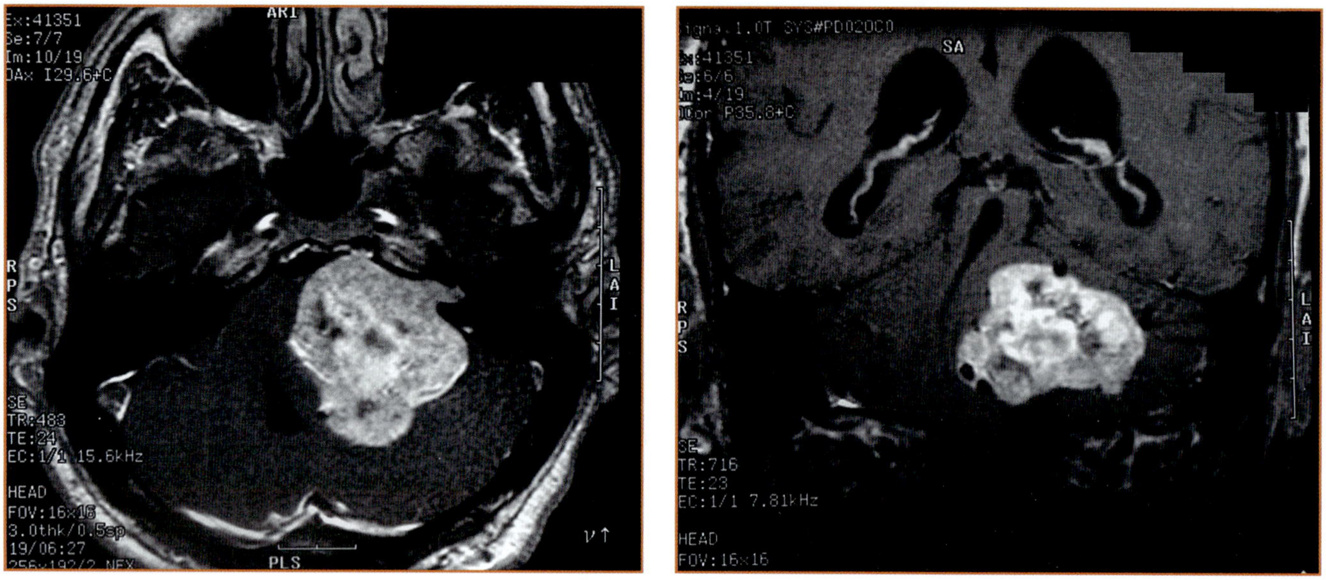

A B

Figure 4–6. Giant acoustic neuroma, left. MRI, T1 weighted with gadolinium contrast, axial (**A**) and coronal (**B**). This brainstem compressive tumor fills the internal auditory canal and causes extensive brainstem and cerebellar compression and displacement. This extreme neural compression causes obstructive hydrocephalus, demonstrated by dilation of the fourth ventricle on axial view and dilation of the cerebral aqueduct, third ventricle (not shown), and lateral ventricles on coronal view. Remarkably, there is minimal widening of the internal auditory canal.

NATURAL HISTORY

Studies following the natural history of acoustic neuromas have all been inherently impartial because of their retrospective nature and implicit selection bias. Nonetheless, a large number of retrospective studies have been published since the advent of MRI detailing individual groups' experiences with conservative management of acoustic neuromas.

A recent, large chart review of 205 patients with tumors less than 2 cm reported nongrowth in 66%, slow growth in 24%, rapid growth in 4%, and tumor regression in 3% with a follow-up ranging from 12 to 120 months.[5] A study that included 53 patients with tumors of sizes 0.2 to 3 cm reported a similar nongrowth percentage of 60%.[6]

At minimum, some studies have reported as little as 9% of acoustic neuromas do not display any significant growth over the follow-up period of patients electing observation.[7] The majority of retrospective studies, however, report rates of tumor nongrowth between 20% and 60%, with the simple average of these studies being approximately 45%.

A meta-analysis of 21 studies comparing 1,345 patients with acoustic neuromas who were initially managed conservatively demonstrated 57% of acoustic neuromas with no growth, with 43% of tumors stable or regressing.[8] Follow-up for all patients ranged from 2 to 5 years.

Mean growth of all tumors followed conservatively has been reported between 1 to 2 mm per year. However, this growth rate is skewed by the presence of the significant number of tumors that do not grow. Of conservatively managed tumors that do demonstrate interval growth, reported mean growth rates have ranged from 4 to 9 mm per year.[6,9,10]

As up to 50 to 60% of tumors followed without treatment do not grow, a large number of newly diagnosed tumors may never progress to requiring any therapeutic intervention. Certainly, tumors which are brainstem compressive or hydrocephalic should be treated proactively, as any additional growth from such tumors can cause significant morbidity or be life threatening. However, tumors that are intracanalicular or cisternal can be observed and reimaged safely within 6 to 9 months with minimal risk.

Conversely, some tumors can have a more aggressive phenotype and significantly faster growth rate, particularly in younger patients, those with neurofibromatosis type II, and those with larger tumors. For this reason, if a patient elects to have the tumor observed rather than treated with radiotherapy or surgery, initial tumor surveillance scan should be performed at 6 to 9 months postdiagnostic scan, in case there should be marked tumor growth beyond the expected mean growth rate. If tumor size is stable, annual MRI rescans are reasonable.

NERVE OF ORIGIN

Schwannomas of the internal auditory canal can arise from any of the nerves residing within this space. It is universally agreed that the probability for the cochlear nerve or the facial nerve to be the nerve of origin for an internal auditory canal schwannoma is exceedingly low, approximately 1% each. The nerve of origin for acoustic neuromas, however, has been extensively debated. Acoustic neuromas have more recently been described as arising in an equally distributed fashion between the inferior and superior vestibular nerves. However, several recent large studies reverse this view and assert the more classical assertion that the vast majority of tumors for which the nerve of origin can be identified, up to 90%, arise from the inferior vestibular nerve.[11–13]

Determination of the nerve of origin in acoustic neuromas, or more generally schwannomas of the internal auditory canal, can have a major impact on preoperative planning and counseling. Although any given nerve of origin does not preclude therapeutic intervention, some interventions are clearly not indicated for some tumors. For instance, if it were known a priori that a schwannoma of the internal auditory canal arose from the facial nerve and the tumor were completely intracanalicular without any evidence of brainstem compression or mass effect, and the patient had completely intact and symmetric facial nerve function, one would be much less inclined to recommend surgical resection. However, if the same tumor in the same clinical scenario was known a priori to be a superior vestibular nerve schwannoma, one would be much more predisposed to recommend a middle fossa craniotomy and hearing conservation approach to resection, as early resection of smaller acoustic neuromas provides the best chance for long term hearing preservation.[14]

Thus, anticipation of the branch of the vestibular nerve, inferior or superior, from which an acoustic neuroma originates can aid in preoperative planning and patient counseling. Patients are at higher risk of both facial nerve injury as well as hearing loss when tumors arising from the inferior vestibular nerve are approached via the middle fossa technique, due to the more extensive nature of dissection from this superiorly based approach, when compared to tumors arising from the superior vestibular nerve.[12,13] The ability to ascertain an inferior rather than superior position to an acoustic tumor does not definitively exclude the option of a middle fossa approach, but such information can be valuable in accurately depicting for the patient the relative risks versus rewards in attempting such an approach, as well as realistically temper the patient's expectations for hearing and facial nerve outcomes.

There are two methods for preoperatively determining whether an acoustic neuroma arises from the inferior or superior vestibular nerve. The most direct method is by simple visualization of the tumor along the inferior internal auditory canal on high-resolution gadolinium-enhanced MRI. This is obviously only possible if the tumor is intracanalicular or extremely small and can be visually localized towards one wall of the internal auditory canal, which in reality is quite rare (Figure 4–7). A less direct but nevertheless useful technique is to evaluate the patient's electronystagmography responses to bithermal caloric stimulation of the vestibular system. A reduced vestibular response implies a superiorly based tumor, as discussed below.

CLINICAL PRESENTATION

Although acoustic neuromas are the most common tumor of the cerebellopontine angle and internal auditory canal, the differential diagnosis for tumors

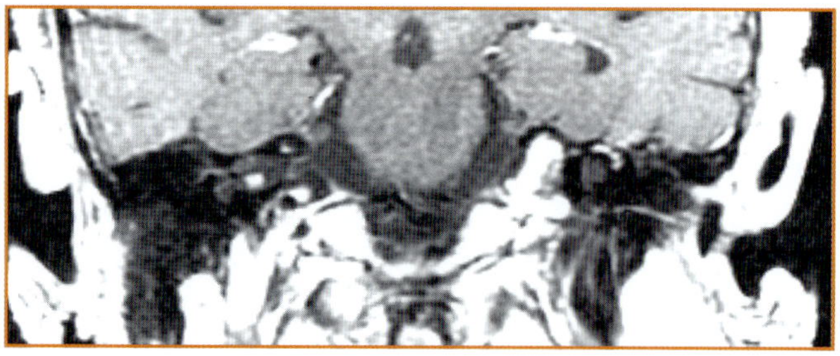

Figure 4–7. Intracanalicular acoustic neuroma, right. MRI, T1 weighted with gadolinium contrast, axial. The enhancing tumor is clearly localized to the inferior half of the internal auditory canal. This degree of localization is not commonly attained on MR imaging and is a function of minimal tumor size and high resolution imaging protocol through the internal auditory canals, with slices ≤1 mm thickness.

Table 4–1. Tumors of the Cerebellopontine Angle, Internal Auditory Canal, and Petrous Apex

Common Name	Formal Name
Acoustic Neuroma	Vestibular Schwannoma
Meningioma	
Glomus Jugulare tumor	Paraganglioma
Epidermoid	Primary Cholesteatoma
Chordoma	
Chondrosarcoma	
Endolymphatic sac tumor	Papillary Adenocarcinoma
Trigeminal Schwannoma	
Facial Schwannoma	
Facial Hemangioma	

in these regions is quite wide, and consideration must be made for the possibility of other tumor types. Table 4–1 lists the differential diagnosis of tumors found in these regions.

Acoustic neuromas account for approximately 90% of tumors of the cerebellopontine angle. Other tumors of the cerebellopontine angle in further descending order of occurrence are meningiomas, epidermoids or primary cholesteatomas of the cerebellopontine angle, and trigeminal schwannomas. In addition, facial schwannomas and facial hemangiomas may present in the internal auditory canal, particularly the lateral fundus region. When considering tumors embedded within the anterior or posterior petrous apex that may extend into the cerebellopontine angle with sufficient growth, the following tumors are also considered: glomus jugulare tumors, chordomas, chondrosarcomas, and endolymphatic sac tumors or papillary adenocarcinomas of the endolymphatic sac. Glomus jugulare tumors that extend to the cerebellopontine angle can account for up to 10% of all cerebellopontine angle tumors when considering both primary cerebellopontine angle tumors and secondary tumors of the temporal bone together.

Tumors that arise in the cerebellopontine angle often present with many of the same symptoms and signs despite the difference in tumor histology. Generally, the cellular nature of such tumors does not determine the clinical presentation, but rather the specificity of tumor location determines the presenting symptoms. Tumor growth adjacent to the cochleovestibular nerve causes unilateral or asymmetric sensorineural hearing loss as the most common presenting symptom. Such hearing loss from cerebellopontine angle tumors is commonly slowly progressive and is rarely sudden in onset. The vast majority of cases of sudden sensorineural hearing loss is of idiopathic or presumptively viral or inflammatory etiology rather than associated with extra-axial neoplasia.

Disequilibrium is also often described by patients, but because of the often slow growing nature of many cerebellopontine angle tumors, such disequilibrium is often of minimal morbidity to the patient or not even noticed at all. For similar reasons, overt vertigo is an uncommon complaint. When present as an inciting complaint, vertigo can suggest a particularly fast growing tumor or one in which there has been rapid or recent enlargement from cystic degeneration or intratumoral hemorrhage causing a sudden reduced unilateral vestibular function.

Because acoustic neuromas are the most common tumors to arise primarily in the internal auditory canal, they have an easier propensity for tumor-mediated compression of functional cochleovestibular nerve fibers within the canal than other cerebellopontine angle tumors, which only enter or invade the internal auditory canal secondarily after initial growth in the cerebellopontine angle. For this reason, acoustic neuromas have a higher rate of auditory and vestibular symptomatology than meningiomas and other tumors of the cerebellopontine angle. A small intracanalicular acoustic neuroma commonly presents with asymmetric SNHL, whereas even quite large meningiomas limited to the cerebellopontine angle with little or no intracanalicular extension can demonstrate normal hearing.

Although the probability and severity of hearing loss is generally proportional to the size of most cerebellopontine angle tumors, large meningiomas of this region can sometimes leaving sensorineural hearing relatively untouched. In such cases, a hearing preservation approach should be attempted, as the patient's hearing can sometimes be preserved, or, even more exceptionally, improved, with resection of the meningioma.

Other less common symptoms and signs of cerebellopontine angle tumors typically occur in cases with greater progression of tumor size, where continued expansion of tumor causes compression of neurovascular structures further from the porus acousticus (Figure 4–8). Facial paresis or paralysis, facial hypoesthesia or trigeminal neuralgia, diplopia, disconjugate gaze, dysphagia, dysphonia, vocal fold paralysis, shoulder weakness, and, rarely, mental status depression or obtundation from hydrocephalus, suggest greater extension of cerebellopontine angle tumor growth.

Unilateral hypoesthesia of the posterior superior external auditory canal, or Hitselberger's sign, has been historically described as a common sign of facial nerve sensory dysfunction in the setting of acoustic neuroma. However, this sign has been infrequently identified in acoustic neuroma patients in our experience. Table 4–2 summarizes findings seen with acoustic neuromas.

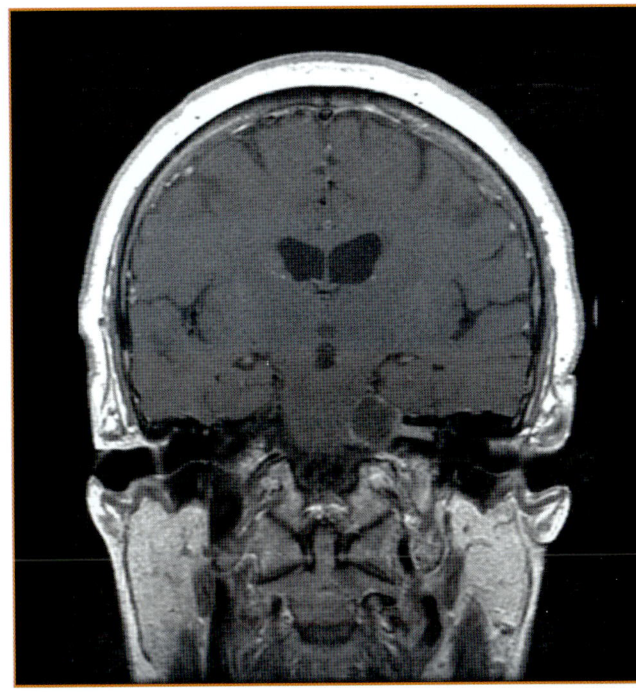

Figure 4–8. Cystic acoustic neuroma, left. MRI, T1 weighted with gadolinium contrast, coronal. This patient presented with a chief complaint of sudden onset left facial hypoesthesia. Further history revealed a long history of slowly progressive hearing loss on the left. Imaging revealed a left acoustic neuroma with significant cystic component in the cerebellopontine cistern, extending superiorly with compression of the trigeminal nerve. The patient's primary complaint likely was caused by rapid expansion of the cisternal component of the tumor, hastened by its cystic nature.

EVALUATION

Audiometry

As the most common presenting symptom of acoustic neuromas is unilateral hearing loss, the most common test used in the diagnosis of acoustic neuromas is clinical audiometry. Unilateral or significantly asymmetric sensorineural hearing loss typifies the audiometric pattern found, as this is the most common, and often only, objective sign in the setting of acoustic neuroma.

What constitutes significant asymmetry is a matter of some debate. Criteria used in our institution that would constitute asymmetry significant enough to recommend further diagnostic evaluation include interaural differences of 10 dB or greater in three or more consecutive tested frequencies or of 15 dB or greater in two or more consecutive tested frequencies. In addition, an interaural difference in speech discrimination score of 15% or greater is

Table 4–2. Presenting Signs and Symptoms of Acoustic Neuromas

Sign/Symptom	Cranial Nerve	Incidence
Asymmetric SNHL	8	Common
Sudden SNHL	8	Uncommon
Unilateral tinnitus	8	Common
Disequilibrium	8	Common
Vertigo	8	Uncommon
Facial paresis	7	Uncommon
Hitselberger's sign	7	Uncommon
Facial hypesthesia	5	Uncommon
Trigeminal neuralgia	5	Rare
Diplopia	6	Rare
Disconjugate gaze	6	Rare
Dysphagia	10	Rare
Dysphonia	10	Rare
Vocal fold paralysis	10	Rare
Shoulder weakness	11	Rare

also considered significant (Figure 4–9). As overall pure-tone thresholds worsen, the size of interaural asymmetry correspondingly increases before being considered significant.

There is no pathognomonic audiometric sign for the presence of acoustic neuroma. However, the presence of a PI-PB rollover in speech detection thresholds implies retrocochlear, or neural rather than sensory, pathology in sensorineural hearing loss. The PI-PB function denotes the performance intensity (PI) function using phonetically balanced (PB) word lists. In patients with normal hearing or hearing loss of cochlear or sensory origin, the measured speech discrimination using phonetically balanced word lists increases with increasing sound level and reaches a maximum or plateaus without degradation at maximally tolerated sound levels. In patients with hearing loss of retrocochlear or neural origin, speech discrimination increases with increasing sound level, reaches a maximum at a given sound level, and then worsens at sound levels above this point.

The standard method for measuring the degree of rollover is by calculating the rollover index: $RI = (PB_{max} - PB_{min})/PB_{max}$, where PB_{max} = maximal speech discrimination score measured and PB_{min} = lowest speech discrimination score measured at a sound level greater than that at the PB_{max}. That is, the rollover index is calculated as the normalized drop in speech discrimination score from the maximal score measured. The rollover index is <0.2 in 85% and 0.2 to 0.4 in 13% of the general population. Thus, rollover has been historically defined as occurring when the rollover index is 0.4 or greater. Our institution typically treats rollover indices of 0.2 or greater with suspicion, in the setting of mild asymmetric sensorineural hearing loss.

This so-called rollover in PI function is thought to be generated by dyssynchrony in neural firing within the auditory nerve.[15] As a result, PI-PB rollover is not specific to acoustic neuromas but can also be attributed to other causes of retrocochlear dysfunction, including auditory neuropathy, multiple sclerosis and other neurodegenerative disorders, neurosyphilis, viral neuropathies, diabetes mellitus, and even age-related hearing loss.[16]

Auditory Brainstem Response

The method of brainstem auditory evoked potentials or auditory brainstem response (ABR) can also be used in the evaluation of acoustic neuroma. ABR test performance is dependent on overall hearing thresholds, which typically must be in the normal to moderate hearing loss level to ensure adequate waveform reproducibility. If hearing thresholds are worse than 70 dB HL at ≥2 kHz, hearing function may be inadequate to reliably produce ABR waveforms.

In the setting of acoustic neuroma evaluation, the most common measurements used are the wave V interaural latency difference, the wave I-V interpeak latency, and, to a lesser extent, the wave I to III interpeak latency. As wave V is typically the most robust of the ABR waveforms and always identified when ABRs are present, the wave V interaural latency difference is most commonly used.

Because of considerable variability in electroencephalographic systems and clinical testing settings, each audiometric center generates its own criteria

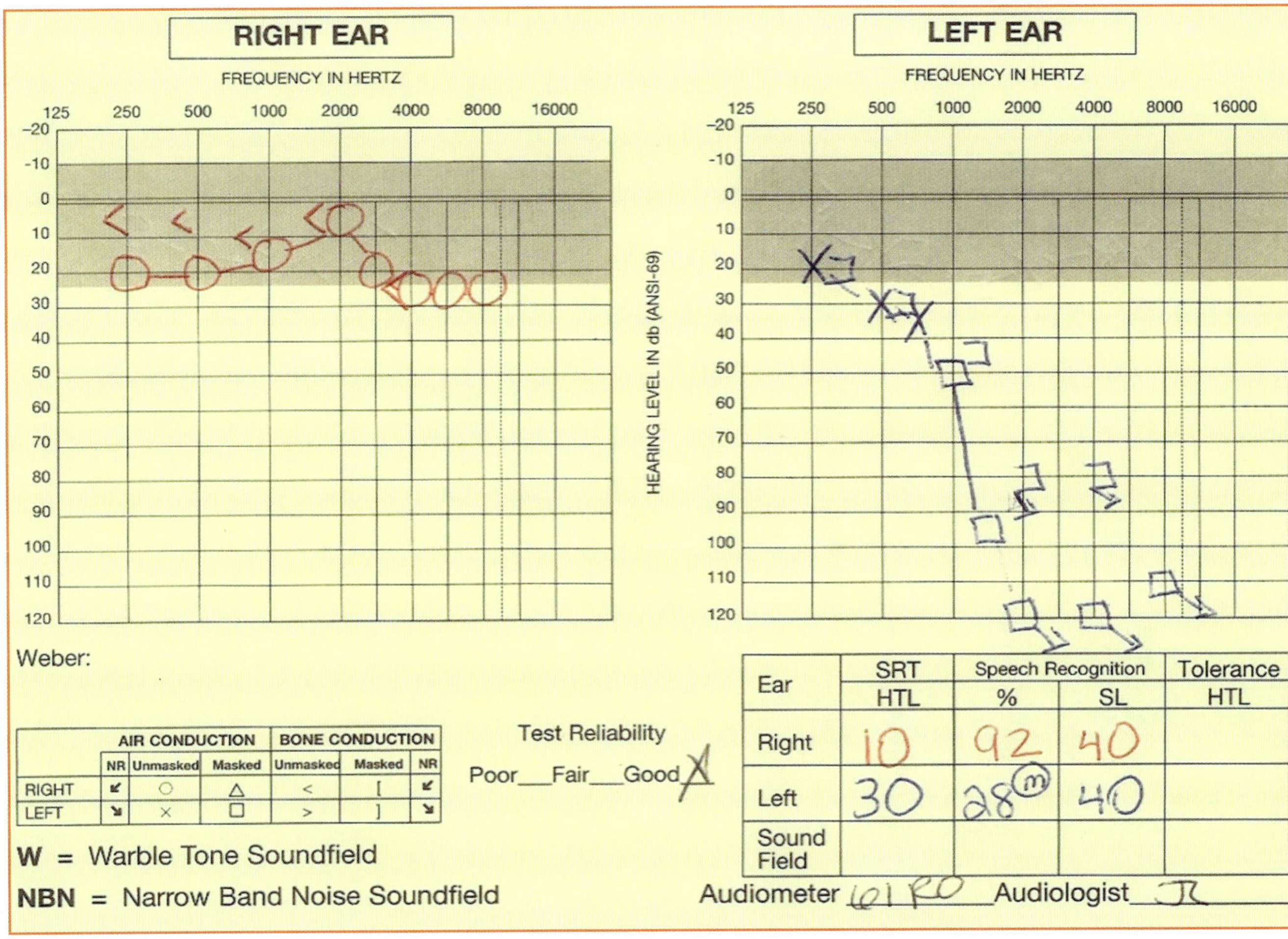

Figure 4–9. Audiogram of patient with left acoustic neuroma. Audiogram demonstrates significant interaural asymmetry at nearly all pure-tone frequencies. Although the patient's speech reception threshold (SRT) is reasonably good in the mild hearing loss range, the speech discrimination score is a dismal 28%, insinuating auditory neural dyssynchrony.

for normative values. In general, however, typical normal values for wave V interaural latency differences are ≤0.2 ms, wave I to V interpeak latencies ≤4.4 ms, and wave I to III interpeak latencies ≤2.5 ms (Figure 4–10).

Prior to the advent of contrast enhanced MRI, ABR was the standard for single modality screening for acoustic neuroma. With increased diagnosis and recognition of smaller acoustic neuromas from MR imaging, it has become clear that ABR as a single modality diagnostic tool is inadequate for anything but larger tumors.

A retrospective study of 111 cases of acoustic neuroma demonstrates an overall ABR sensitivity of 95%. However, when stratified by tumor size, sensitivity drops, using wave V interaural latency difference as. For tumors greater than 2 cm in maximal dimension, sensitivity was 100%; for tumors 1.1 to 2 cm, sensitivity was 98%; and for tumors ≤1 cm, sensitivity was only 89%.[17]

A more recent retrospective study of 676 patients with acoustic neuroma, however, suggests that associating responses in ABR with ENG caloric testing and clinical audiometry can reduce false negative rates to 1% in diagnosis of acoustic neuroma.[18] The study is hampered by selection bias due to its retrospective nature and study base in a tertiary referral center.

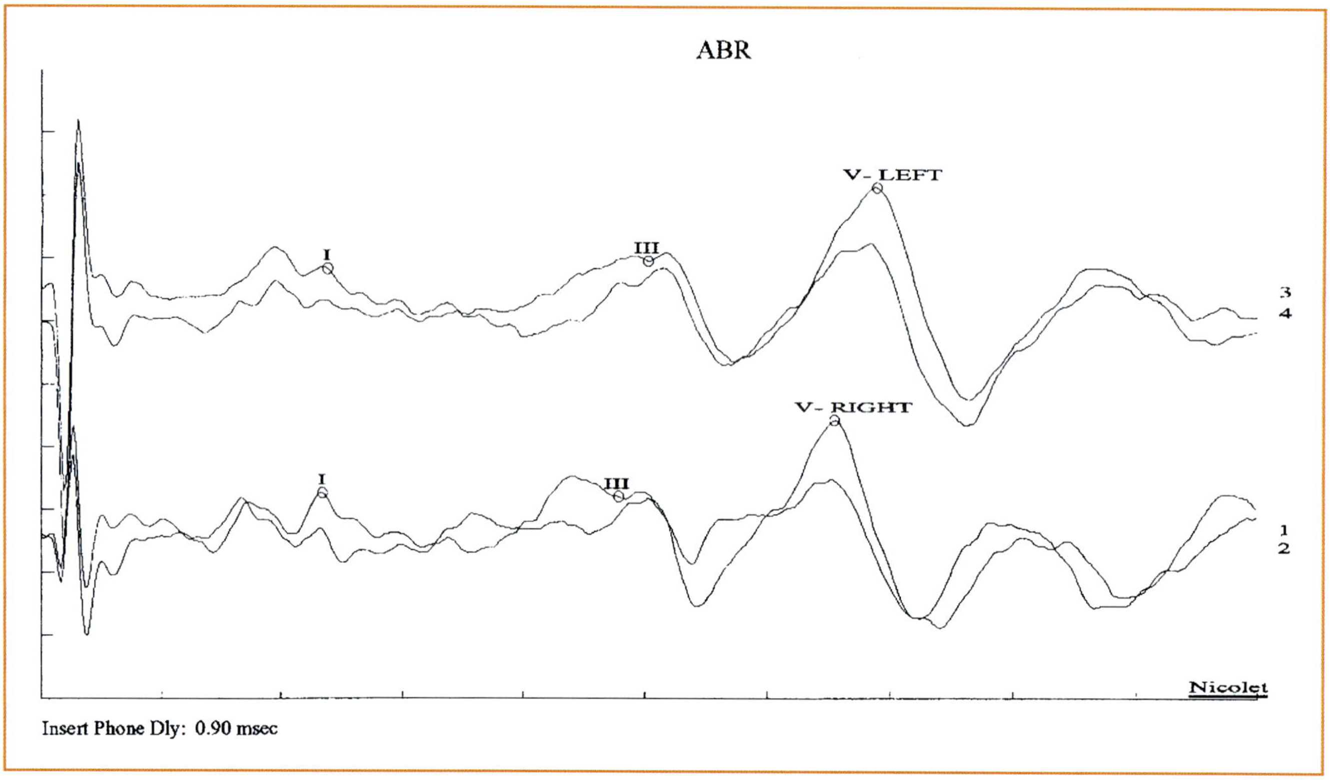

Figure 4–10. Auditory brainstem response of a patient with left acoustic neuroma. Evoked responses on the right are normal, whereas left evoked responses demonstrate delayed wave I to III interpeak latency of 2.8 ms (normal ≤2.5 ms) and delayed wave I to V interpeak latency of 4.7 ms (normal ≤4.4 ms). Wave V interaural latency difference is 0.4 ms (normal ≤0.2 ms), which is the most constant ABR abnormality noted in the setting of acoustic neuroma.

The largest prospective study comparing MRI and ABR enrolled 312 patients with asymmetric SNHL and demonstrated cerebellopontine angle lesions on MR imaging in 31, or 10%. Of these, ABR was abnormal in 22 and normal in 9, giving a false negative rate of 29%. Calculated separately was an ABR false positive rate of 77%, yielding an overall sensitivity of 71% and specificity of 74%. Based on these results, the author recommends abandoning ABR completely as a screening tool for asymmetric SNHL.[19]

In contrast to the relative imprecision of standard ABR measurements in evaluating for small acoustic neuromas, a new method of ABR measurement, the "stacked ABR," appears to provide significant improvement in both sensitivity and specificity. The stacked ABR technique involves sequential high pass acoustic stimulation to generate derived band ABR waveforms. Each derived band ABR waveform essentially corresponds to stimulation of frequency-specific regions of the auditory nerve. Temporal alignment of each derived band ABR waveform along its wave V maxima and subsequent summation yields the "stacked ABR," representing wave V neural activity with deletion of any frequency-dependent phase shift.

This ABR technique displays sensitivity to detection of small acoustic neuromas in comparison of summated wave V amplitude to normative values rather than in assessing interaural latency differences. In selecting a normalized stacked wave V amplitude of 0.74, a sensitivity of 95% and specificity of 88% can be achieved for evaluation of small acoustic neuromas or those that otherwise yield normal values in standard ABR benchmarks.[20]

The technique of derived band ABR generation and stacked ABR summation is relatively new and, probably much more so than standard ABR, is extremely system and operator dependent. Normative values for stacked wave V amplitudes must be generated for individual testing centers, as the sensitivity and specificity of this technique in screening for small acoustic neuromas is exquisitely dependent on this metric.

Electronystagmography (ENG)

High-resolution gadolinium-enhanced T1 images of the internal auditory canal can sometimes localize a small intracanalicular acoustic tumor to the upper or lower half of the internal auditory canal, implying a superiorly or inferiorly based tumor. However, radiographic localization is rarely achieved.

Electronystagmography with bithermal caloric stimulation can aid in differentiation superior from inferior vestibular tumors. A normal, symmetric caloric response between affected and non-affected sides can indicate either an inferior vestibular tumor or a superior vestibular tumor that has not physiologically affected responses from the horizontal semicircular canal. An abnormal, asymmetric response with unilateral weakness on the tumor side, however, typically indicates a superiorly based vestibular tumor with paresis of its attendant horizontal semicircular canal. Appropriately asymmetric responses on caloric testing, with the tumor side displaying unilateral weakness, suggest a more direct access to the superiorly based tumor and possibly less risk of injury to the facial and cochlear nerves when approached through a middle fossa craniotomy (Figure 4–11).

As with all electrophysiological studies, variations in equipment and operators make it advisable to generate normative values for use in each center.

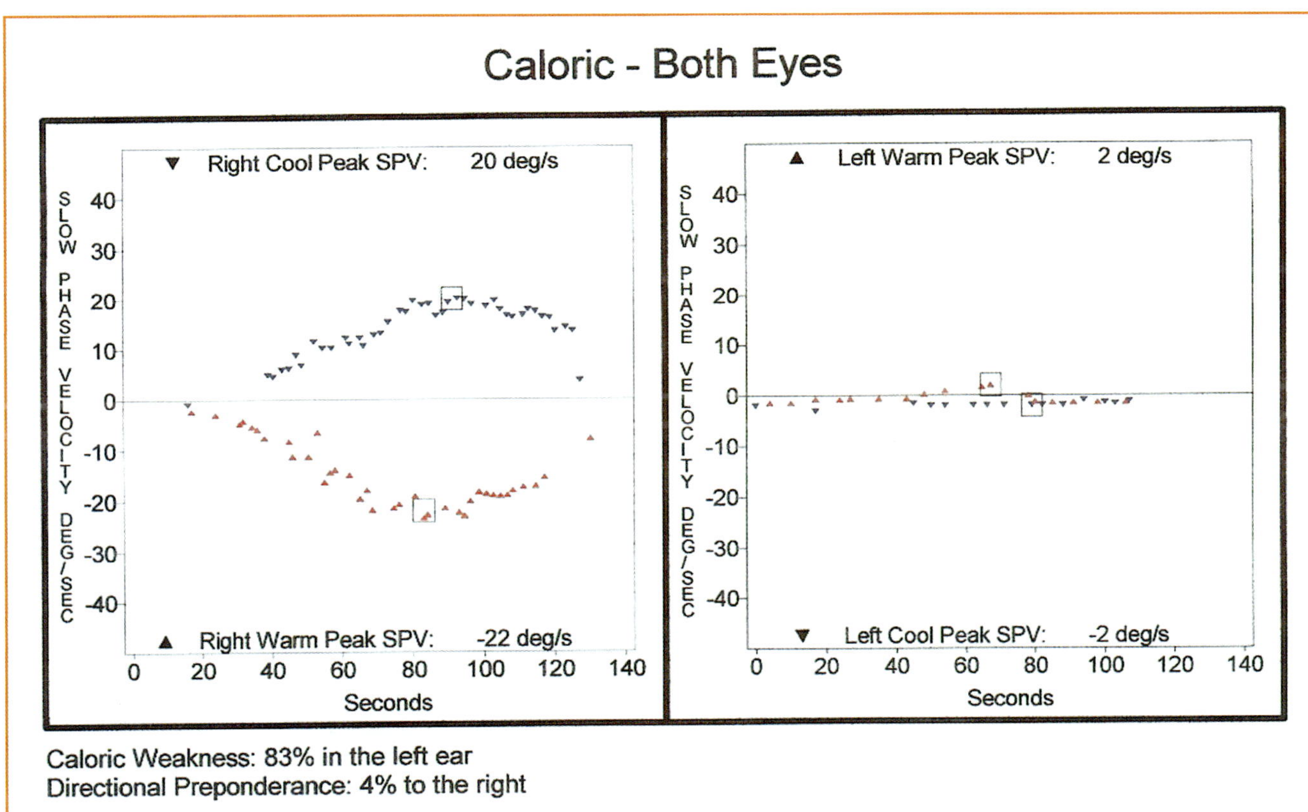

Figure 4–11. Electronystagmography of a patient with left acoustic neuroma. This patient has a significant reduced vestibular response on the left, suggesting a superiorly based tumor.

However, reduced vestibular response on bithermal caloric stimulation is typically accepted for unilateral weakness falling between 20 to 30%. Directional preponderance is not a reliable diagnostic or prognostic indicator and is not used.

Electroneuronography (ENOG)

Electroneuronography, or evoked electromyography, of the facial nerve is of minimal benefit in the preoperative evaluation of internal auditory canal tumors. Abnormal reduction in facial nerve compound muscle action potential amplitude correlates generally with increasing acoustic neuroma tumor size, but it does not provide predictive value for postoperative facial nerve outcome.[21] In this setting of large acoustic tumors, multiple factors, both tumor and surgeon specific, beyond reduced electroneuronographic activity can affect postoperative facial nerve outcome (Figure 4–12).

Some suggest that electroneuronography be routinely performed for intracanalicular tumors to screen for the possibility of facial neuroma. A retrospective review of intracanalicular facial neuromas demonstrated a range of CMAP reduction from 33 to 100%, despite 40% having normal facial function preoperatively.[22] Subsequent studies, however, have failed to demonstrate similar stratification (Figures 4–13A and 4–13B).

IMAGING

The gold standard for evaluation of asymmetric SNHL and acoustic neuroma, or internal auditory canal and cerebellopontine angle lesions in general, is magnetic resonance imaging. In this sense, diagnosis of acoustic neuroma is essentially radiographic: if an acoustic neuroma is not identified on high-resolution gadolinium-enhanced MRI, it is not present.

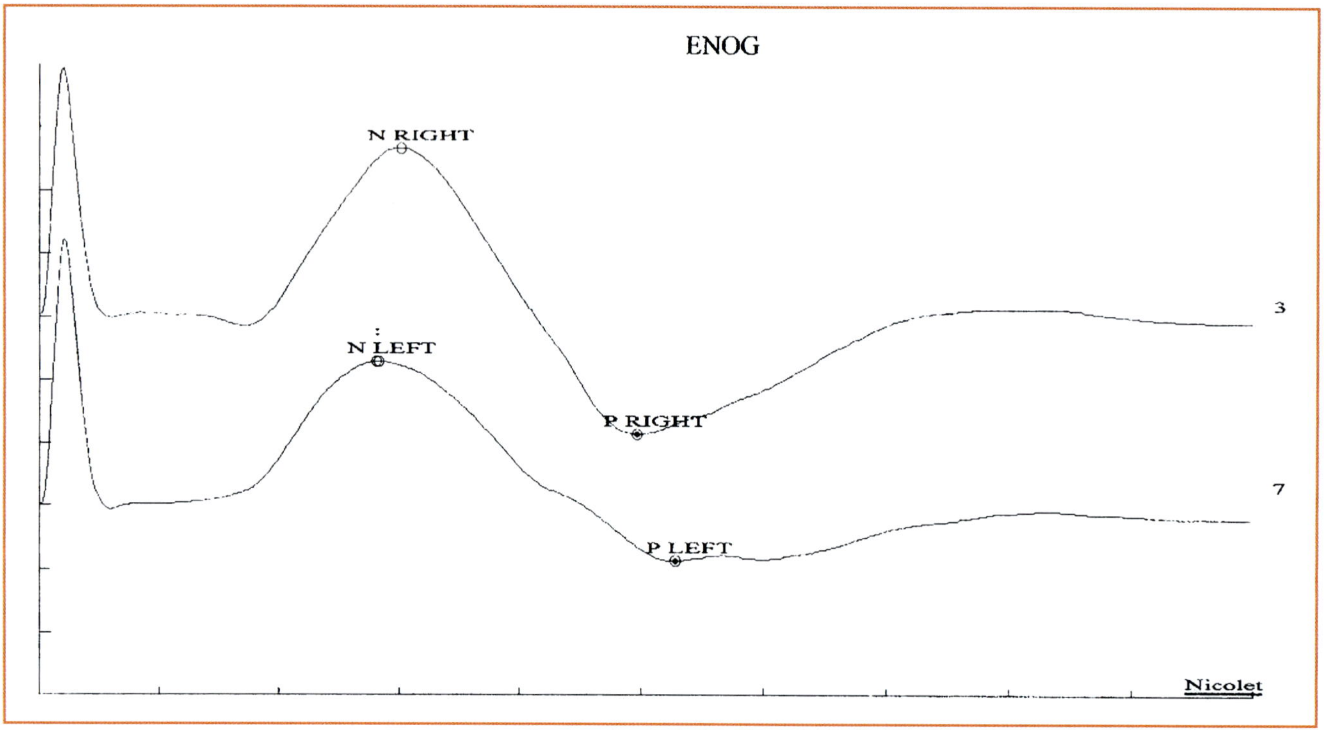

Figure 4–12. Electroneuronography of a patient with left acoustic neuroma. The compound muscle action potential of each side is calculated as the maximal change in potential from zenith N to nadir P. The CMAPs between sides are compared and the CMAP of the weaker side is reported as a percentage of the CMAP of the stronger side.

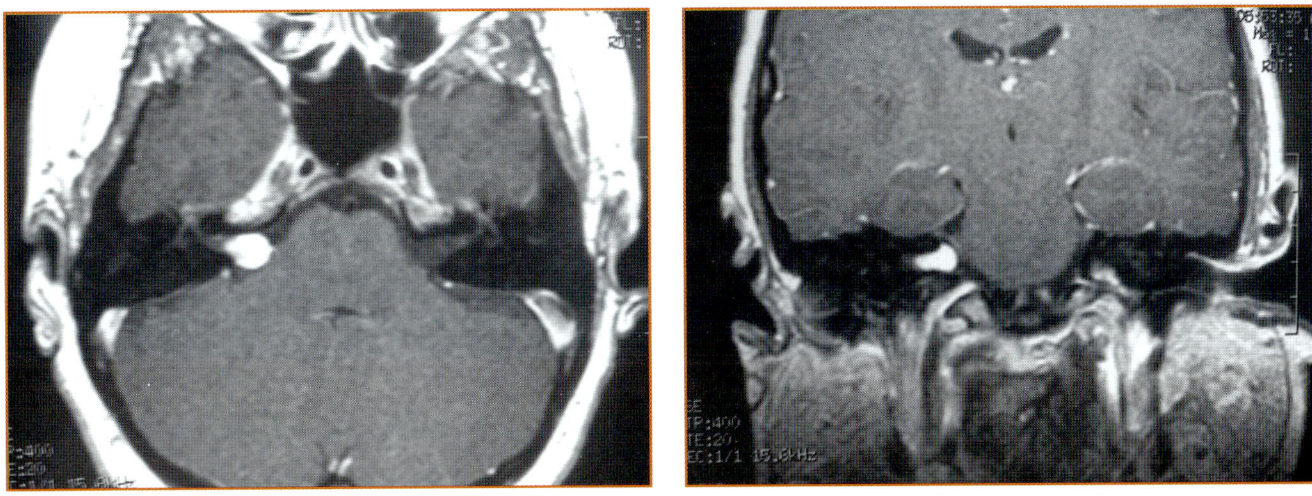

A B

Figure 4–13. Facial schwannoma, right. MRI, T1 weighted with gadolinium contrast, axial (**A**) and coronal (**B**). This patient presented with asymmetric SNHL and normal facial nerve function. Imaging revealed what appeared to be an acoustic neuroma. Intraoperatively, the tumor appeared densely integrated into the contour of the facial nerve, and every surface of the tumor was stimulated with the facial nerve stimulator at lowest settings. The tumor was not resected. The radiographic appearance of facial schwannomas can be indistinguishable from that of acoustic neuromas. Intraoperative facial nerve monitoring and active stimulation are invaluable tools in this setting.

Plain Film Radiography

Prior to CT and MRI, the subtle signs of a widened internal auditory canal seen on plain films and later x-ray tomography provided the only radiographic clues to the presence of an acoustic tumor. These techniques were positive only in cases in which very large tumors had deformed the surrounding temporal bone architecture. Needless to say, they have been supplanted long ago by more sensitive imaging modalities (Figure 4–14).

Computed Tomography (CT)

CT of the skull base provided a significant leap forward in the imaging of cerebellopontine angle lesions. Contrast enhanced CT could routinely image large tumors of the cerebellopontine angle, CPA. Air contrast CT improved sensitivity further but was extremely uncomfortable for the patient. Despite these incremental improvements, CT remained ineffective to reliably identify smaller tumors and intracanalicular tumors (Figure 4–15).

Magnetic Resonance Imaging (MRI)

The advent of magnetic resonance imaging ushered in the modern era of radiographic diagnosis of acoustic neuromas and cerebellopontine angle lesions in general. MRI provides exquisite anatomical detail of intracranial structures and generates unrivaled contrast of tissue signal within the central nervous system.

Early implementations of MRI were limited by the relatively long acquisition times and relatively poor spatial resolution in comparison to x-ray based tomographic imaging. However, the latest MR imaging modalities take advantage of significantly increased magnetic field strength and proprietary computational techniques to generate the most detailed images of intracranial and intratemporal structures available.

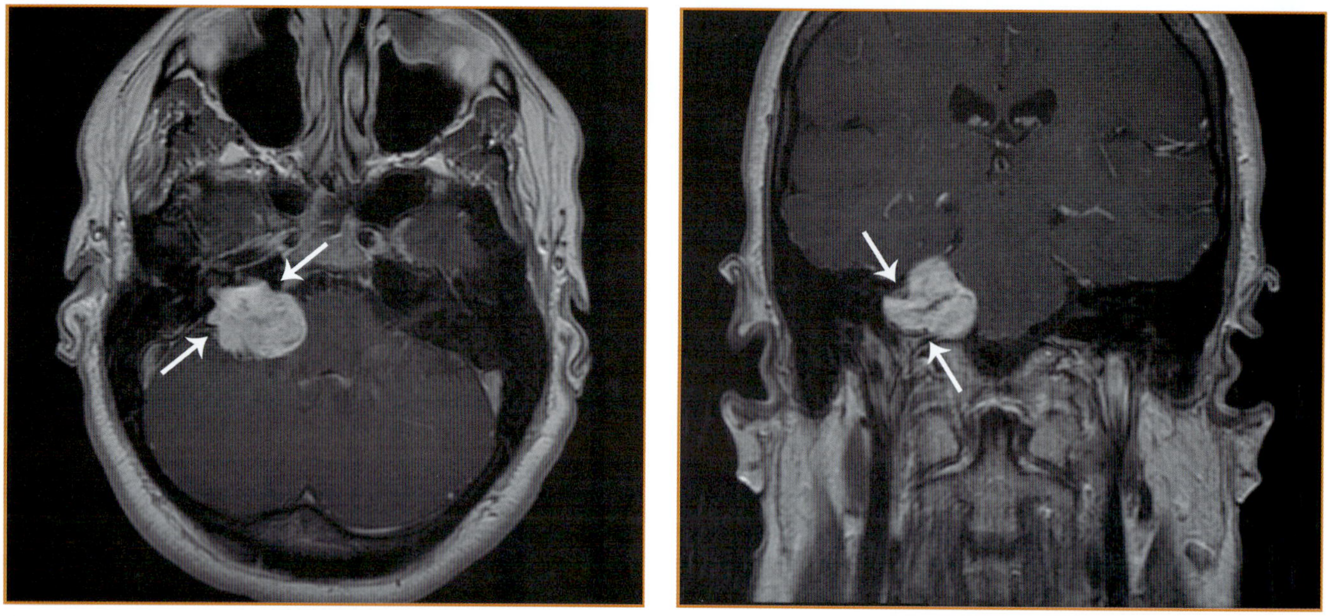

A B

Figure 4–14. Large acoustic neuroma with internal auditory canal expansion, right. MRI, T1 weighted with gadolinium contrast, axial (**A**) and coronal (**B**). This tumor exhibited significant bony widening of the internal auditory canal. White arrows call attention to the tumor indentations denoting the location of the porus acousticus. The tumor anterolateral to the porus is intracanalicular, which on axial projection appears as wide as the cisternal component of the tumor.

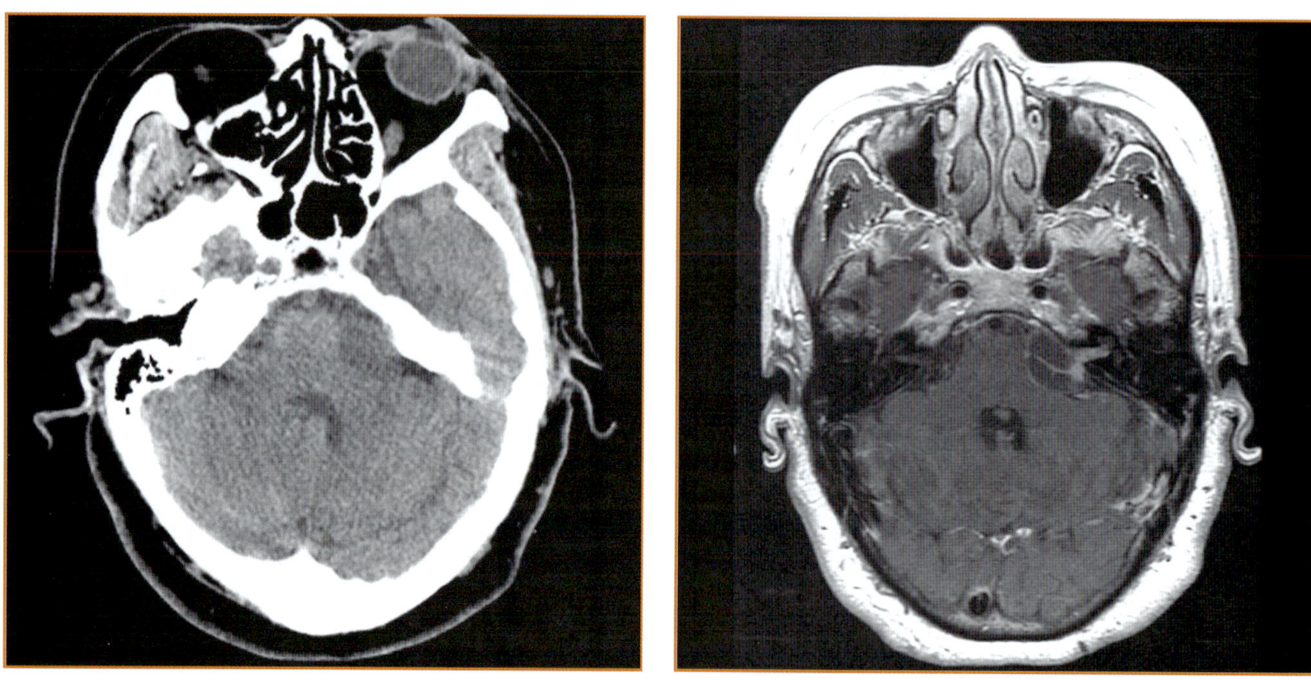

A B

Figure 4–15. Medium acoustic neuroma, left. CT head, axial (**A**). MRI, T1 weighted with gadolinium contrast, axial (**B**). The patient presented to her primary care physician with complaint of sudden onset unilateral facial hypoesthesia. A head CT was obtained, which was read as normal. Further workup with high-resolution contrast-enhanced MRI clearly revealed a left acoustic neuroma with solid intracanalicular component and cystic cisternal component. On repeat evaluation, the head CT suggests a hypodense lesion in the left cerebellopontine cistern with mild displacement of the pons contralaterally. However, the poor sensitivity of CT in detecting the acoustic neuroma in this case is clearly illustrated.

Fast spin echo T2-weighted MR protocols can also be used to image acoustic neuromas. This technique takes advantage of the cisternography-like appearance to T2-weighted images: neural soft tissue has relatively low T2 signal intensity, juxtaposed against the brilliant high signal intensity of surrounding CSF. Both large and small acoustic neuromas can be readily identified using this pseudocisternography technique.

Fast spin echo T2-weighting sequences have been described as equally sensitive at intracanalicular tumor identification as the more accepted gadolinium-enhanced T1 standard protocol.[23]

Similar heavily T2-weighted T2 pseudocisternography protocols can be achieved using other sequences exploiting constructive interference steady-state (CISS) to achieve extremely rapid slice acquisition and high resolution. These protocols, which come under colorful and proprietary names such as 3D-Fast-Imaging-Employing-Steady-sTate-Acquisition (3D-FIESTA), True-Fast-Imaging-with-Steady-Precession (TrueFISP), True-Fast-Field-Steady-Precession (TrueFFSP), Balanced-Fast-Field-Echo (Balanced FFE), Balanced-Spoiled-steady-state-Acquisition-Rewinded-Gradient-Echo (Balanced SARGE, BASG), Periodically-Rotated-Overlapping-ParallEL-Lines-with-Enhanced-Reconstruction (PROPELLER), DRIven-Equilibrium (DRIVE), and Coherent-Oscillatory-State-acquisition-for-Manipulation-of-Image-Contrast (COSMIC), all use variations of a balanced gradient echo waveform to product high liquid/solid tissue contrast and ultrafast slice acquisition for sub-millimeter spatial resolution, thus enhancing detection of smaller tumors (Figure 4–16).

Despite these recent advances in MR imaging sequences, a high resolution, axial and coronal, pre- and

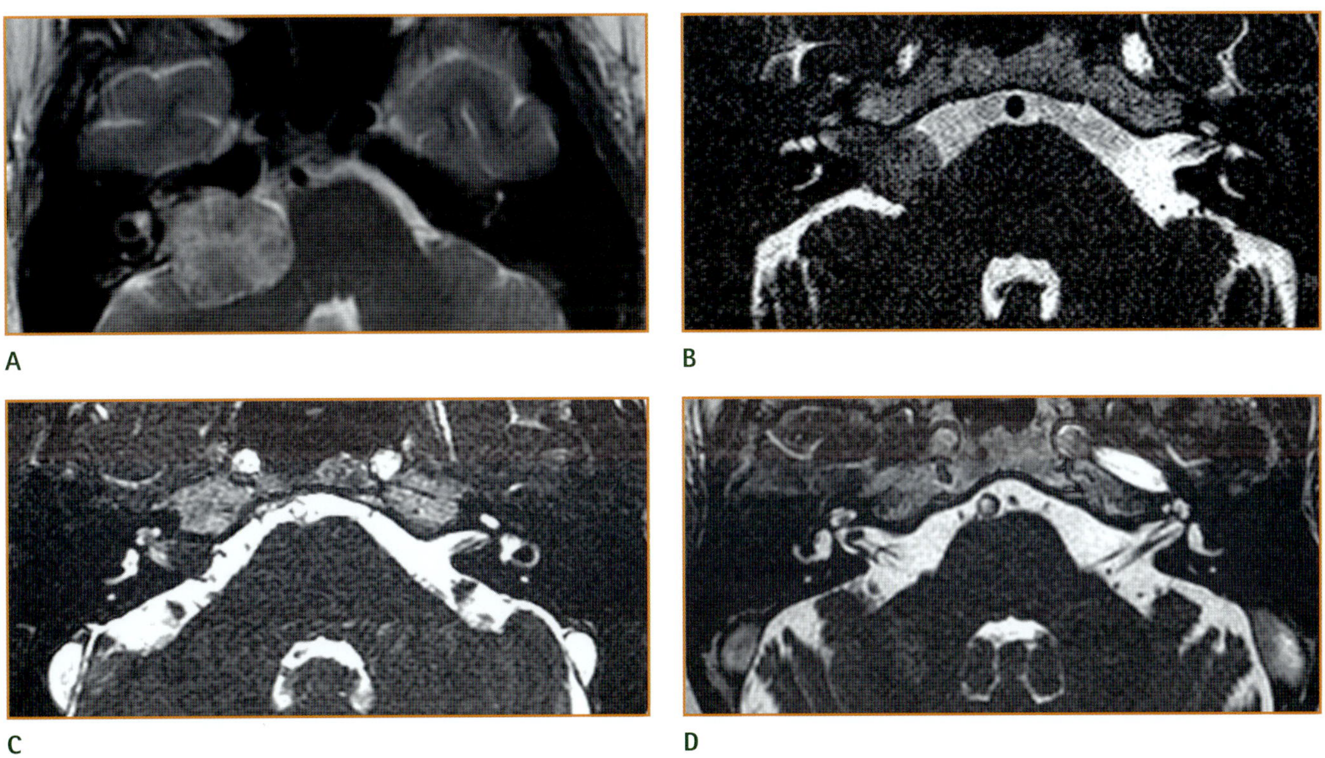

Figure 4–16. Constructive interference steady state imaging protocols for MRI. Large right acoustic neuroma in FSE T2 (**A**), medium right acoustic neuroma in DRIVE (**B**), small right acoustic neuroma in 3D-FIESTA (**C**), and very small right acoustic neuroma in 3D-FIESTA (**D**). The appearance of the final, tiny acoustic neuroma in (**D**) is equivocal using a pseudocisternography technique. Its presence was separately verified using gadolinium-enhanced T1-weighted images (see Figure 4–18), illustrating the continued reliance on contrast-enhanced high-resolution T1 imaging as the gold standard for radiographic diagnosis.

post-gadolinium enhanced T1 imaging protocol through the internal auditory canal and cerebellopontine angle region is still accepted as the gold standard imaging protocol for acoustic neuroma evaluation.

Because of the distinctive imaging signal characteristics of histologically different tumors, MRI can be an invaluable tool in helping to differentiate between such tumors and acoustic neuromas. The unique signal characteristics of the most common cerebellopontine angle and internal auditory canal lesions are summarized in Table 4–3.

Table 4–3. Imaging Characteristics of CPA/IAC Lesions

MRI	T1	T2	Gad	CT	Comments
acoustic neuroma	iso	iso	(+)	contrast enhancing	
meningioma	iso	iso	(+)	intratumoral calcification	dural tail
cholesterol granuloma	↑	↑ / mixed	-	smooth expansion	
epidermoid	↓	↑	± peripheral enhancement	smooth expansion	DWI bright
mucocele	variable (dependent on protein content)	↑	peripheral enhancement	smooth expansion	
fat (pseudolesion)	↑	↓	–	check contralateral side; correlate location c MRI	use fat suppression T1
mucus (pseudolesion)	variable (dependent on protein content)	↑	–	preservation of septae	
arachnoid cyst (pseudolesion)	↓	↑	–	CT cisternogram to differentiate with epidermoid	DWI dark
chordoma	iso	↑ (Ca++ areas dark)	(+)	skull base erosion; contrast enhancing	midline; notochordal basiocciput, basisphenoid
chondrosarcoma	iso	↑ (Ca++ areas dark)	(+)	skull base erosion; contrast enhancing	paramedian; petroclival synchondrosis
fibrous dysplasia	iso	mixed	mixed (+)	ground glass; otic capsule spared, EAC stenosis	definitive on CT
ossifying hemangioma	iso	↑	(+) ?	intratumoral calcification; ill-defined bony margin	geniculate ganglion (facial)
endolymphatic sac tumor	mixed	mixed	(+)	locally destructive	posterior to labyrinth
trigeminal neuroma	iso	↑	(+)	smooth remodeling of apex	Meckel's cave
cavernous sinus hemangioma	iso	very ↑	(+)	bony erosion when large	similar to trigeminal neuroma
plasmacytoma/multiple myeloma	iso	↓	(+)	skull base erosion; contrast enhancing	
metastasis	iso	iso	central enhancement	skull base erosion; contrast enhancing	

Following definitive treatment, postoperative MR imaging should again be performed with high resolution T1 axial and coronal protocol with gadolinium enhancement. However, when surgical reconstruction is performed using fat grafts, the postoperative appearance of the surgical reconstruction can potentially mask any recurrence of tumor, as T1 fat signal is hyperintense in a fashion similar to gadolinium-enhanced tissue. To minimize such confusion, postoperative MR imaging following translabyrinthine resection (or any other treatment employing fat graft wound reconstruction) should be performed utilizing chemical shift imaging techniques for fat signal suppression, such as the fat-saturation technique (presaturation of fat proton signal) (Figure 4–17).

TREATMENT

The treatment of acoustic neuromas falls into three broad categories: (1) observation with serial imaging, (2) radiotherapy, and (3) surgical resection.

Observation

As 20 to 60% of all acoustic neuromas show little to no growth on serial MR imaging, the approach of observation with serial imaging can be a reasonable one, dependent on either patient or tumor characteristics.

Patient characteristics for which conservative management can be advised included: advanced age, multiple or serious medical co-morbidities for which there is increased surgical risk, normal hearing, patient prerogative, and "asymptomatic" presentation, that is, incidental radiographic diagnosis of an acoustic neuroma in a scan performed for other purposes.

Tumors that are small and cause no risk of brainstem compression can be watched safely. Tumors that exhibit stability and little or no growth over time can continue to be watched without intervention. However, treating the tumor as early as possible gives the best chance of preserving residual hearing, as most acoustic neuromas invariably yield a progressive hearing loss. In addition, tumors over 2 cm that are resected with microsurgery have a much lower chance of preserving residual or serviceable hearing compared to tumors under 2 cm.[14] Removal of smaller tumors also increases the chance of excellent postoperative facial nerve function for similar reasons, as dissection of larger tumors places the facial nerve at increasing risk (Figure 4–18).

Tumors that exhibit moderate or fast growth should be treated in a timely fashion once such growth has been identified, and ideally before there is onset of new or significant symptoms, for reasons stated above. In addition, tumors that demonstrate slow growth over time but which have, during that time, become brainstem touching or brainstem compressive tumors, should be considered for intervention, as they likely will continue to grow.

Radiotherapy

Radiotherapy as primary treatment of acoustic neuromas is a physically noninvasive option for treatment. For a more complete description of the radiobiology and radiation-based therapeutic options for management of acoustic neuroma, please see Chapter 10.

Radiotherapeutic protocols can take on many forms and can be thought of in a few different ways: fractionated versus single dose radiotherapy, and non-conformal versus highly conformal or stereotactic radiotherapy. Table 4–4 summarizes this therapy.

For all intents and purposes, Gamma Knife, CyberKnife, and other stereotactic treatment modalities, rather than conventional external beam radiotherapy, are now considered the gold standard of radiotherapy options for acoustic neuroma management.[24,25] The upper limit of tumor size that can be safely treated by stereotactic radiotherapeutic means is commonly accepted as 3 cm maximal diameter.

SURGERY

Translabyrinthine Approach

Arguably the most common and familiar avenue to the cerebellopontine angle employed by neurotologists is the translabyrinthine approach. As the name

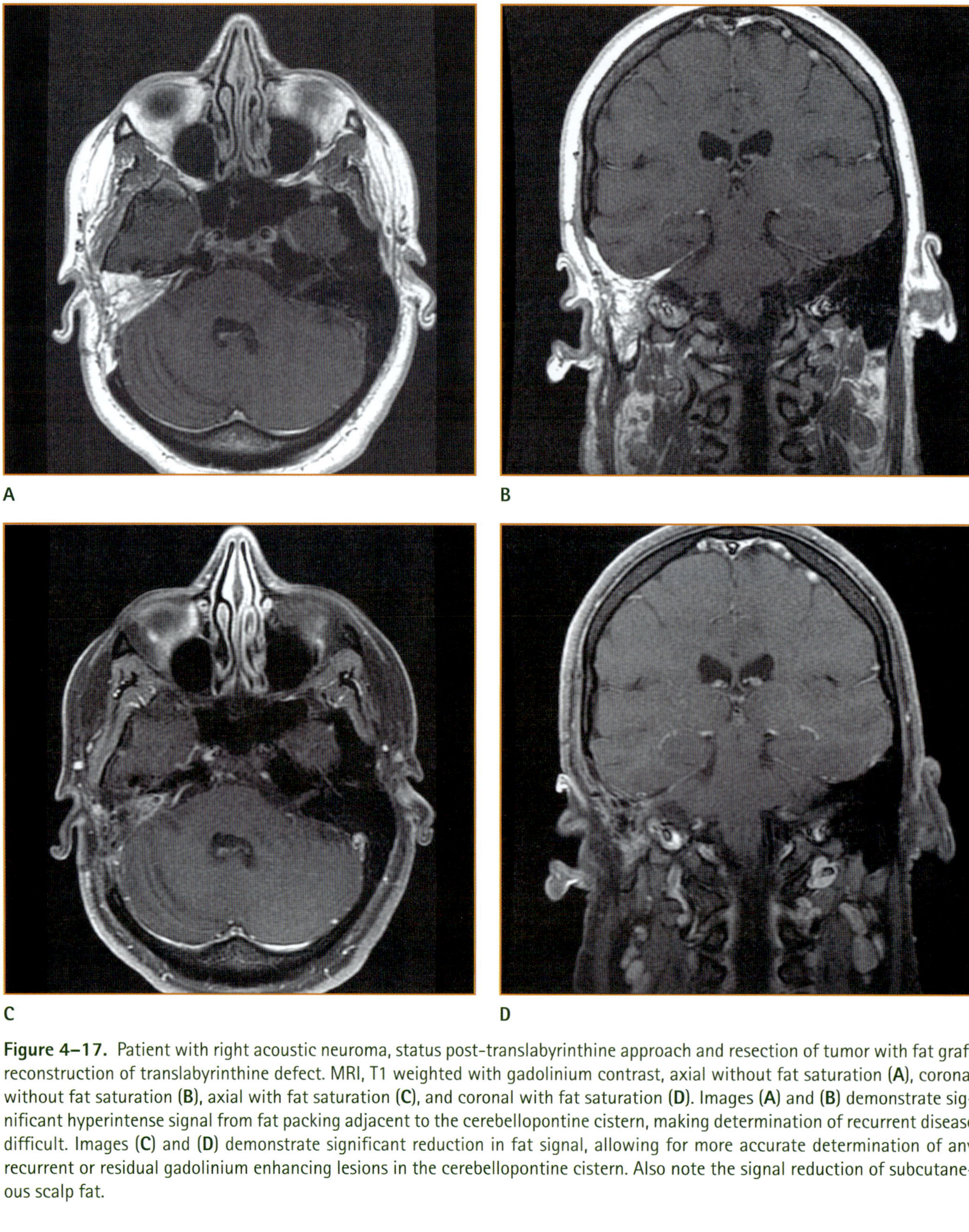

Figure 4–17. Patient with right acoustic neuroma, status post-translabyrinthine approach and resection of tumor with fat graft reconstruction of translabyrinthine defect. MRI, T1 weighted with gadolinium contrast, axial without fat saturation (**A**), coronal without fat saturation (**B**), axial with fat saturation (**C**), and coronal with fat saturation (**D**). Images (**A**) and (**B**) demonstrate significant hyperintense signal from fat packing adjacent to the cerebellopontine cistern, making determination of recurrent disease difficult. Images (**C**) and (**D**) demonstrate significant reduction in fat signal, allowing for more accurate determination of any recurrent or residual gadolinium enhancing lesions in the cerebellopontine cistern. Also note the signal reduction of subcutaneous scalp fat.

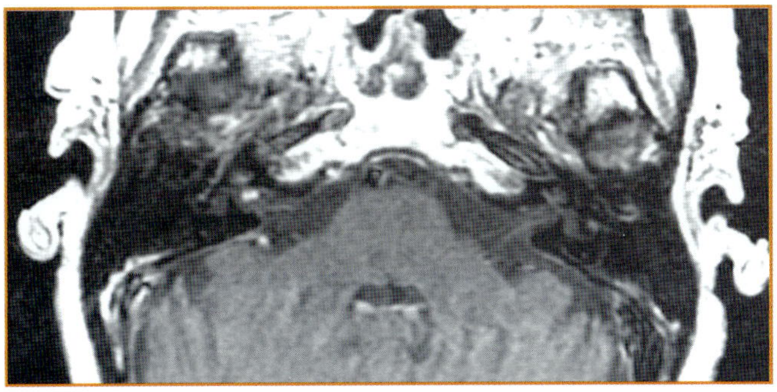

Figure 4–18. Intracanalicular acoustic neuroma, right. MRI, T1 weighted with gadolinium contrast, axial. This tumor was found incidentally in a patient without cochleovestibular or facial symptoms. It has been followed with serial imaging with contrast-enhanced MRI for three years without growth.

Table 4–4. Radiotherapy Modalities

	Fractionated	Single Dose
Non-conformal/ Minimally Conformal	External Beam Radiotherapy	N/A
Conformal/Stereotactic	CyberKnife/other LINAC	Gamma Knife

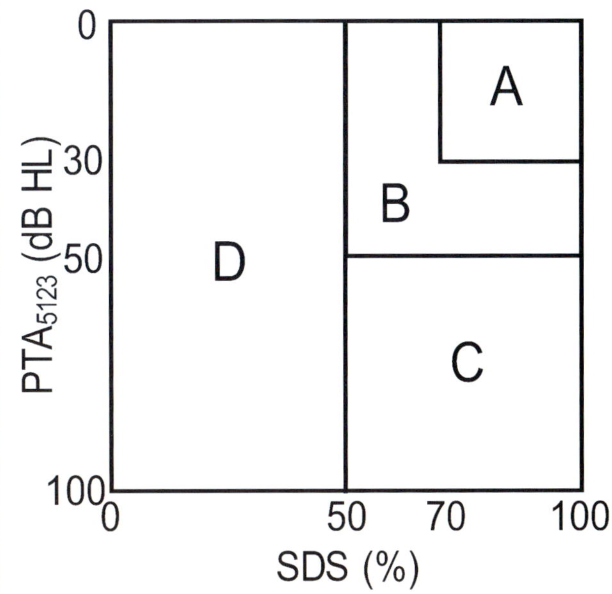

Figure 4–19. American Academy of Otolaryngology-Head and Neck Surgery Committee on Hearing and Equilibrium hearing classification. Hearing can be classified into four classes: A, B, C, and D. Classes A and B constitute "serviceable" hearing, where a hearing conservation approach to tumor resection may be considered if appropriate. Classes C and D constitute "non-serviceable" hearing, where hearing preservation is not attempted. (Adapted from: Committee on Hearing and Equilibrium guidelines for the evaluation of hearing preservation in acoustic neuroma (vestibular schwannoma.) (American Academy of Otolaryngology-Head and Neck Surgery Foundation, Inc. *Otolaryngol Head Neck Surg.* 1995;113(3):179–180.)

implies, the translabyrinthine approach is a transtemporal approach which traverses the labyrinth or posterior otic capsule to reach the internal auditory canal and intracranial vault. In so doing, the removal of the labyrinth causes complete loss of both auditory and vestibular function from that inner ear.

Surgically induced anacusis may at first seem to be a condition that few patients would be willing to accept. However, as a large fraction of patients with acoustic neuromas continue to present with significantly diminished hearing and speech discrimination ipsilaterally, the loss of the remainder of such nonserviceable levels of hearing does not add any additional morbidity for such patients. Patients with hearing class C or D, and some would argue B, based on 1995 AAO-HNS Committee on Hearing and Equilibrium guidelines for evaluation of hearing preservation in acoustic neuroma, are generally considered to have nonserviceable hearing and would be appropriate candidates for a hearing destructive skull base approach such as the translabyrinthine craniotomy[26] (Figure 4–19).

In addition, a subset of patients will characterize vertigo or disequilibrium as their chief complaint, above and beyond any associated hearing loss. The ongoing episodic vertigo or persistent disequilibrium can markedly affect their function at work and home and markedly diminish their societal interaction. In such patients, the destruction of the vestibular end organ in conjunction with the division of the vestibular nerve at the site of the tumor can ensure a quicker and more complete resolution to such debilitating balance symptoms, offering a solution that other nondestructive approaches or nonsurgical treatments cannot. Thus, the translabyrinthine approach continues to be the workhorse for removal of medium, large, and even small acoustic neuromas for which postoperative anacusis is not a barrier to treatment for the patient.

The surgical technique is described in great detail in Chapter 2.

Ultimate limitations for tumor exposure are: superiorly, the tentorium cerebelli and superior petrosal sinus; posteriorly, the posteriormost retraction of contracted sigmoid sinus; inferiorly, the jugular bulb, which cannot and should not be uncovered of its overlying bone, as the dural folds over the jugular bulb are quite thin and can be easily damaged if unroofed; anteriorly, the vertical facial nerve and external auditory canal (Figure 4–20). Although the external auditory canal can be resected and the middle ear and ear canal overclosed, this extension to the lateral dissection does not aid in improving anterior exposure as long as the vertical facial nerve remains in position. Performing an anterior facial nerve transposition, infratemporal fossa A approach, or transotic or transcochlear approach will increase anterior exposure intracranially. However, such dissection is very rarely warranted, as the cerebellopontine angle anterior to the porus acousticus can almost always be accessed directly through an unmodified translabyrinthine craniotomy.

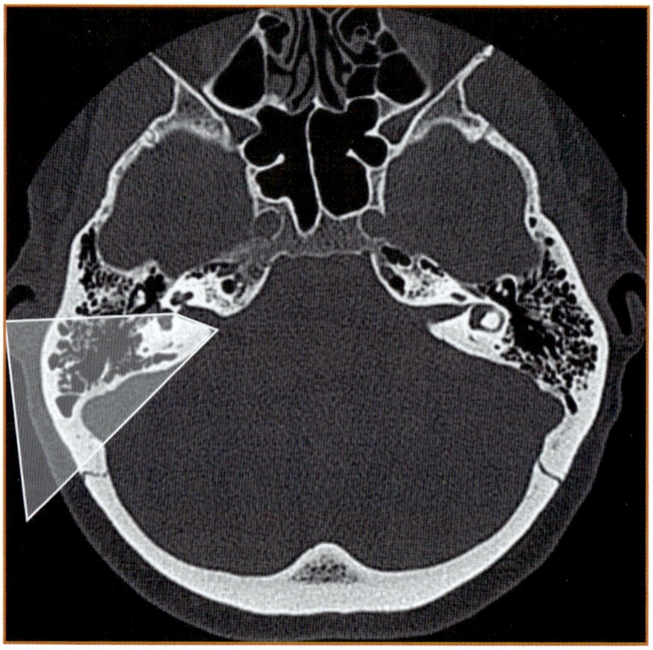

A

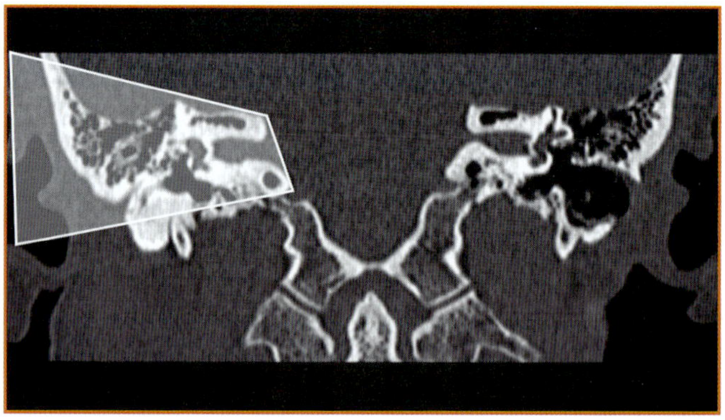

B

Figure 4–20. Translabyrinthine craniotomy for access to the internal auditory canal and cerebellopontine angle, axial **(A)** and coronal **(B)** schematic.

Thus, even very large tumors can be resected through this approach. The only significant limitation of this approach to the cerebellopontine angle, compared to a retrosigmoid or suboccipital approach is the native location of the jugular bulb: a normal or low jugular bulb will allow equally effective access to the cerebellopontine angle via translabyrinthine approach as retrosigmoid. However, a high-riding jugular bulb can severely limit the access to the inferior cerebellopontine angle and can put the lower cranial nerves at significant risk of injury if blind dissection behind the jugular bulb is required.

The translabyrinthine approach, although somewhat time consuming, offers far and away the best access to both the internal auditory canal and cerebellopontine angle compartments through one craniotomy. The field of view and proximity to the internal auditory canal, from fundus to porus, is unmatched. A natural plane of dissection between the facial nerve and vestibular nerves, via Bill's bar, can be easily developed at the fundus. The entire course of the facial nerve, from root entry zone to stylomastoid foramen, is within the dissection cavity. This may seem counterintuitive as an advantage, but knowing, and visualizing, the entire course of the facial nerve is always safer than dissection adjacent to the nerve without complete confidence in its exact location. Finally, the translabyrinthine approach typically involves less brain retraction than a retrosigmoid approach.

Retrosigmoid Approach

The retrosigmoid approach is a suboccipital approach commonly employed by neurosurgeons to access the posterior fossa. Acoustic neuromas were historically always accessed by Neurosurgery via a unilateral or bilateral medial suboccipital approach to avoid contamination of a sterile surgical field by opening the more forwardly placed mastoid air cells. A medially placed suboccipital craniotomy was not ideal to accessing the cerebellopontine cistern, as significant cerebellar retraction was necessary.

The modern retrosigmoid approach places the suboccipital craniotomy as far anteriorly and laterally as possible, minimizing cerebellar retraction and also minimizing the depth of the surgical dissection from the craniotomy.[29] Mastoid air cells are always encountered, but this has not led to any increase in postoperative wound infection or meningitis as previously feared. As long as mastoid aeration is thoroughly addressed prior to closure, the rate of postoperative CSF leak is also comparable to other approaches.

The great strength of the retrosigmoid approach is the ability to fully visualize the entire pontine cistern from clivus to foramen magnum. As such, this approach is the most appropriate for extremely large tumors over 4 cm, brainstem compressive tumors, large tumors with significant inferior extension, and tumors in which the jugular bulb has been identified preoperatively as being particularly high, thereby constricting inferior access to the cerebellopontine angle when viewed through a translabyrinthine craniotomy.

The retrosigmoid approach is also employed when a hearing conservation approach to tumor removal is desired. Tumor removal via the retrosigmoid is not limited by size but rather by location: when employed in a hearing conservation technique, the retrosigmoid approach does not provide for direct visualization to the lateral third to half of the internal auditory canal. Thus, the approach is inadequate for tumors with significant lateral extension into the internal auditory canal, as tumor dissection in the fundus will be blind and potentially dangerous both for preservation of hearing and facial function. Fortunately, it is uncommon for patients with serviceable hearing to present with tumors extending far beyond the internal auditory canal, and as such most can be approached via a subtemporal technique. In contrast, patients with large posterior fossa meningiomas and serviceable hearing are best handled via a retrosigmoid approach: these tumors rarely extend significantly into the internal auditory canal, and decompression of the cochleovestibular nerve in the cerebellopontine angle routinely results in conserved sensorineural hearing and, exceptionally, in reversal of this hearing loss.

Surgical Technique

The patient is positioned for retrosigmoid approach supine or in lateral decubitus position on the operating table and rotated 180 degrees from anesthesia. If the patient is supine, the ipsilateral shoulder is bumped, and the head is turned maximally away from the side of surgery and maximally flexed with chin to contralateral shoulder. The head may be secured with Mayfield pins or taped securely onto the operating table.

The montage of facial nerve monitoring electrodes is applied ipsilaterally, and electrodes for intraoperative ABR are also placed, along with insert earphones in ears bilaterally. These are placed in a nonsterile fashion, as the ear is draped out of the surgical field. For tumors with extensive inferior or superior extension, laryngeal, palatal, sternocleidomastoid, trapezius, hypoglossal, and motor trigeminal monitoring electrodes can be employed as well.

The scalp is shaved and cleansed adequately for a curvilinear incision approximately four fingerbreadths behind and two to three fingerbreadths above the postauricular crease. As the external auditory canal does not have to be prepared within the sterile field, the horizontal plane at the level of the external auditory canal is marked out onto the postauricular scalp. This plane estimates the level of the transverse sinus, which defines the superior border of the retrosigmoid craniotomy. The planned surgical field is circumscribed by segmented sheets of clear drape, and the field is sterilely prepared.

A curvilinear incision is made behind the ear and positioned to be bisected by the plane denoting the transverse sinus. The incision is carried down to the sternocleidomastoid and suboccipital musculature and raised forward to the external auditory canal. The suboccipital musculature is divided and mastoid and occipital periosteal attachments are elevated and retracted. This is often easiest to achieve by developing and raising an inferiorly based, inverted U-shaped musculoperiosteal flap. The asterion and surrounding mastoid, occipital, and parietal cortices are exposed. The asterion is the point on posterior cranium defined by the confluence of the temporal mastoid, parietal, and occipital cortices. This point delineates the junction of the transverse sinus to the sigmoid sinus beneath.

As with the translabyrinthine approach, mannitol infusion is started at the beginning of the case to ensure adequate osmotic diuresis and reduction in intracranial pressure. Hyperventilation to 25 to 28 cm H_2O is conducted to assist in lowering intracranial pressure.

Drilling commences 1 cm posterior and 1 cm inferior to the asterion. A 4 cm × 4 cm parallelogram shaped craniotomy is fashioned with walls parallel to the transverse sinus and sigmoid sinus. Cutting burs are used to remove the bulk of bone, with diamond burs used to finish bony removal above the dura. Care is taken to avoid injury to dura, as this must be closed primarily at the conclusion of the case to prevent CSF leak. Mastoid air cells are often entered along the anterior border of the craniotomy, and this region can be exenterated of all posterior mastoid air cells to obtain better visualization of the bony skeleton of the sigmoid sinus. Following completion of the craniotomy and posterior mastoidectomy, remaining mastoid air cells are thoroughly occluded with bone wax to minimize postoperative risk of CSF rhinorrhea or otorrhea. The craniotomy bone flap is gently elevated off the underlying dura and held in saline.

The occipital dura is incised along the anterior and superior borders of the craniotomy, leaving a healthy edge of dura beyond the sigmoid and transverse sinus borders onto which the dural flap can be sewn at closure. For large tumors, significant intracranial pressure can cause cerebellar protrusion through the dural opening. Therefore, it is important to find the anterior cerebellar edge and retract the cerebellum posteriorly to open and drain the cerebellopontine cistern as quickly as possible, as doing so will allow rapid decompression of cerebrospinal fluid and avoid undue cerebellar herniation. In cases in which extremely large tumors cause hydrocephalus, preemptive measures such as ventriculostomy placement prior to craniotomy are warranted.

Once the posterior fossa has been decompressed, the cerebellum can be more easily retracted posteriorly to fully reveal the pontine cistern from tentorium cerebelli superiorly to foramen magnum inferiorly. Thus, with appropriate cerebellar retraction, cranial nerves 5 through 12 can be visible exiting the brainstem via this approach. Large tumors and those with significant superior or inferior extension can be confidently resected due to direct visualization of the trigeminal and lower cranial nerves.

The brain-tumor interface is identified and tumor elevated away from the cerebellum. The tumor envelope is checked for facial EMG activity with the facial nerve stimulator, and after assuring no facial nerve activity over the superficial face of the envelope, this area is cauterized with bipolar electrocautery and resected. The central tumor volume is debulked using sharp and blunt dissection, with frequent mapping with the facial nerve stimulator to avoid dissection near the facial nerve. After adequate central debulking, the tumor walls are elevated off the surrounding cerebellum and collapsed to the center.

Tumor walls are checked for facial EMGs, and all clear regions are resected. The tumor is gently elevated off of the underlying brainstem. As the brainstem comes into view, the root entry zones of the facial and cochleovestibular nerves are identified and preserved. The tumor is gently dissected off of both nerves in a medial to lateral fashion toward the porus acousticus.

With sufficient tumor debulking, the posterior face of the petrous temporal bone can be readily accessed. The operculum, or petrous bone medial to the vestibular aqueduct overlying the internal auditory canal posteriorly, is drilled away.

In a hearing conservation approach, drilling should be kept medial to the vestibular aqueduct, as entry into the aqueduct and endolymphatic sac injury will lead to hearing loss. This limits internal auditory canal exposure to the medial half to two-thirds. If hearing conservation is not a goal, then the vestibular aqueduct can be transected and the entire internal auditory canal exposed out to the fundus.

The internal auditory canal dura is then incised along the posterior face, cheating inferiorly, and the contents exposed. The intracanalicular tumor is slowly dissected away from the underlying nerves. Without exposure of the fundus, Bill's bar cannot be identified, and hence the natural plane of dissection between the superior vestibular nerve and the facial nerve cannot be easily developed. Tumor and vestibular nerve dissection must proceed in a relatively blind fashion off of the underlying facial and cochlear nerves. To minimize shearing forces on the cochlear nerve at its modiolar attachment, medial to lateral dissection is attempted in a hearing conservation approach. This is not always possible, however, due to the often tight adherence of tumor to the facial and cochlear nerves at the porus.

Following tumor removal, Valsalva maneuvers are performed and the intracranial vault is checked for bleeding. The retracted cerebellum is gently released. The posterior fossa dura is primarily closed; a duraplasty is performed if necessary to span any gap in dural repair. The bone flap is replaced, and overlying muscle and soft tissue reapproximated. The skip flap is closed in layers in a watertight fashion. A snug mastoid dressing is applied. The wound is checked daily for signs of subcutaneous CSF collection, wound leak, otorrhea, or rhinorrhea. The dressing is changed once and removed after one week.

Far and away the biggest advantage to the retrosigmoid approach is the ability to access the entire pontine cistern from tentorium cerebelli to foramen magnum (Figure 4–21). Thus, the largest tumors can be approached by this technique, and the ability to control the overlying cerebellar tissue and visualize all posterior fossa cranial nerves is unmatched. This approach also offers the only option for hearing conservation for tumors with significant extracanalicular or cerebellopontine angle extension. The rate of CSF leak from the retrosigmoid approach is low and comparable to that of other approaches for acoustic neuromas.

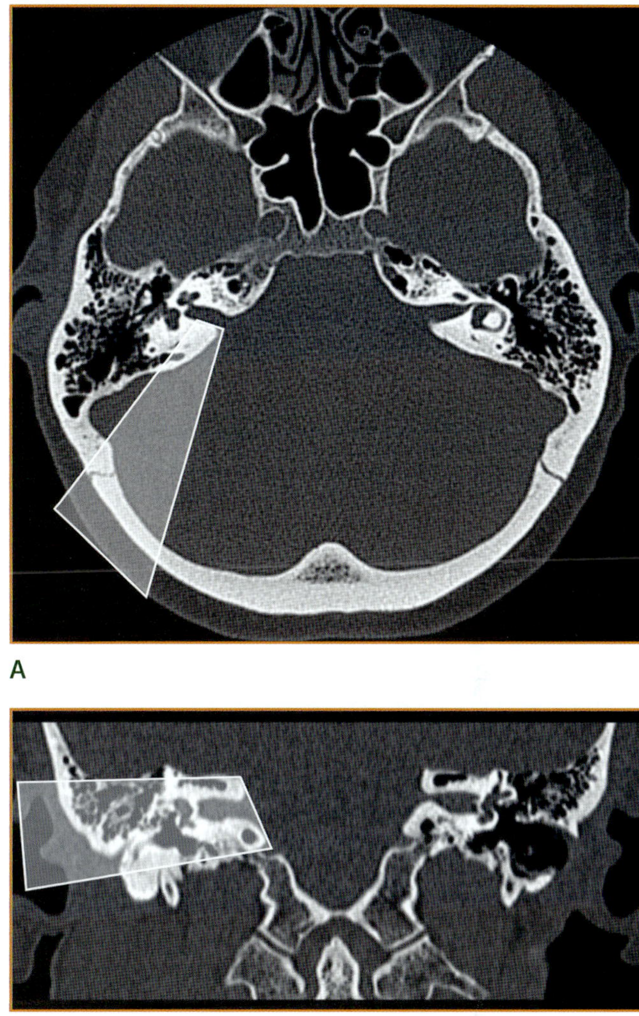
A

B

Figure 4–21. Retrosigmoid craniotomy for access to the internal auditory canal and cerebellopontine angle, axial (**A**) and coronal (**B**) schematic.

The biggest significant disadvantage to this approach, although one often still debated, is the relatively higher incidence of postoperative and chronic headaches as compared to other approaches. All acoustic neuroma patients with preoperative headaches are at higher risk for chronic postoperative headaches, although those who undergo retrosigmoid craniotomy tend to rate their postoperative headaches as both more frequent and more severe than those undergoing translabyrinthine or subtemporal craniotomies.[29,30]

Middle Fossa Approach

The standard middle fossa approach or subtemporal approach for acoustic neuroma surgery is only applicable for tumors that remain intracanalicular.

Tumors that extend just beyond the porus acousticus into the cerebellopontine angle can sometimes be completely resected with certainty, but tumors greater than 1.5 cm in maximal dimension are not amenable to total tumor removal via middle fossa craniotomy without modifications to this approach.

The great advantage to the middle fossa approach is the ability to visualize the entire internal auditory canal and resect tumors completely with good hope for hearing preservation. The retrosigmoid approach just covered is the only other standard technique for tumor removal in which hearing preservation is possible. However, the retrosigmoid approach does not permit visualization of the lateral third to half of the internal auditory canal if performed in a hearing preservation manner.

The patient is positioned on the operating table supine and rotated with head 180 degrees from Anesthesia. The head is turned and secured with maximal rotation away from the side of tumor, up to 80 to 90 degrees if possible.

Preparation for a middle fossa or subtemporal craniotomy begins with adequate scalp shaving, four fingerbreadths above the root of the helix and four fingerbreadths wide, centered over the external auditory canal. Skin is thoroughly cleansed with alcohol, and mastisol or benzoin adhesive applied. Segmented sheets of 1000 drape or other occlusive draping are placed circumferentially around the temporal skin and ear.

In addition to the montage of facial nerve monitoring electrodes, electrodes for intraoperative ABR must be placed, along with insert earphones in ears bilaterally. The ipsilateral mastoid or lobule electrode and the ipsilateral insert earphone can either be placed preoperatively in a nonsterile fashion with the external auditory canal prepped outside the surgical field or intraoperatively in a sterile fashion with the ear remaining in the sterile surgical field.

Mannitol infusion and hyperventilation are started at the beginning of the case to ensure adequate osmotic diuresis and reduction in intracranial pressure prior to dural elevation and temporal retraction.

The skin incision is planned in a curvilinear fashion over the temporal scalp and extends to the preauricular crease just superior to the tragus. The incision is taken down to the temporalis muscle fascia, taking care to avoid the superficial temporal artery and vein. A wide temporalis muscle fascia graft and a small amount of additional temporalis muscle are harvested for later reconstruction of the middle fossa floor defect. The temporalis muscle is divided below the arc of the superior temporal line, leaving a cuff of muscle and temporalis muscle fascia onto which the muscle flap can be sewn during closure. The temporalis muscle flap is elevated off of the temporal fossa and folded inferiorly over the zygomatic root.

The subtemporal craniotomy is created by fashioning a bone window 4 cm square, centered over or slightly anterior to the external auditory canal, with the inferior side along the inferior temporal line. The craniotomy is created with a 3- or 4-mm cutting bur and final cuts over the dura are finished with a similar-sized diamond bur. The bone flap is gently elevated off of the middle fossa convexity dura, and any residual ledge of squamosal bone inferiorly is removed flush to the middle fossa floor. Mastoid air cells are often encountered inferiorly. These air cells are waxed over to minimize entry of irrigation fluid into the mesotympanum via the mastoid air cells, which can alter ABR waveforms and, in particular, shift wave latencies.

The middle fossa dura is gently elevated off of the middle fossa floor and dissected posteriorly to the petrous ridge and anteriorly to the foramen spinosum and middle meningeal artery.

Dural dissection is carried in a posterior to anterior direction to avoid traction injury on the greater superficial petrosal nerve medially. The greater superficial petrosal nerve can often be identified using the facial nerve monitor by direct electrical stimulation on the nerve and antidromic conduction to the geniculate ganglion. Brisk bleeding is often encountered along the anterior most extent of dural dissection, although this can be confidently controlled with firm application of surgicel packing along the dural-bone interface.

Dura is elevated medially to the arcuate eminence, which typically delineates the superior most elevation of bone along the middle fossa floor. As the dura is elevated further medially, the bony contour of the middle fossa floor takes a shallow dive and plateaus onto a flat medial plane of bone, the meatal plane.

The general position of the internal auditory canal is estimated prior to drilling of the middle fossa floor. There are minimal landmarks present on the somewhat nondescript middle fossa floor. As a result, many authors have suggested many techniques of providing a general estimation of the internal auditory canal's location.

In the most straightforward sense, the position and orientation of the internal auditory canal roughly approximates the axis of the external auditory canal extended medially. This axis can be further refined by removing the lateral middle fossa floor or tegmen tympani, exposing the epitympanic space and ossicles which lie directly between the external auditory canal and internal auditory canal. If this technique is performed, irrigation fluid may enter the mesotympanic space, causing a conductive hearing loss intraoperatively and altering ABR responses. In addition, the surgeon must remember to reconstruct the tegmen tympani prior to closure or encephalocele and postoperative conductive hearing loss may result.

The axis of the internal auditory canal can be best estimated by bisecting the angle subtended by the long axis of the arcuate eminence and the long axis of the greater superficial petrosal nerve and extending this line onto the meatal plane.[30,31] This result gives the most consistent localization of the internal auditory canal than any other method but requires positive identification of both the greater superficial petrosal nerve and the arcuate eminence.

If the greater superficial petrosal nerve cannot be reliably identified, the axis of the internal auditory canal can be approximated by subtending a 60-degree angle anterior to the arcuate eminence alone.[31,32] The angle subtended by the axes of the greater superficial petrosal nerve and arcuate eminence is typically roughly 120 degrees, although the symmetry between subtended angles is actually more consistent than is the accuracy of the subtended angle being close to 60 degrees.[32,33]

If the greater superficial petrosal nerve is identified, it can be followed in a retrograde fashion to the geniculate ganglion, uncovering the meatal foramen from which the labyrinthine segment of the facial nerve can be followed medially to the fundus of the internal auditory canal.[33,34] The internal auditory canal can be skeletonized medially to the petrous ridge. This approach is one of the more technically challenging approaches in that the facial nerve must be decompressed along its entire course medial to the mesotympanum. However, if done properly and safely, this medial facial nerve decompression can lower the rate of delayed postoperative facial paresis or paralysis, as discussed in the section on translabyrinthine approaches.

Morphometric analyses of the middle fossa floor can sometimes aid in establishing the location of the internal auditory canal. The medial most portion of the vestibule is always 28 mm or less from inner table of the temporal squamosa when measured along the transverse bitemporal line.[34,35] However, this rule is often ineffective, as the petrous ridge often falls within 28 mm of the inner table of the temporal squamosa. The internal auditory canal lumen can be estimated to be approximately 10 mm anteriomedial to the apex of the superior semicircular canal in a direction parallel to the petrous ridge and superior petrosal sinus.[35] The location of the geniculate and cochlea can be estimated by locating the apex of the superior semicircular canal and measuring 5 mm anterolaterally perpendicular to the axis of the greater superficial petrosal nerve and 10 mm anteromedially parallel to the axis of the greater superficial petrosal nerve.[36]

In the last two cases, a distinction must be made between the arcuate eminence and the superior semicircular canal: the former, while roughly denoting the location of the superior semicircular canal, can be shifted several millimeters or rotated several degrees from the latter and therefore must be taken down completely in order to confidently blue line the apex of the superior semicircular canal. Failure to do so renders the above measurements ineffective.

Finally, the surgeon can simply choose the most medial face of the meatal plane and begin drilling. As the outline of the internal auditory canal is developed, drilling is directed posterior and anterior to the axis of the internal auditory canal, remaining medial. As the contour of the internal auditory canal is developed medially, dissection can be extended slowly laterally, taking into consideration the relative locations of the vestibule posteriorly and cochlea anteriorly, utilizing some of the techniques above.

The contour of the internal auditory canal should be developed as circumferentially as possible.

Medially, up to 270 degrees of dissection may be possible, with excellent delineation of the porus dura. Laterally, circumferential dissection is limited by the cochlea anteriorly and vestibule posteriorly, obviously neither of which should be violated. With good dural and brain retraction, it is possible to dissect the superior face of the bone and fully uncover the fundus from this approach.

The eggshell-thin bone overlying the internal auditory canal is gently elevated, and the internal auditory canal dura incised from porus to fundus, along the posterior superior aspect to minimize risk to the facial nerve. The intracanalicular facial nerve is identified and electrically stimulated to confirm functional integrity. Tumor dissection should be carried from a medial to lateral direction if possible, to minimize traction of the cochlear nerve. In addition, papaverine soaked pledgets may be used to minimize vasospasm of the intracanalicular microvasculature. The intracanalicular tumor is then dissected off of surrounding nerve and resected.

Reconstruction begins with the middle fossa floor defect. Petrous apex air cells, both anterior and posterior, should be thoroughly waxed to avoid CSF leak through the mesotympanum. A muscle plug is placed in the bony defect of the internal auditory canal. If the tegmen tympani has been removed or the arcuate eminence taken down and mastoid air cells opened, these defects must be repaired with a bone graft or bone cement to prevent encephalocele and CSF leak. The temporalis muscle fascia graft is applied to cover the dissected middle fossa floor, and the retracted temporal lobe and dura slowly released onto the reconstructed floor.

Any remaining lateral mastoid air cells should be waxed over. If there has been injury to the convexity dura, this should be appropriately repaired as well. The temporal squamosal bone flap is replaced, and the temporalis muscle flap reapproximated and closed along the superior temporal line. The skin is closed in layers to provide a secure, watertight seal.

The wound is cleansed and dressed with a mastoid pressure dressing. As with the previous approaches, the dressing is changed once on postoperative day three and kept in place for a total of one week. The wound is checked daily for any sign of CSF otorrhea, CSF wound leak, or CSF fluid collection.

The greatest advantage to the middle fossa approach is the ability to provide a hearing conservation approach and fully visualize the entire internal auditory canal. However, this approach, without modification, does not provide adequate posterior fossa exposure and hence is not appropriate for tumors extending more than 3 to 5 mm beyond the porus acousticus (Figure 4–22).

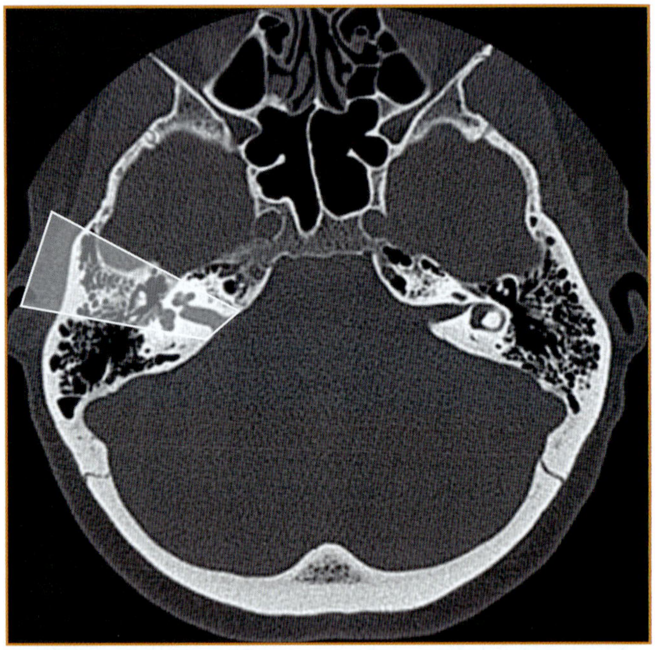

A

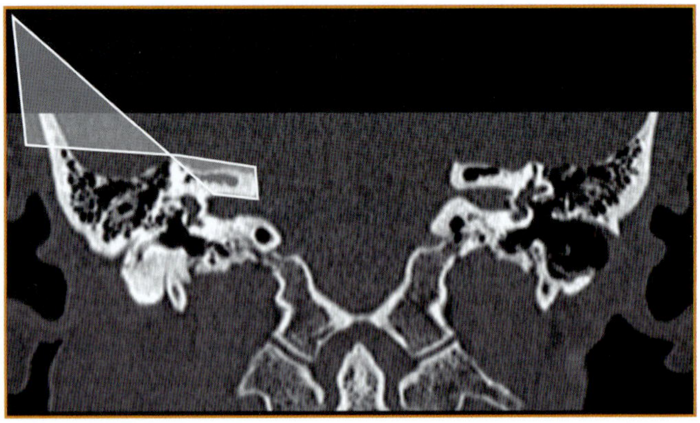

B

Figure 4–22. Middle fossa craniotomy for access to the internal auditory canal and cerebellopontine angle, axial (**A**) and coronal (**B**) schematic.

As the approach to the internal auditory canal is completely extradural, drilling of the middle fossa floor does not introduce bone dust into the intracranial space, potentially limiting the amount of dural irritation and chronic headaches that may plague the retrosigmoid approach. Retraction of the temporal lobe introduces the risk of aphasia, dependent on the side of tumor and the patient's handedness, not present in the other approaches. Patients of advanced age may be at higher risk of CSF leak because of greater attenuation of their dura; conversely, age-related cortical volume loss can allow for easier compression middle fossa contents and less aggressive dural retraction.

Nonstandard Approaches

Beyond the three standard approaches to the cerebellopontine angle and internal auditory canal described above, modifications to these approaches exist, each of which has its own advantages and disadvantages. The modified translabyrinthine exposure compromises lateral internal auditory canal exposure for an attempt at hearing preservation. The extended middle fossa approach expands the utility of the subtemporal approach to the internal auditory canal to include access to the posterior fossa, but with added risk of extended dural elevation and sinus division (Figure 4–23).

Staged Resection

Staged resection should be considered for management of extremely large tumors in patients who are appropriate surgical candidates. Although staged resection protocols expose the patient to the risks of repeat craniotomy and general anesthesia, the rate of long-term facial nerve function appears to be

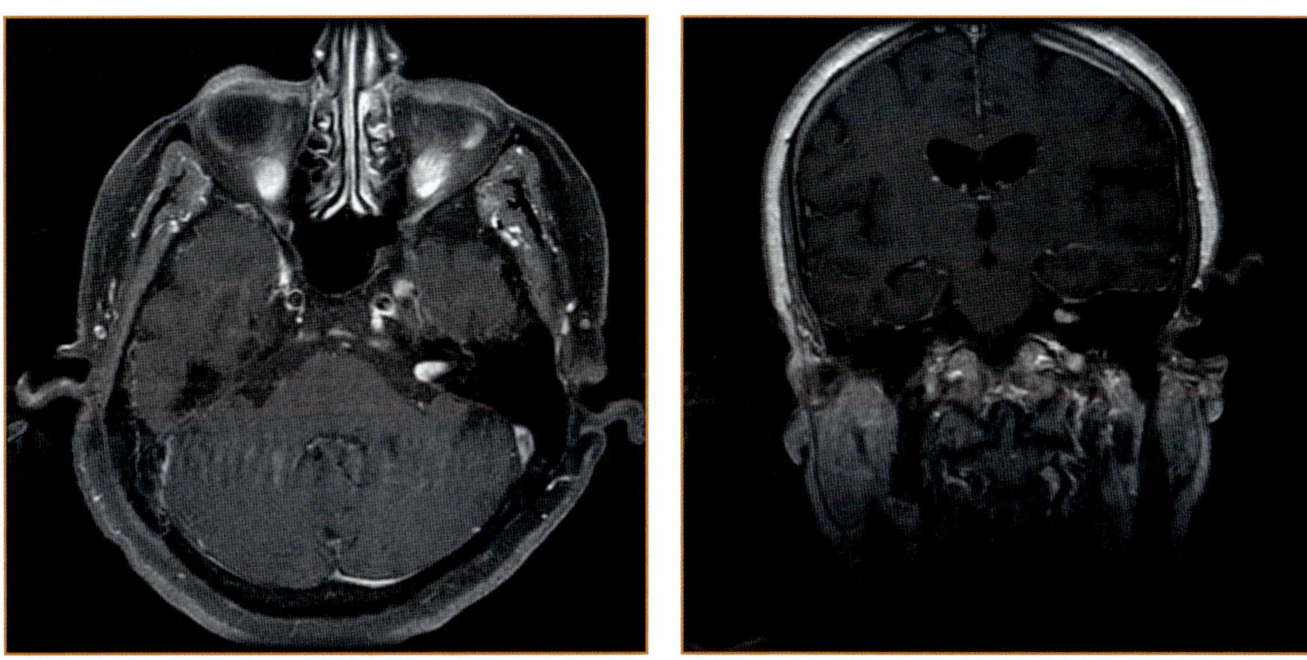

A B

Figure 4–23. Small acoustic neuroma, left. MRI, T1 weighted with gadolinium contrast, axial **(A)** and coronal **(B)**. This tumor can be fully accessed via a standard middle fossa approach. If the small cisternal component is not directly visible via this approach, the approach can be extended by dividing the superior petrosal sinus and tentorium cerebelli to improve access to the cerebellopontine cistern and posterior fossa.

significantly improved compared to that obtained from single stage resection. Long-term facial nerve preservation rates, either House Brackmann grade I or II, following single staged resection of acoustic neuromas >3 cm range from 30 to 60%, whereas two or even three staged resection protocols yield a long-term HBG I or II rate of 94% in a study of 34 patients undergoing planned multiple staged resection.[37]

Staged resection can be performed either through the same craniotomy, that is, translabyrinthine-translabyrinthine, or more commonly through different craniotomies, that is, retrosigmoid-translabryinthine. The utilization of different craniotomies takes full advantage of each approach's strengths. Initial resection via retrosigmoid approach provides the greatest visualization of the prepontine cistern and posterior fossa, most helpful for extremely large tumors. The cerebellopontine angle component of tumor is fully debulked and decompressed off of the brainstem. The initial resection stage forgoes drillout of the internal auditory canal, minimizing the risk of meningeal irritation from subarachnoid bone dust and long-term headaches as well as preserving the bony dissection plane of the internal auditory canal for the later stage. The staged resection via translabyrinthine craniotomy passes through intact transmastoid and translabyrinthine dissection planes and allows for best visualization of the facial nerve within the internal auditory canal (Figure 4–24).

The staged resection is typically timed 4 to 6 months following initial tumor resection. This latency period allows for sufficient patient recovery from the initial craniotomy and allows for relaxation and often reconstitution of the previously attenuated facial nerve fibers, a result commonly seen on subsequent stages.

Endoscopic Craniotomy

Endoscopic resection of acoustic neuromas and other cerebellopontine angle lesions via a minimally invasive posterior fossa "keyhole" craniotomy has been described. This method attempts to minimize the morbidity of the larger retrosigmoid craniotomy. The miniaturized craniotomy does not allow for direct microscopic visualization of the posterior fossa, therefore endoscopes are necessary to attain adequate imaging of neurovascular structures. This approach is not routinely performed for tumor resection, as impaired access can compromise patient safety in the setting of significant or uncontrolled bleeding during tumor removal. However, endoscopic posterior fossa craniotomy is suitable for cases involving minimal or no tissue resection, such as trigeminal neurovascular decompression procedures. More detail can be found on this approach in Chapter 3 (Table 4–5).

INTRAOPERATIVE NEURAL MONITORING

In all cases of surgical resection within the cerebellopontine angle and internal auditory canal, intraoperative neural monitoring of the facial nerve is performed and takes advantage of active monitoring techniques. That is, rather than simply passive monitoring of electromyographic activity, the surgeon can employ electrified dissection instruments to map out the course of the facial nerve simultaneously during tumor dissection. Active monitoring aids in intraoperative tumor dissection and also can be used for prognostic value. Postdissection facial compound muscle action potentials at or greater than 240 µV evoked with minimal stimulus intensity at or less than 0.05 mA near the root entry zone generally suggest excellent long term postoperative facial function of House-Brackmann Grade I or II.[38]

Intraoperative neural monitoring is technically possible for all cranial nerves and warranted in extremely large cerebellopontine angle tumors. This is further described in Chapter 11.

COMPLICATIONS

Complications following stereotactic radiotherapy for acoustic neuroma occur at generally low rates and tend to occur in a delayed fashion several months following treatment. Earlier Gamma Knife treatment protocols using the higher prescribed peripheral isodose of 16 gray demonstrated unacceptably high rates of facial paralysis and trigeminal neuralgia, each approximately 25%. At currently

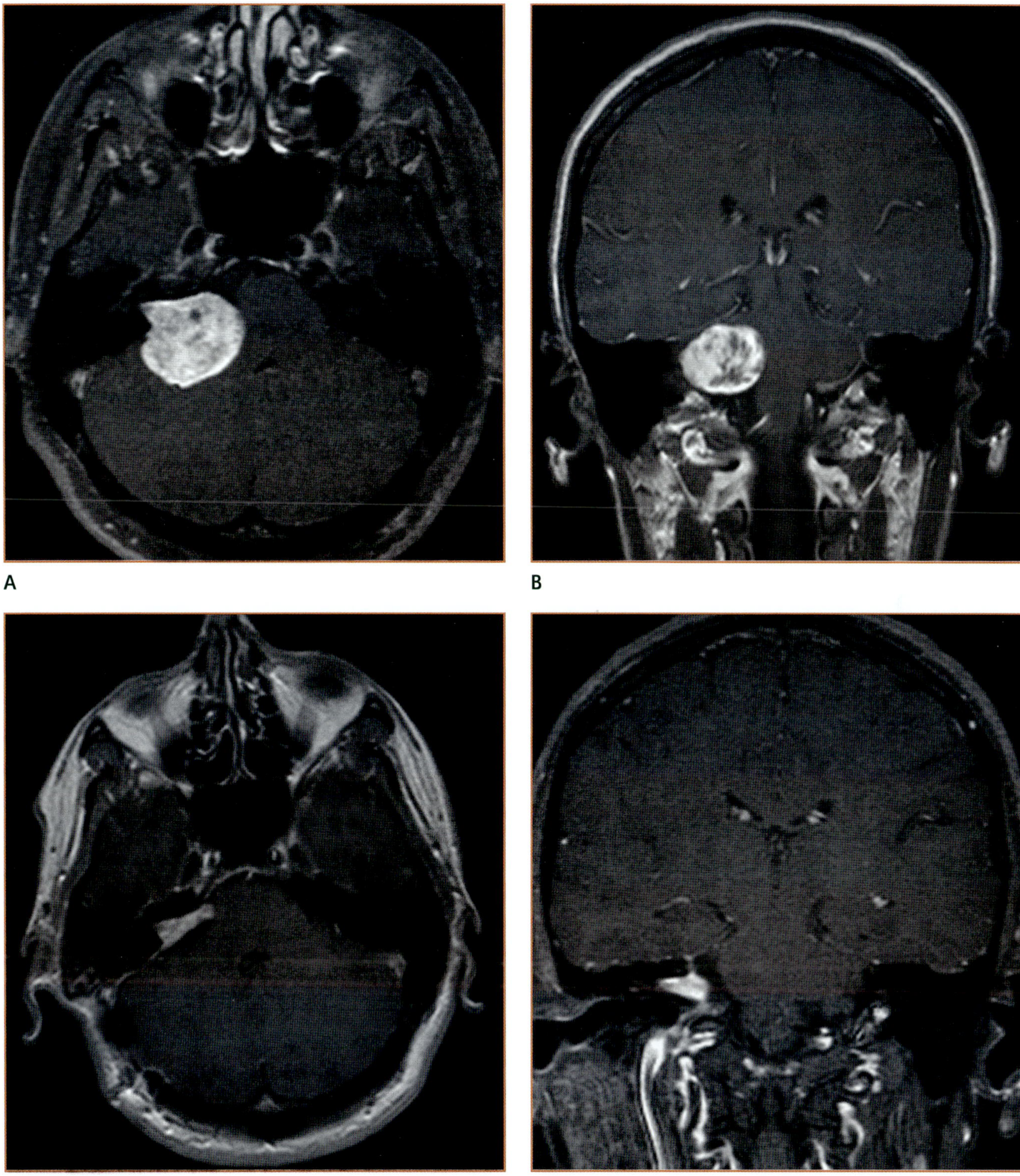

Figure 4–24. Staged resection of large acoustic neuroma, right. MRI, T1 weighted with gadolinium contrast, axial before 1st stage (**A**), coronal before 1st stage (**B**), axial before 2nd stage (**C**), coronal before 2nd stage (**D**). The patient underwent staged resection of a large acoustic neuroma with brainstem and cerebellar compression and internal auditory canal widening (**A** and **B**). Following the 1st stage retrosigmoid approach, the patient had complete clearance of all cerebellopontine angle component and had only residual in the internal auditory canal (**C** and **D**). Following 2nd stage translabyrinthine approach, she had complete resection of tumor and intact and symmetric facial nerve function postoperatively.

Table 4–5. Surgical Approaches for Acoustic Neuroma

Approach	Advantages	Disadvantages
Translabyrinthine	- closer to tumor - entire course of the facial nerve accessible - meatal foramen decompression - minimal brain retraction - direct view of brainstem - almost any size tumor - familiar transmastoid anatomy	- anacusis - fat graft reconstruction - inferior cisternal access limited if there is high-riding jugular bulb
Retrosigmoid	- best exposure of the posterior fossa - any size tumor - fast exposure - chance for hearing preservation - no separate graft needed	- greater cerebellar retraction - fundus of IAC not in direct view - tangential view of brainstem - deeper hole, farther from tumor - postoperative headache
Middle Fossa	- chance for hearing preservation - only approach that exposes entire IAC without violating otic capsule - no separate graft site needed	- intracanalicular tumors only - temporal lobe retraction - facial nerve is superior and at risk with dissection of inferior tumors

prescribed peripheral isodoses of 12 to 13 gray at the 50% isodose line, the rate of long-term facial dysfunction is 1% and that of long term trigeminal neuralgia is 3%. Post-treatment hydrocephalus has been reported in up to 2% of Gamma Knife patients.

In contrast, postoperative complications tend to occur immediately following surgery. The most common postoperative complications are CSF leak (10%), permanent facial nerve injury (2 to 4%), meningitis (1%), other cranial nerve deficits (1%), and postoperative hydrocephalus (0.3%). These results, however, are biased against microsurgery, as they include patients with all sizes of tumor, including those tumors greater than 3 cm for which stereotactic radiotherapy is contraindicated, and for which all postoperative complications have greater risk due to increased tumor size and extent of dissection.

Postoperative headache is common, and long-term complaints of daily headache can continue in up to 30% of patients following surgery, in patients who underwent retrosigmoid approaches more frequently than those undergoing other approaches.

Though not technically a complication, post-treatment hearing loss rates between radiotherapeutic and surgical options are often compared. Hearing preservation approaches are only attempted for patients with preoperative serviceable hearing, that is, AAO-HNS class A or B hearing with greater than 50% speech discrimination scores and greater than 50 dB HL pure-tone thresholds averaged between 512 Hz and 3 kHz. In these patients, success of postoperative hearing preservation is directly correlated to size of tumor. Generally, tumors larger than 2 cm in diameter have a low likelihood of long-term serviceable hearing preservation regardless of treatment modality. Long-term preservation of serviceable hearing following resection of large tumors varies from 6 to 17%.[38–40]

Surgically resected tumors that are smaller than 2 cm generally have a better chance for long-term hearing preservation, while some studies for intracanalicular tumors show slightly better rates, up to 50% but not typically higher.[12,14,39,40]

A comparative analysis comparing all microsurgical and Gamma Knife series reported in the 1990s showed equivalence in overall hearing preservation rates between patients treated with microsurgery and those treated with Gamma Knife: of patients with pretreatment serviceable hearing, 44% in each group maintained serviceable hearing post-treatment.[41]

More devastating, but exceedingly rare, are pontomedullary complications which may develop following surgical resection of acoustic neuromas. Injury to adjacent vascular structures, such as the posterior inferior cerebellar artery (PICA) and anterior inferior cerebellar artery (AICA) can cause catastrophic postoperative complications. Vascular injury to PICA causes corresponding neural infarction leading to lateral medullary syndrome or Wallenberg syndrome, characterized by gait ataxia, vertigo, ipsilateral vagal and glossopharyngeal dysfunction causing vocal cord paralysis and dysphagia, ipsilateral Horner's sign, ipsilateral loss of pain and temperature sensation from the face, and contralateral loss of pain and temperature sensation from the body. AICA vascular injuries cause lateral pontine infarction and AICA syndrome, characterized by ipsilateral facial paralysis, ipsilateral SNHL and vestibular weakness, in addition to variable features of Wallenberg syndrome deficits.

OUTCOMES

Prior to microsurgical techniques, the primary outcome measurement in treatment of acoustic neuroma was survival rather than tumor control. Surgical resection resulted in mortality rates of 40%. With the advent of modern microsurgical techniques and instrumentation, coupled with the modern trend toward earlier diagnosis and greater percentage of small and medium-sized tumors rather than large and hydrocephalic tumors, mortality rates for acoustic neuroma surgery now are 1% or less.

In the modern era, outcome measurements following microsurgery have focused on tumor control rates, long-term facial nerve function, and preservation of serviceable hearing, when applicable. With the emergence of a nonsurgical option for primary treatment of acoustic neuroma, the arena of discussion now centers on comparison of tumor control rates between microsurgical and radiotherapeutic alternatives.

Radiotherapy as primary treatment for acoustic neuroma has several advantages. The inherently lower risk of a noninvasive treatment modality makes this option particularly well suited for older patients or the medically infirm, for whom a craniotomy and intracranial tumor dissection, possibly along the brainstem and multiple neurovascular structures, poses significant risk of morbidity and mortality.

Published tumor control rates for Gamma Knife and LINAC based systems are comparable to those of microsurgery. However, a central and critical argument to published tumor controls rates following radiotherapy is the definition of tumor control itself. In many published series of primary radiotherapy for acoustic neuroma, tumor control is defined as either minimal growth over follow up period or "resection-free" control rate.[25,42] These metrics of tumor control favorably bias outcomes from radiotherapeutic management: as the majority of acoustic neuromas grow at rates of 1 to 2 mm per year, treated tumors may continue to grow as part of the natural history of the tumor, irrespective of radiation treatment, and still be considered tumor control. Even in comparison of hearing preservation and complication rates, comparison between the microsurgical and radiotherapy literature is difficult because of variable criteria used for measuring hearing preservation.

To our best understanding, it appears that rates of major post-treatment complications: namely, facial nerve paralysis and loss of serviceable hearing in attempted hearing preservation techniques, are comparable between microsurgical and radiotherapy treatment regimes.

Patients electing radiotherapy gain the advantage of lower immediate post-treatment complication rates at the expense of possible latent complications and possible continued slow tumor growth. Patients electing microsurgical resection inherit greater perioperative and immediate postoperative risks with the benefit of lower rates of latent complication and clearer postoperative prognosis on tumor control, especially when total or near total resection is performed. Further comparison in tumor control rates is not realistically possible until uniform reporting measures for tumor control are instituted between the microsurgical and radiotherapy communities (Table 4–6).

Table 4–6. Treatment Outcomes

Measure	Microsurgery	Stereotactic Radiotherapy
Tumor Control	90–95%	"90–98%"[†]
Facial Nerve Paralysis	2–4%	1–2%
Hearing Preservation	40–50% for tumors <2 cm	40–70%
CSF Leak	10%	N/A
Meningitis	1%	N/A
Trigeminal Neuralgia	N/A	3%
Post Treatment hydrocephalus	<1%	2%
Based on:	all tumor sizes	tumors <3 cm

[†]Definition of tumor control varies by study, and can include "minimal growth" and "resection-free control," among others.

SUMMARY

Acoustic neuromas are the most common intracranial tumor encountered and treated by the neurotologist. A rich historical legacy and graduated improvements in understanding of tumor biology, natural history, diagnostic evaluation, and treatment options has resulted in exceptionally high tumor control and marked reductions in perioperative morbidity and mortality.

Many acoustic neuromas do not need to be treated, but criteria exist for which intervention is warranted: large size or brainstem compressive nature, radiographically demonstrated tumor growth, or uncontrolled or unmanageable symptoms such as disabling vertigo or disequilibrium.

Many options for acoustic neuroma management are available. A comprehensive understanding of the strengths and deficiencies of each therapeutic option, as well as an appreciation for the limitations in the current literature comparing outcomes from each of these treatment modalities, can ensure thorough patient education and a team approach to identification of the most appropriate treatment plan for each individual.

REFERENCES

1. Neely JG. Hearing conservation surgery for acoustic tumors—a clinical-pathologic correlative study. *Am J Otol.* 1985;suppl:143–146.
2. Rouleau GA, Merel P, Lutchman M, et al. Alteration in a new gene encoding a putative membrane-organizing protein causes neuro-fibromatosis type 2. *Nature.* 1993; 363(6429):515–521.
3. Trofatter JA, MacCollin MM, Rutter JL, et al. A novel moesin-, ezrin-, radixin-like gene is a candidate for the neurofibromatosis 2 tumor suppressor. *Cell.* 1993;72(5):791–800.
4. Welling DB, Packer MD, Chang LS. Molecular studies of vestibular schwannomas: a review. *Curr Opin Otolaryngol Head Neck Surg.* 2007;15(5):341–346.
5. Al Sanosi A, Fagan PA, Biggs ND. Conservative management of acoustic neuroma. *Skull Base.* 2006;16(2):95–100.
6. Wiet RJ, Zappia JJ, Hecht CS, O'Connor CA. Conservative management of patients with small acoustic tumors. *Laryngoscope.* 1995;105(8 pt 1):795–800.
7. Charabi S, Tos M, Thomsen J, Charabi B, Mantoni M. Vestibular schwannoma growth--long-term results. *Acta Otolaryngol Suppl.* 2000;543:7–10.
8. Smouha EE, Yoo M, Mohr K, Davis RP. Conservative management of acoustic neuroma: a meta-analysis and proposed treatment algorithm. *Laryngoscope.* 2005;115(3): 450–454.
9. Nedzelski JM, Canter RJ, Kassel EE, Rowed DW, Tator CH. Is no treatment good treatment in the management of acoustic neuromas in the elderly? *Laryngoscope.* 1986; 96(8):825–829.
10. Strasnick B, Glasscock ME, 3rd, Haynes D, McMenomey SO, Minor LB. The natural history of untreated acoustic neuromas. *Laryngoscope.* 1994;104(9):1115–1119.
11. Komatsuzaki A, Tsunoda A. Nerve origin of the acoustic neuroma. *J Laryngol Otol.* 2001;115(5):376–379.
12. Jacob A, Robinson LL Jr., Bortman JS, Yu L, Dodson EE, Welling DB. Nerve of origin, tumor size, hearing preservation, and facial nerve outcomes in 359 vestibular schwannoma resections at a tertiary care academic center. *Laryngoscope.* 2007;117(12):2087–2092.
13. Khrais T, Romano G, Sanna M. Nerve origin of vestibular schwannoma: a prospective study. *J Laryngol Otol.* 2008; 122(2):128–131.
14. Doyle KJ, Shelton C. Hearing preservation in bilateral acoustic neuroma surgery. *Am J Otol.* 1993;14(6):562–565.
15. Miranda TT, Pichora-Fuller MK. Temporally jittered speech produces performance intensity, phonetically balanced rollover in young normal-hearing listeners. *J Am Acad Audiol.* 2002;13(1):50–58.
16. Shirinian MJ, Arnst DJ. PI-PB rollover in a group of aged listeners. *Ear Hear.* 1980;1(1):50–53.
17. Zappia JJ, O'Connor CA, Wiet RJ, Dinces EA. Rethinking the use of auditory brainstem response in acoustic neuroma screening. *Laryngoscope.* 1997;107(10):1388–1392.

18. Bozorg Grayeli A, Refass A, Smail M, et al. Diagnostic value of auditory brainstem responses in cerebellopontine angle tumours. *Acta Otolaryngol.* 2008;128(10):1096–1100.
19. Cueva RA. Auditory brainstem response versus magnetic resonance imaging for the evaluation of asymmetric sensorineural hearing loss. *Laryngoscope.* 2004;114(10): 1686–1692.
20. Don M, Kwong B, Tanaka C, Brackmann D, Nelson R. The stacked ABR: a sensitive and specific screening tool for detecting small acoustic tumors. *Audiol Neurotol.* 2005; 10(5):274–290.
21. Kartush JM, Niparko JK, Graham MD, Kemink JL. Electroneurography: preoperative facial nerve assessment for tumors of the temporal bone. *Otolaryngol Head Neck Surg.* 1987;97(3):257–261.
22. Syms CA, 3rd, House JR, 3rd, Luxford WM, Brackmann DE. Preoperative electroneuronography and facial nerve outcome in acoustic neuroma surgery. *Am J Otol.* 1997; 18(3):401–403.
23. Shelton C, Harnsberger HR, Allen R, King B. Fast spin echo magnetic resonance imaging: clinical application in screening for acoustic neuroma. *Otolaryngol Head Neck Surg.* 1996;114(1):71–76.
24. Kondziolka D, Lunsford LD, McLaughlin MR, Flickinger JC. Long-term outcomes after radiosurgery for acoustic neuromas. *N Engl J Med.* 1998;339(20):1426–1433.
25. Flickinger JC, Kondziolka D, Niranjan A, Lunsford LD. Results of acoustic neuroma radiosurgery: an analysis of 5 years' experience using current methods. *J Neurosurg.* 2001;94(1):1–6.
26. Committee on Hearing and Equilibrium guidelines for the evaluation of hearing preservation in acoustic neuroma (vestibular schwannoma). American Academy of Otolaryngology-Head and Neck Surgery Foundation, Inc. *Otolaryngol Head Neck Surg.* 1995;113(3):179–180.
27. Sargent EW, Kartush JM, Graham MD. Meatal facial nerve decompression in acoustic neuroma resection. *Am J Otol.* 1995;16(4):457–464.
28. Bloch DC, Oghalai JS, Jackler RK, Osofsky M, Pitts LH. The fate of the tumor remnant after less-than-complete acoustic neuroma resection. *Otolaryngol Head Neck Surg.* 2004;130(1):104–112.
29. Smith MF, Lagger RL. Hearing conservation in acoustic neurilemmoma surgery via the retrosigmoid approach. *Otolaryngol Head Neck Surg.* 1984;92(2):168–175.
30. Ryzenman JM, Pensak ML, Tew JM Jr. Headache: a quality of life analysis in a cohort of 1,657 patients undergoing acoustic neuroma surgery, results from the acoustic neuroma association. *Laryngoscope.* 2005;115(4):703–711.
31. Garcia-Ibanez E, Garcia-Ibanez JL. Middle fossa vestibular neurectomy: a report of 373 cases. *Otolaryngol Head Neck Surg.* 1980;88(4):486–490.
32. Fisch U, Mattox D. *Microsurgery of the Skull Base.* Stuttgart; New York: Thieme; 1988.
33. Maina R, Ducati A, Lanzino G. The middle cranial fossa: morphometric study and surgical considerations. *Skull Base.* 2007;17(6):395–403.
34. House WF, Gardner G, Hughes RL. Middle cranial fossa approach to acoustic tumor surgery. *Arch Otolaryngol.* 1968;88(6):631–641.
35. Cohadon F, Castel JP. [Angles of incidence in some anatomical studies of the routes of surgical approach to the internal auditory canal]. *Rev Laryngol Otol Rhinol (Bord).* 1968;89(11):643–658.
36. Kartush JM, Kemink JL, Graham MD. The arcuate eminence. Topographic orientation in middle cranial fossa surgery. *Ann Otol Rhinol Laryngol.* 1985;94(1 pt 1):25–28.
37. Patni AH, Kartush JM. Staged resection of large acoustic neuromas. *Otolaryngol Head Neck Surg.* 2005;132(1):11–19.
38. Neff BA, Ting J, Dickinson SL, Welling DB. Facial nerve monitoring parameters as a predictor of postoperative facial nerve outcomes after vestibular schwannoma resection. *Otol Neurotol.* 2005;26(4):728–732.
39. Lassaletta L, Fontes L, Melcon E, Sarria MJ, Gavilan J. Hearing preservation with the retrosigmoid approach for vestibular schwannoma: myth or reality? *Otolaryngol Head Neck Surg.* 2003;129(4):397–401.
40. Yates PD, Jackler RK, Satar B, Pitts LH, Oghalai JS. Is it worthwhile to attempt hearing preservation in larger acoustic neuromas? *Otol Neurotol.* 2003;24(3):460–464.
41. Kaylie DM, Horgan MJ, Delashaw JB, McMenomey SO. A meta-analysis comparing outcomes of microsurgery and gamma knife radiosurgery. *Laryngoscope.* 2000; 110(11):1850–1856.
42. Chopra R, Kondziolka D, Niranjan A, Lunsford LD, Flickinger JC. Long-term follow-up of acoustic schwannoma radiosurgery with marginal tumor doses of 12 to 13 Gy. *Int J Radiat Oncol Biol Phys.* 2007;68(3):845–851.

CHAPTER 5

Neurofibromatosis Type II and Auditory Brainstem Implant

Rodney C. Diaz and Jeremy D. Meier

INTRODUCTION

Neurofibromatosis type II (NF2) presents unique challenges to the neurotologist. The hallmark and clinically defining feature of NF2 is the presence of bilateral acoustic neuromas or vestibular schwannomas. Many other central tumors may also be present in this disease, limited not only to the intracranial vault but along the spinal axis as well. Limiting disease progression while preserving function remains the top priority. The risks and implications with observation versus treatment for the vestibular schwannoma are magnified in NF2 due to its bilateral presentation and progressive nature of the disease.

PATHOPHYSIOLOGY

Neurofibromatosis type II can be a potentially devastating disease. Fortunately, it is relatively rare, with an estimated birth incidence of 1 in 25,000 to 1 in 50,000.[1,2] NF2 is inherited in an autosomal dominant fashion, although 50% of cases arise from de novo mutations with no prior family history.[3] There is no sex or ethnic predilection for NF2. The mean age of presentation is 25 years, although most patients have had symptoms present for 5 to 7 years prior to formal diagnosis.

Biallelic mutations of the NF2 gene are responsible for the generation of both the sporadic form of acoustic neuromas as well as the familial form of bilateral acoustic neuromas seen in neurofibromatosis type II, from which the gene receives its name[4,5] (Figure 5–1). The NF2 gene, located on the long arm of chromosome 22, 22q12, encodes for the tumor suppressor protein schwannomin, more commonly known as merlin (Table 5–1).

The merlin protein obtains its name from its relative homology to the <u>m</u>oesin, <u>e</u>zrin, and <u>r</u>adix<u>in</u> proteins. It is a 69 kDa protein that, like its namesakes, localizes to the cell membrane and appears to manage cellular proliferation by inhibiting multiple cell signaling pathways controlling extracellular matrix interactions, cytoskeletal organization, actin polymerization, regulation of growth factors, cell cycle proteins, apoptosis cascades, Schwann cell-axonal interaction, and cell-cell adhesion during tissue fusion.[6] Although high levels of merlin protein are found in many tissues during embryonic development, in adult tissues merlin is highly expressed in Schwann cells, neurons, meningeal cells, and lens, explaining the propensity for neoplastic disease in these tissues in NF2.[7] Loss of function of the merlin protein on both alleles allows for tumorogenesis leading to the formation of schwannomas, meningiomas, ependymomas, retinal hamartomas, and posterior subcapsular lenticular opacities commonly found in NF2.

The hallmark of NF2 is the presence of bilateral vestibular schwannomas, but schwannomas of any of the cranial nerves is possible. Approximately 50% of NF2 patients will demonstrate presence of non-vestibular schwannomas. The majority of these originate from the trigeminal nerve (70%) and the oculomotor nerve (15%). Schwannomas originate from the remainder of the cranial nerves IV, VI,

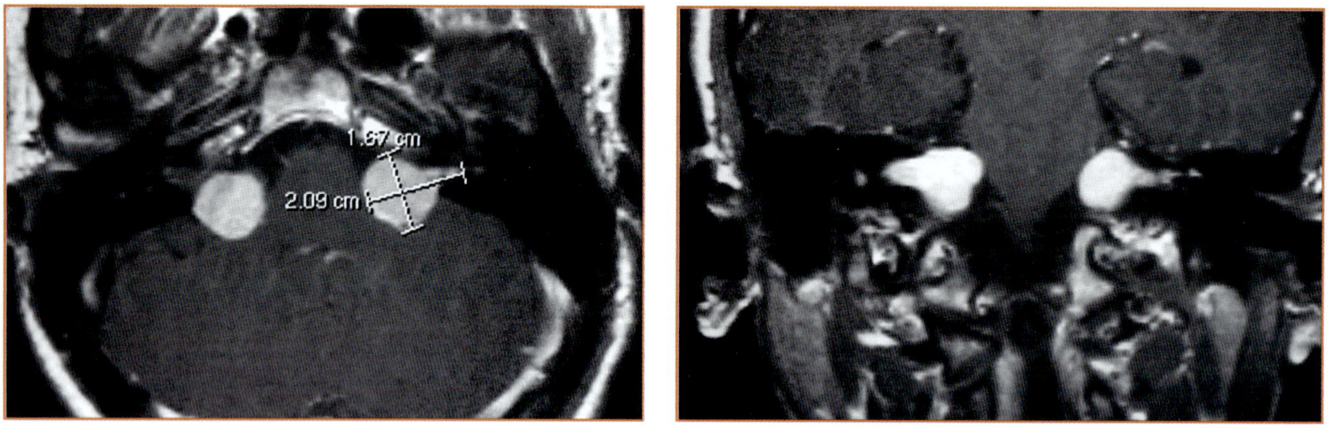

A B

Figure 5–1. Bilateral vestibular schwannomas. MRI, T1 weighted with gadolinium contrast, axial (**A**) and coronal (**B**). This patient was diagnosed with NF2 upon demonstration of bilateral vestibular schwannomas on MRI. The schwannomas are each medium in size and touch but do not significantly compress the brainstem.

Table 5–1. Comparison of Neurofibromatosis Type II and Type I

Criteria	NF Type II	NF Type I
Also known as:	Central Neurofibromatosis	Peripheral Neurofibromatosis
Medical eponym	Wishart-Gardner-Eldridge Syndrome	von Recklinghausen Syndrome
Birth prevalence	1:25,000–1:50,000	1:3000–1:4000
Mean age of diagnosis	25 (symptoms of 5+ years)	childhood
Sex predilection	M = F	M = F
Ethnic predilection	none	none
Chromosome	22q12.2	17q11.2
Gene	NF2	NF1
Gene class	tumor suppressor	tumor suppressor
Gene product	merlin, schwannomin	neurofibromin
Protein function	cytoskeletal	GTPase-activating enzyme
Inheritance	AD by inheritance AR at gene level	AD

IX, X, XI, and XII in approximately 1 to 4 % each in NF2 patients.[8] Schwannomas of the olfactory and optic nerves have not been reported in NF2, although olfactory ensheathing cell tumors have been reported, as have optic nerve meningiomas.[9]

Up to 90% of NF2 patients will have spinal tumors found on full spine MRI.[10] Although many of these spinal tumors are slow growing, up to one-third of these patients will need to have surgical resection of one or more spinal tumors at some point.[10]

Although frequently confused with neurofibromatosis type I (NF1), NF2 was first recognized as a distinct disease in 1981. Neurofibromatosis type I, also known as von Recklinghausen's disease, is also an autosomal dominant disease resulting from mutations located on chromosome 17. The NF1 gene product is involved in modulation of distinctly different signal transduction pathways from those of merlin, thereby confirming on a genetic basis the clinical differentiation between neurofibromatosis type I and neurofibromatosis type II. The NF1 gene encodes a GTPase-activating protein called neurofibromin, which is involved in regulation of the proto-oncogene ras.[11] Loss of functioning neurofibromin leads to increased ras activity and tumorogenesis, especially in neurocutaneous tissues.

Nerve sheath neoplasms are characteristics of both NF1 and NF2 disorders. However, NF1 typically produces neurofibromas and malignant peripheral nerve sheath tumors, whereas NF2 leads to schwannomas. Cutaneous findings such as café au lait spots and subcutaneous neurofibromas are much more common in NF1 than NF2 but can be found in both syndromes. Dermal or subcutaneous nerve sheath tumors in both syndromes are derived, at least partially, from Schwann cells and are clinically and histologically similar. However, NF1 neurocutaneous tumors are neurofibromas, which have a mixed cellular population, whereas NF2 neurocutaneous tumors can be either neurofibromas or schwannomas, which maintain a singular cellular population from the nerve sheath.

CLINICAL PRESENTATION

The Manchester criteria for diagnosis of NF2 describe four possible scenarios for clinical diagnosis. The first, and most common, scenario involves the presence of bilateral vestibular schwannomas. The second scenario involves identification of a first-degree relative with NF2 and the presence of a unilateral vestibular schwannoma or any two of the following lesions: meningioma, schwannoma, glioma, neurofibroma, or posterior subcapsular lenticular opacities. The third scenario involves the presence of a unilateral vestibular schwannoma with any two of the following lesions: meningioma, schwannoma, glioma, neurofibroma, or posterior subcapsular lenticular opacities. Finally, the fourth scenario involves the presence of multiple meningiomas and a unilateral vestibular schwannoma or any two of the following lesions: schwannoma, glioma, neurofibroma, or cataract is the fourth possible clinical criteria[12] (Table 5–2).

Historically, patients with NF2 were identified in large family cohorts, within which the clinical severity of the disease process remained relatively uniform. Some family cohorts were burdened with significant and aggressive disease progression, whereas other groups afflicted with NF2 had family members who maintained relatively good function and low mortality over long periods of time.

Neurofibromatosis type II thus can be divided into two clinical or phenotypic subgroups.[13] The Wishart subtype is the more severe of the two groups,

Table 5–2. Diagnostic Criteria for Neurofibromatosis Type II and Type I

Neurofibromatosis Type II
Bilateral acoustic neuromas
OR
1st degree relative with NF II
Unilateral acoustic neuroma or any two of the following: meningioma, glioma, neurofibroma, schwannoma, presenile cataract
OR
Unilateral acoustic neuroma
Any two of the following: meningioma, glioma, neurofibroma, schwannoma, presenile cataract
OR
Multiple meningiomas
Unilateral acoustic neuroma or any two of the following: meningioma, glioma, neurofibroma, schwannoma, presenile cataract
Neurofibromatosis Type I
TWO OR MORE:
Six or more post-pubertal café-au-lait macules >15 mm
Two or more neurofibromas, any type, or one plexiform neurofibroma
Freckling in axillary or inguinal regions
Optic glioma
Two or more Lisch nodules (iris hamartomas)
Osseous lesion with or without pseudoarthrosis
1st degree relative with NF I by the above criteria

with a typical age of onset in the late teens or early twenties. Patients with this subtype are afflicted with bilateral vestibular schwannomas and multiple intracranial and spinal tumors. The Gardner subtype is the milder of the two groups, with disease typically presenting in older patients and with a significantly decreased incidence of multiple intracranial tumors (Figures 5–2 and 5–3).

A third form of NF2, termed segmental NF2, is sometimes considered and results from somatic

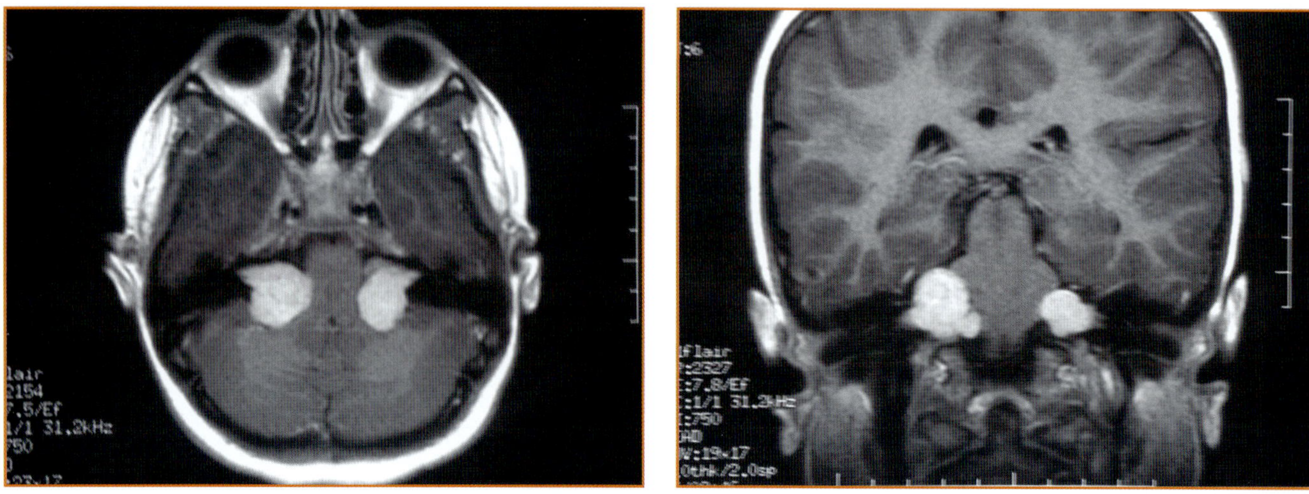

A B

Figure 5–2. Bilateral vestibular schwannomas. MRI, T1 weighted with gadolinium contrast, axial (**A**) and coronal (**B**). This patient was diagnosed with NF2 upon demonstration of bilateral vestibular schwannomas on MRI. The schwannomas are each large in size and cause moderate brainstem compression.

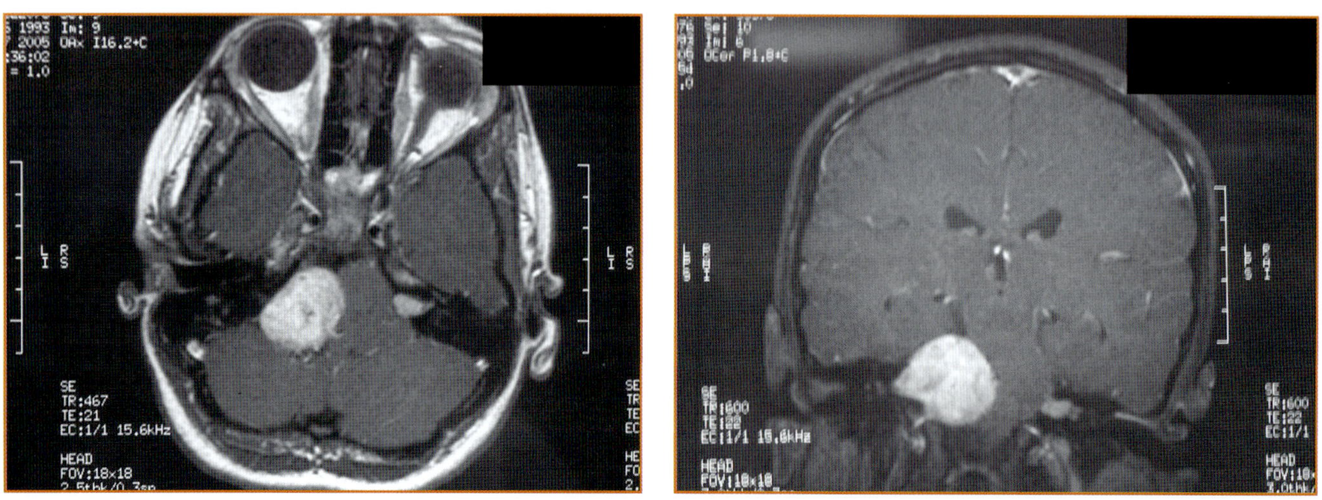

A B

Figure 5–3. Bilateral vestibular schwannomas. MRI, T1 weighted with gadolinium contrast, axial (**A**) and coronal (**B**). This patient was diagnosed with NF2 upon demonstration of bilateral vestibular schwannomas on MRI. The schwannomas are huge on the right and small or intracanalicular on the left, with the right tumor causing significant brainstem and cerebellar compression. This patient and the patient in Figure 5–2 are twin sisters who were both diagnosed with NF2 at the age of 12. Because of their early onset of symptoms and diagnosis as well as large tumor size at initial presentation, they have the Wishart subtype of NF2.

mosaicism, in which the genetic mutation occurs during embryogenesis and thereby affects only a portion of the patient's somatic cells. Bilateral vestibular schwannomas may not be present with this subtype of NF2. Phenotypically, this form closely resembles the clinical progression seen in Gardner subtype NF2 and can be considered part of this, more indolent, group.

The phenotypic distinction between Wishart and Gardner subtypes has been shown to correlate to specific genotypic disturbances. Patients with the Wishart or "severe" variant of NF2 typically have constitutional nonsense or frameshift truncation mutations in the NF2 gene. Patients with the Gardner or "mild" variant of NF2 typically have constitutional missense mutations, splice site mutations, large deletions, or the aforementioned somatic mosaicism (Table 5–3).

EVALUATION

Evaluation for suspected NF2 begins with a thorough history and physical examination, as clinical characteristics often greatly aid in diagnosis and stratification of disease severity. Most patients present in the second to fourth decade of life. However, almost one-fifth present under 15 years of age, typically in the Wishart subtype.[14]

Table 5–3. Categorization of Severity in Neurofibromatosis Type II

Gardner Subtype	Wishart Subtype
"INDOLENT"	"AGGRESSIVE"
later onset of symptoms	early onset of symptoms
smaller tumors	larger tumors
few tumors	many tumors
slower growing tumors	faster growing tumors
hearing loss related to tumor size	hearing loss not related to tumor size
fewer disabilities, stable symptoms	deafness, blindness, paralysis, death by 40
missense mutations splice site mutations large deletions somatic mosaicism	nonsense mutations frameshift mutations

Workup for suspected NF2 patients always includes an audiogram, as hearing loss is the most common symptom. Up to 40% of patients do not present with bilateral vestibular schwannomas and will subsequently develop only unilateral hearing loss.[12] However, unlike sporadic vestibular schwannomas in which asymmetric hearing loss is the rule, unilateral or bilateral sensorineural hearing loss may be found. Poor speech discrimination, consistent with retrocochlear pathology, is frequently present.

Auditory brainstem response (ABR) testing can be performed but is frequently unreliable. Interaural differences cannot be depended on due to the presence of possible bilateral tumors. The utility of ABR has diminished as MRI technology and costs have improved.

Tinnitus, disequilibrium, vertigo, facial paresis, and facial hypesthesia are often present, as would be the case for any tumor of the internal auditory canal or cerebellopontine angle. Schwannomas of the lower cranial nerves are relatively uncommon in NF2, but when they are present, corresponding signs and symptoms of lower cranial nerve dysfunction are common on physical examination.[8,13] Although present in up to 90% of patients, spinal tumors are often asymptomatic.

As with sporadic unilateral vestibular schwannoma, gadolinium-enhanced high-resolution T1-weighted MRI of the internal auditory canal and cerebellopontine angle remains the gold standard imaging modality for diagnosis of NF2 vestibular schwannomas. Heavily T2-weighted fast spin echo imaging can also be performed to exploit the pseudocisternographic imaging characteristics of this modality, but extremely small intracanalicular vestibular schwannomas may be missed. Similarly, constructive interference steady state (CISS) imaging techniques such as 3D-FIESTA, TrueFISP/FFSP, Balanced FFE, PROPELLER, DRIVE, and COSMIC imaging protocols can provide fast acquisition, high resolution, and high tissue/liquid contrast and can aid in adjunctive assessment of the internal auditory canal and cerebellopontine angle (Figure 5–4).

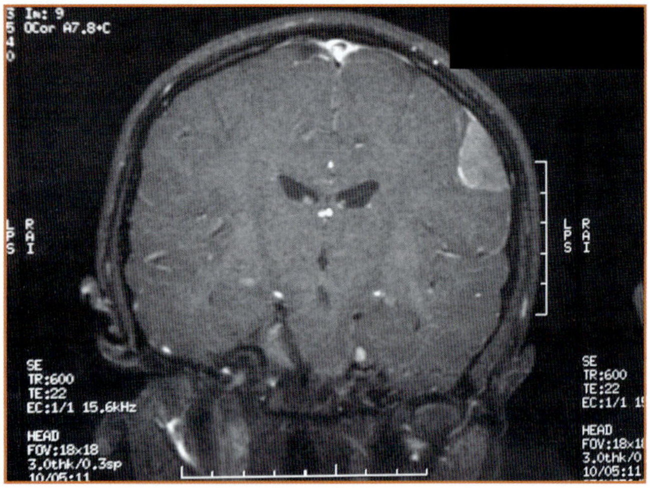

Figure 5–4. Left parietal convexity meningioma. MRI, T1 weighted with gadolinium contrast, coronal. This image is from the same patient as in Figure 5–3.

Imaging of the entire central neural axis, including brain and full length spinal column, with gadolinium-enhanced MRI is warranted, given the previously stated high incidence of primary spinal tumors in NF2. Spinal disease should be monitored in conjunction with serial monitoring of intracranial lesions, although the majority of spinal lesions will not require intervention (Figure 5–5).

With the identification of the NF2 gene, genetic testing is available for possible as well as clinically diagnosed NF2 patients. However, the clinical utility of genetic testing above and beyond clinical diagnosis has not yet been established definitively. The presence of multiple central tumors, and hence the clinical diagnosis, can be readily established with appropriate imaging. For patients with an established diagnosis of NF2, disease severity can often also be established clinically, based on age of presentation, size of tumors, and number of tumors. Patients with an unclear diagnosis of possible mild or segmental NF2, with positive family history and only one tumor, may have a false negative genetic analysis if tested for constitutional mutations, as such patients may have somatic mosaicism. These patients need tumor biopsy for subtype diagnosis at the genetic level.

MANAGEMENT OPTIONS

Options for treatment of NF2 patients are discussed primarily in reference to intracranial and intraspinal lesions. Treatment of lenticular and neurocutaneous lesions should be undertaken as appropriate to the standard of care management for those systems. All NF2 patients should therefore be referred to ophthalmology and dermatology for initial specialist evaluation and appropriately followed and treated by these specialists for such extracranial pathology.

The treatment algorithm for vestibular schwannomas in a patient with NF2 is much more complicated than for a patient with a sporadic unilateral vestibular schwannoma. Bilateral tumors and the expectation that new intracranial tumors will develop throughout the patient's life lead to complex management and decision making in NF2 cases. The timing of intervention and the treatment modality are controversial. Ultimately, there is no cure for NF2. The goals of treatment are: (1) to keep the patient safe from life threatening intracranial and intraspinal tumor expansion, and (2) to delay or prevent the occurrence of cranial neuropathies that arise either as a result of the disease or its treatment.

Therapeutic options for intracranial and intraspinal lesions include observation, stereotactic radiotherapy, or microsurgery.

Observation

A period of watchful waiting at the initial diagnosis or in the early phases of NF2 is sometimes warranted, particularly when intracranial tumors are small or the clinical presentation suggests a mild subtype of disease.

Auditory and facial nerve function following surgical resection of CPA tumors is traditionally worse in NF2 patients than in those with sporadic unilateral vestibular schwannomas. Therefore, many surgeons have recommended postponing resection until the patient's hearing is no longer serviceable. This recommendation can only be made if the existing CPA tumors do not pose a threat to the patient's

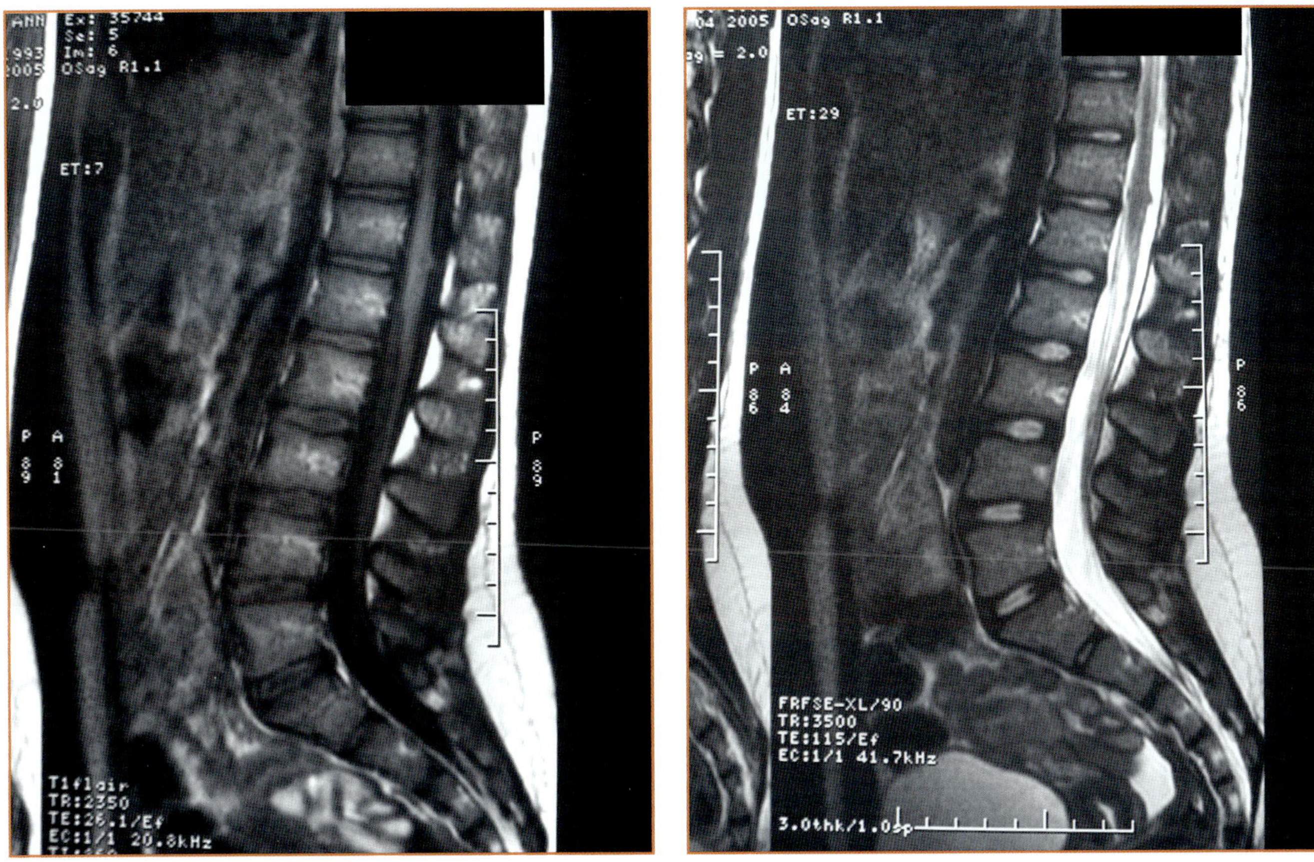

A B

Figure 5–5. Spinal lesions. MRI, proton density (PD) weighted (**A**) and fast spin echo (FSE) T2 weighted (**B**), sagittal. A small spinal lesion is noted on the cord between T12 and L1. These images are from the same patient as in Figure 5–2.

health or life based on tumor size and degree of brain and brainstem compression. In cases where one or more tumors demonstrate significant brainstem compression, and in all cases of hydrocephalic disease, immediate surgical resection, or at minimum staged surgical debulking of tumor, is warranted (Figure 5–6).

Patients with tumors in an only hearing ear or with a low likelihood of hearing preservation, such as bilateral tumors both larger than 2 cm, may be watched closely every 6 to 12 months.[13,15] Once American Academy of Otolaryngology-Head and Neck Surgery (AAO-HNS) class C or D hearing loss occurs and hearing is no longer considered serviceable, the tumor on that side is removed. A decision to delay surgery beyond the time frame when surgical resection is first indicated (based on the audiometric criteria above) may increase the risk of injury to the facial nerve, as risk of postoperative facial nerve weakness is directly correlated to tumor size.

Radiation Therapy

As long-term data accumulate, stereotactic radiotherapy is becoming a more accepted treatment. In patients who are medically infirm or otherwise poor candidates for surgical resection and for patients who do not wish to have surgery, stereotactic radiation is a good option.

Stereotactic radiotherapy can damage hearing and increases facial nerve injury at a later resection.

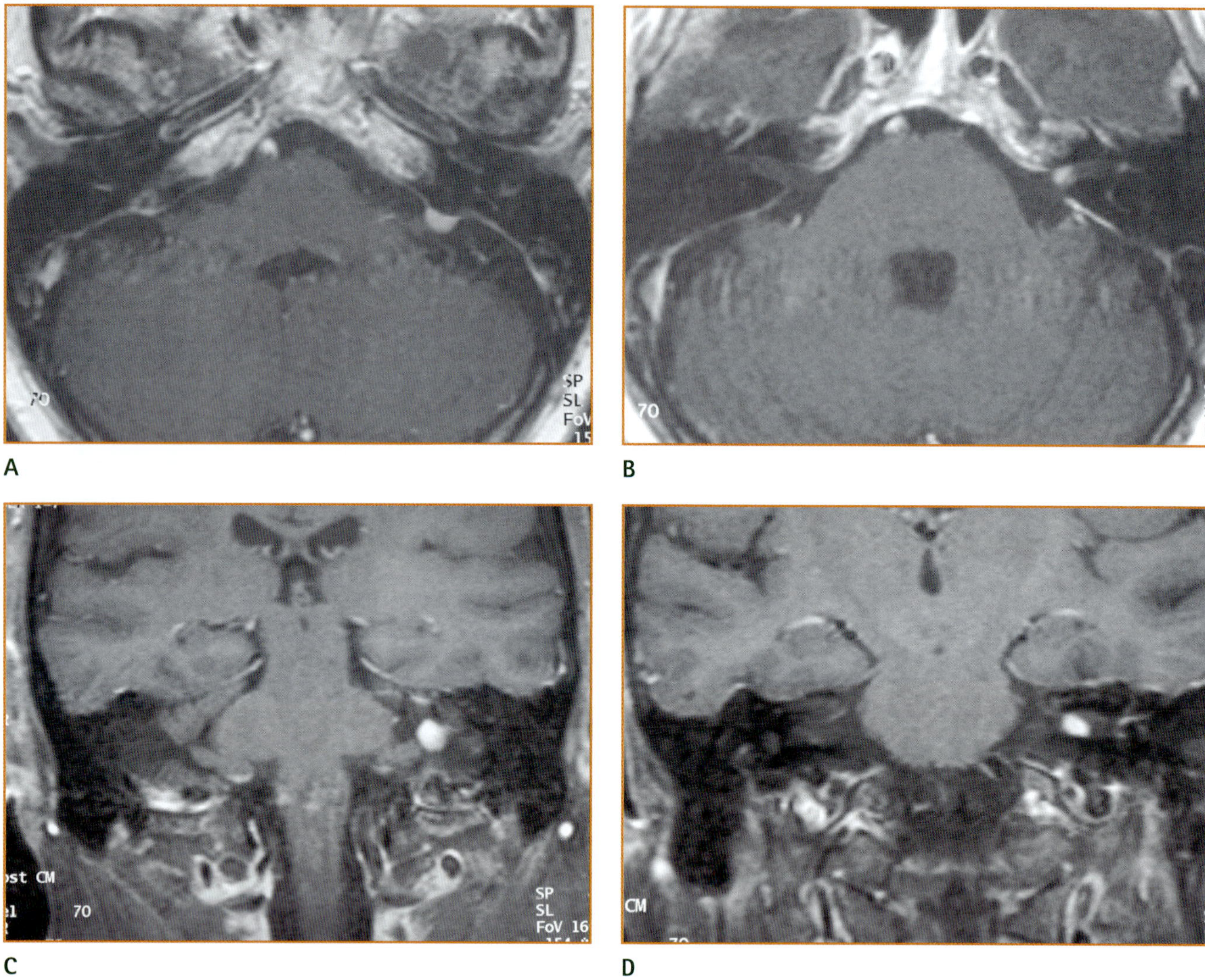

Figure 5–6. Meningioma and vestibular schwannoma on ipsilateral side, left. MRI, T1 weighted with gadolinium contrast, axial **(A)** and **(B)** and coronal **(C)** and **(D)**. This patient demonstrated two separate tumors in the ipsilateral region: a cerebellopontine angle meningioma with characteristic dural tails **(A)** and **(C)**, and an internal auditory canal vestibular schwannoma just medial to the porus acousticus **(B)** and **(D)**. The lesions were resected with preservation of hearing, confirming their independent nature and histologic classifications.

Further studies comparing the long-term results of stereotactic radiation to standard surgical resection in the NF2 population are needed.

Stereotactic radiotherapy for spinal tumors must be performed by linear accelerator based machines, as the Gamma Knife system does not allow for stereotactic treatment lower than the foramen magnum.

Surgery

When hearing loss is significant or the tumor is causing brainstem compression, the decision to operate is more straightforward. However, in other instances, when to proceed with surgery is not as clear. Some authors recommend rigorous screening in at risk individuals with the hope of making an early diagnosis followed by surgical resection.[15] Those who recommend this approach suggest that early surgical resection allows for a greater chance of hearing preservation and facial nerve function.

Measureable hearing can be preserved in approximately 70% of ears in NF2 patients undergoing hearing conservation approaches, whereas approximately 80% of NF2 patients undergoing bilateral hearing conservation approaches maintain some measure of hearing bilaterally after one year.[15,16] Hearing preservation rates are best for tumors ≤1.5cm, with overall preservation of serviceable hearing, that is, AAO-HNS class A or B hearing, in approximately 50% of appropriately chosen cases.[17]

The surgical approach varies depending on the tumor location and the patient's hearing status. The translabyrinthine approach provides the best visualization of the facial nerve but destroys any residual hearing. The retrosigmoid approach can preserve hearing but carries a slightly higher risk of facial nerve injury. The middle fossa approach is the most appropriate approach for attempts at hearing conservation but is limited to tumors smaller that 1 to 1.5 cm in maximal dimension.

Other surgical options include middle fossa decompression to relieve pressure on the auditory nerve or tumor debulking. Both of these options may prevent or prolong hearing loss development, but leave residual tumor behind. Some feel that tumor debulking may actually increase the risk of hearing loss. However, this belief is not shared by all.[18]

HEARING REHABILITATION AND AUDITORY BRAINSTEM IMPLANT

Maintaining the patient's native hearing for as long as possible provides greater benefit than current options of hearing restoration following surgical resection and ablation of hearing. As hearing decreases, hearing aids can provide temporary benefit. Once hearing is lost, rehabilitation includes either cochlear implantation or auditory brainstem implantation.

Cochlear implantation in NF2 patients can be effective so long as the cochlear nerve is preserved at the conclusion of resection.[19] When the cochlear nerve has been preserved, a small series suggests that cochlear implantation provides better communication skills than auditory brainstem implants.[20] This is not often the case, however, and if the cochlear nerve is severed at the time of surgery, auditory brainstem implantation is often performed at that time as well.

In a collaborative effort by the House Ear Institute, Cochlear Corporation, and Huntington Medical Research Institutes, the multichannel auditory brainstem implant (ABI) gained FDA approval in 1993. There are now several ABI implants. The ABI can be implanted during the removal of the first tumor to give the patient exposure to the sound quality of the implant prior to removal of the tumor on the contralateral side. Also, if the first implant is unsuccessful the second side may be implanted.

Although other companies make similar devices, the Cochlear Corporation ABI has 21 platinum disk contacts placed in three rows on a silastic carrier pad. The ABI functions by electrically stimulating the cochlear nuclear complex, which consists of the dorsal and ventral cochlear nuclei. The platinum disk is attached to a receiver stimulator that is placed in a well identical to the placement of the receiver stimulator of the cochlear implant.

Like conventional cochlear implants, all ABI implants have an external speech processor that contains a microphone and speech processor. The speech processor converts speech into electrical signals that are sent across the skin to the internal receiver stimulator that, in turn, sends impulses to individual electrode contacts.

Because of the difficulty in reliably placing the silastic carrier pad over the cochlear nuclei, or shifting of the pad postoperatively, performance with the implant varies from only nonauditory sensation to improvement in lip-reading ability. Postoperatively, ABI patients are strongly encouraged to participate in aural rehabilitation to improve communication. Sign language instruction for the patient and family prior to tumor removal should be suggested to ease communication if the ABI is unsuccessful.

In a 1998 study, Otto et al[21] reported a majority of patients with the implant were able to distinguish temporal cues and stress patterns in closed set hearing testing (patients have a list of words from which they choose the word they think they hear). The ABI improved lip-reading. A report by Kanowitz et al,[22] showed better performance in patients using the Nucleus 24 ABI version than patients using the Nucleus 22 version. However, no open-set speech discrimination (patients attempt to repeat words with nothing but auditory cues) was found either study. In all subjects, performance was better with the sound provided by the ABI that with lip-reading alone. Both studies concluded that the ABI is a safe and effective way to provide auditory sensation to most patients with NFII.

CONCLUSION

With greater understanding of the cellular pathways regulated by merlin, targeted therapy at the cellular level may eventually play a role in treating NF2. Current treatment options include surgery and radiotherapy.

Neurofibromatosis type II provides one of the most challenging scenarios for clinical management in neurotology and skull base surgery. Surgical management of each tumor presents a technical challenge in and of itself, but the competing goals of minimizing hazard from tumor burden and maintaining maximal sensory function for as long as possible present the true dilemma in this disease. Each patient presents unique circumstances that require individualized treatment algorithms. Fundamentally however, in most cases patient safety takes ultimate priority, at the expense of sensory function.

REFERENCES

1. Evans DG, Huson SM, Donnai D, et al. A genetic study of type 2 neurofibromatosis in the United Kingdom. I. Prevalence, mutation rate, fitness, and confirmation of maternal transmission effect on severity. *J Med Genet.* 1992;29(12):841–846.
2. Evans DG, Moran A, King A, Saeed S, Gurusinghe N, Ramsden R. Incidence of vestibular schwannoma and neurofibromatosis 2 in the North West of England over a 10-year period: higher incidence than previously thought. *Otol Neurotol.* 2005;26(1):93–97.
3. Hanemann CO. Magic but treatable? Tumours due to loss of merlin. *Brain.* 2008;131(pt 3):606–615.
4. Rouleau GA, Merel P, Lutchman M, et al. Alteration in a new gene encoding a putative membrane-organizing protein causes neuro-fibromatosis type 2. *Nature.* 1993; 363(6429):515–521.
5. Trofatter JA, MacCollin MM, Rutter JL, et al. A novel moesin-, ezrin-, radixin-like gene is a candidate for the neurofibromatosis 2 tumor suppressor. *Cell.* 1993;72(5):791–800.
6. Welling DB, Packer MD, Chang LS. Molecular studies of vestibular schwannomas: a review. *Curr Opin Otolaryngol Head Neck Surg.* 2007;15(5):341–346.
7. Baser ME, Evans DG, Gutmann DH. Neurofibromatosis 2. *Curr Opin Otolaryngol Neurol.* 2003;16:27–33.
8. Fisher LM, Doherty JK, Lev MH, Slattery WH 3rd. Distribution of nonvestibular cranial nerve schwannomas in neurofibromatosis 2. *Otol Neurotol.* 2007;28(8):1083–1090.
9. Yasuda M, Higuchi O, Takano S, Matsumura A. Olfactory ensheathing cell tumor: a case report. *J Neurooncol.* 2006; 76(2):111–113.
10. Mautner VF, Tatagiba M, Lindenau M, et al. Spinal tumors in patients with neurofibromatosis type 2: MR imaging study of frequency, multiplicity, and variety. *AJR Am J Roentgenol.* 1995;165(4):951–955.
11. Yohay K. Neurofibromatosis types 1 and 2. *Neurologist.* 2006;12(2):86–93.
12. Baser ME, Friedman JM, Wallace AJ, Ramsden RT, Joe H, Evans DG. Evaluation of clinical diagnostic criteria for neurofibromatosis 2. *Neurology.* 2002;59(11):1759–1765.
13. Neff BA, Welling DB. Current concepts in the evaluation and treatment of neurofibromatosis type II. *Otolaryngol Clin North Am.* 2005;38(4):671–684, ix.
14. Evans DG, Birch JM, Ramsden RT. Paediatric presentation of type 2 neurofibromatosis. *Arch Dis Child.* 1999;81(6): 496–499.
15. Brackmann DE, Fayad JN, Slattery WH 3rd, et al. Early proactive management of vestibular schwannomas in neurofibromatosis type 2. *Neurosurgery.* 2001;49(2):274–280; discussion 280–273.
16. Slattery WH 3rd, Fisher LM, Hitselberger W, Friedman RA, Brackmann DE. Hearing preservation surgery for neurofibromatosis Type 2-related vestibular schwannoma in pediatric patients. *J Neurosurg.* 2007;106(4 suppl): 255–260.
17. Doyle KJ, Shelton C. Hearing preservation in bilateral acoustic neuroma surgery. *Am J Otol.* 1993;14(6): 562–565.
18. Samii M, Matthies C, Tatagiba M. Management of vestibular schwannomas (acoustic neuromas): auditory and facial nerve function after resection of 120 vestibular schwannomas in patients with neurofibromatosis 2. *Neurosurgery.* 1997;40(4):696–705; discussion 705–696.
19. Lustig LR, Yeagle J, Driscoll CL, Blevins N, Francis H, Niparko JK. Cochlear implantation in patients with neurofibromatosis type 2 and bilateral vestibular schwannoma. *Otol Neurotol.* 2006;27(4):512–518.

20. Vincenti V, Pasanisi E, Guida M, Di Trapani G, Sanna M. Hearing rehabilitation in neurofibromatosis type 2 patients: cochlear versus auditory brainstem implantation. *Audiol Neurootol.* 2008;13(4):273–280.
21. Otto SR, Shannon RV, Brackmann DE, Hitselberger WE, Staller S, Menapace C. The multichannel auditory brainstem implant: performance in twenty patients. *Otolaryngol Head Neck Surg.* 1998;118(3 pt 1):291–303.
22. Kanowitz SJ, Shpairo WH, Golfinos JG, Cohen NL, Roland JT. Auditory brainstem implantation in patients with neurofibromatosis type 2. *Laryngoscope.* 2004;114(12): 2135–2146.

CHAPTER 6

Lesions of Petrous Apex

Christopher Linstrom, Raj Murali, and Dan Sdrulla

INTRODUCTION

Lesions of the petrous apex are relatively rare, but must be considered as part of the differential diagnosis in a patient presenting with hearing loss, tinnitus, vertigo, disequilibrium, otalgia, or headache. Furthermore, the combination of any unilateral otologic complaint with weakness or paralysis of the abducens nerve (CN VI) suggests a lesion of the petrous apex. The focus of this chapter is the clinical presentation, investigation, and treatment of the common lesions of the petrous apex.

ANATOMY

The petrous (πέτρα; Greek meaning stone) portion of the temporal bone has a shape resembling a pyramid. Following the long axis of the temporal bone, the apex is situated anterior and medial, whereas the base is posterior and lateral. Structures lateral to the petrous apex include the otic labyrinth, the carotid artery and the eustachian tube. These structures form the base of the petrous apex.[1] The petrous apex also abuts the internal auditory canal (IAC), and a small notch in the most superior and medial edge of this pyramid identifies Dorello's canal, that houses the sixth cranial nerve (abducens). A small depression of the anterosuperior surface of the petrous apex identifies Meckel's cave that houses the trigeminal ganglion. The arcuate eminence, also found on the superior surface of the petrous pyramid, serves as an approximate landmark for the superior semicircular canal. Pneumatization of the petrous apex may occur; however, the degree may vary from side to side. Air cell tracts that pass from the middle ear either above or below the cochlea are thought to invaginate into the apex when pneuamatization occurs. Variable amounts of fatty marrow may be present within the cancellous bone of the petrous apex.[2]

PATHOPHYSIOLOGY

The pathophysiology of lesions found in the petrous apex is determined by the nature of the lesion. Cholesterol granulomas, epidermoids, and vascular abnormalities such as aneurysms arise within the apex itself. Other anomalies, such as cerebrospinal fluid cysts, encephaloceles, and meningiomas grow towards the petrous apex from nearby structures. Metastatic spread of cancer to the petrous apex is also encountered. Common primary sources of metastatic disease to the petrous temporal bone include cancer of the breast, kidney, prostate, and malignant melanoma. Several of these lesions are considered in greater detail under the differential diagnosis of lesions of the petrous apex.

CLINICAL PRESENTATION AND PHYSICAL EXAMINATION

The clinical history of lesions found within the petrous apex is often subtle compared to the radiologic findings. For example, patients with lesions of the petrous apex may only have vague otologic complaints (such as aural fullness) until the lesion impinges on critical structures resulting in hearing loss, tinnitus, or facial weakness. Patients may also complain of facial pressure or pain, paresthesias of the face, headaches, or visual complaints, such as diplopia.

A complete otologic and head and neck examination should be done with a focus on cranial nerves II to XII. A microscopic examination of the tympanic membrane is necessary. Clinical tests of balance should be performed. A minimal clinical examination of hearing includes a tuning fork examination and an audiogram. A 512-Hz tuning fork test will usually suffice, though more frequencies may be tested. There should be congruence between the tuning form examination and the audiometric findings.

If the patient complains of pulsatile tinnitus, it is important to auscultate the neck (carotid), periauricular region, retromastoid area, and the periorbital region in a quiet room, such as an audiometric booth. In addition, the patient should hold his or her breath during auscultation so that any bruit may not be hidden under respiratory noise.

EVALUATION

Audiometric

All patients with otologic complaints should have an audiometric battery of tests as deemed appropriate. In rare cases, an auditory brainstem response (ABR) may demonstrate either a lack of a wave I or, more commonly, an increase in wave I to III latency on the affected side. The abnormality on the ABR may revert after the lesion has been treated.

Radiologic

Patients with unilateral otologic complaints such as hearing loss, tinnitus, fullness, or pressure should be evaluated for a retrocochlear lesion with an appropriate study. For most patients, the study of choice is an MRI without and with gadolinium enhancement. It is the test of choice for the detection of retrocochlear pathology. Many lesions of the petrous apex are incidentally discovered by screening MRI that is done for other reasons.

A word of caution is indicated. As previously discussed, the degree of pneumatization of each petrous apex in an individual may vary from side to side. The petrous apex is pneumatized in approximately 30% of temporal bones.[3] The inexperienced radiologist may fail to realize this fact and may misread the fatty signal from bone marrow in a pneumatized and marrow-containing petrous apex as a cyst or other neoplasm. This may create a diagnostic and therapeutic dilemma for the physician and create stress for the patient. Correlating clinical findings with radiographic interpretation is therefore of utmost importance. If there are no complaints such has facial pain, hypoesthesia, hearing loss, tinnitus, or dizziness and no objective signs of disease on physical examination, both physician and patient may be reassured that the increased signal on the T1-weighted image is from bone marrow or may represent an incidental finding. A quick look at the other petrous apex or other marrow-containing areas of the skull may also be of assistance. A T1-weighted image with fat suppression will also demonstrate that a suspected lesion is marrow fat. Ultimately, the film should be reviewed by an experienced neuroradiologist in conjunction with the surgeon.

Once a lesion in or near the petrous apex has been discovered, additional imaging studies will likely be obtained. In an excellent review of radiographic imaging of the petrous apex, Curtin and Som postulate five questions that should be asked to properly identify a lesion of the petrous apex[2] (Table 6–1). These questions may usually be answered by complementary studies of the petrous apex. If the patient has had a magnetic resonance image (MRI), then a computed tomography (CT) would be the next test of

Table 6–1. Five Questions that Should Be Asked to Properly Identify a Lesion of the Petrous Apex

Is the abnormality arising in the petrous apex or from contiguous areas? (Is the lesion expansile, infiltrative, or destructive)
Are the bony walls of the apex and the septations in the air cells smoothly remodeled? (eg, cholesterol granuloma, cholesteatoma, or mucocele) or destroyed (metastatic lesions)
What are the MR imaging signal characteristics of the lesion?
Is there enhancement of the internal "matrix" of the lesion? (Does the central part of the lesion have a blood supply?)
What is the relationship of the lesion to the carotid artery? (Is it bowed to the side, is the canal effaced, is it an aneurysm of the petrous carotid artery?)

choice. CT with a bone algorithm yields excellent information about bone and the soft-tissue/bone/air interface but is far less sensitive and specific than MRI in detecting soft tissue neoplasia.

Additional studies, such as MR angiography or MR venography may be necessary to determine extent of disease or possibility of aneurysm.

DIFFERENTIAL DIAGNOSIS

The differential diagnosis of lesions of the petrous apex is vast. Lesions may be benign or malignant, expansile or erosive, and may arise from nearby structures or metastatic spread.

Although a wide differential diagnosis should be entertained, the lesions most commonly encountered will be cholesterol granulomas, cholesteatomas, and mucoceles, whereas encephaloceles/meningoceles and aneurysms are less commonly seen.

Many sources differ in the classification and nomenclature of lesions of the petrous apex. These lesions will be presented as well as a brief description of the more common lesions.[2,4,5] Lesions in the petrous apex and CPA have certain imaging characteristics that may aid in the diagnosis as well. A summary table of these findings can be found in Table 6–2.

INFLAMMATORY/INFECTIOUS/CYSTIC

Cholesterol Granuloma

Manasse reported a case of "granulation tumor with foreign body cells" of the petrous apex in 1894. The term "cholesterin or cholesterol granuloma" has been used since that report.[6]

By far, the most common clinical entity that will be encountered within the petrous apex is cholesterol granuloma. The second most common lesions are cholesteatomas. The pathophysiology of these two lesions is discussed below.

Cholesterol granulomas have been produced in animal studies by two mechanisms: (1) The introduction of irritants into the middle ear cleft and (2) The isolation of a bony air-filled cavity that normally communicates with the atmosphere.[7]

Beaumont[8] produced cholesterol granuloma in the chick humerus by obstructing the foramen pneumaticum (the connection with the respiratory system) with a muscle pedicle. Histologic examination revealed no associated loss of blood or infection. Surgical trauma as a causative factor was excluded because an identical procedure performed on the contralateral humerus without complete occlusion of the foramen pneumaticum did not result in cholesterol granuloma formation. These findings support the "obstruction-vacuum" hypothesis of cholesterol granulomas.

Friedman[9] was able to develop cholesterol granulomas by injecting sterile suspensions of cholesterol into the middle ear of the guinea pig. He proposed that the blood breakdown product cholesterol incited a foreign body reaction. Sadé and Teitz[10] dispute the necessity for hemorrhage as a predisposing factor for cholesterol granuloma formation.

A second major theory for the pathogenesis of cholesterol granuloma is the "exposed marrow" hypothesis. The marrow-filled cavities of the petrous apex are eroded as air cells develop. This erosion may cause hemorrhage into the air cells with subsequent degradation into blood products such as cholesterin, thereby resulting in an inflammatory reaction and cyst development. The expansion of the cyst results from continued bleeding within the marrow cavities.

Table 6–2. Imaging Characteristics of Petrous Apex Lesions

MRI	T1	T2	Gad	CT
cholesterol granuloma	↑	↑ / mixed	-	smooth expansion
epidermoid	↓	↑	± peripheral enhancement	smooth expansion
mucocele	variable (dependent on protein content)	↑	peripheral enhancement	smooth expansion
fat (pseudolesion)	↑	↓	-	check contralateral side; correlate location c MRI
mucus (pseudolesion)	variable (dependent on protein content)	↑	-	preservation of septae
arachnoid cyst (pseudolesion)	↓	↑	-	CT cisternograms to differentiate with epidermoid
fibrous dysplasia	iso	mixed	mixed (+)	ground glass; otic capsule spared, EAC stenosis
ossifying hemangioma	iso	↑	+ ?	intratumoral calcification; ill defined bony margin
trigeminal neuroma	iso	↑	+	smooth remodeling of apex
cavernous sinus hemangioma	iso	very ↑	+	bony erosion when large
plasmacytoma/multiple myeloma	iso	↓	+	skull base erosion; contrast enhancing
metastasis	iso	iso	+	skull base erosion; contrast enhancing

These authors reported a small retrospective series of four patients with aggressive cholesterol granulomas in the mastoid. In all cases, there was a nearby blood source. The authors note that an "obstruction-vacuum" postulate alone would not have explained the source of the hemorrhage, and a blood source must have supplied these aggressive lesions.[11,12]

Cholesterol granulomas appear as granulation tissue or may occur as cystic masses that are brown, green, or glistening yellow. Cholesterol granuloma is not a precursor of cholesteatoma. An MRI +/− contrast is the required preoperative evaluation. It will be bright on both T1 and T2-weighted images, characteristic of cholesterol granulomas.

Major factors predisposing to the formation of cholesterol granuloma are summarized in Table 6–3.

Table 6–3. Major Factors Predisposing to Formation of Cholesterol Granulomas

Obstruction of the ventilation of an air-filled bony cavity that normally equilibrates the atmosphere.
Obstruction of drainage.
Reaction to a foreign body such as cholesterol.
Bone marrow products including blood leading to cholesterol cysts.
Hemorrhage.

Epidermoid/Cholesteatoma

Cholesteatoma, or more properly keratoma, is not a true neoplasm but rather the accumulations of a living matrix of keratinizing squamous epithelium and its cellular debris in an enclosed space. It may be classified as congenital, (arising de novo within the anatomical location) or acquired. Acquired cholesteatomas may be subdivided as primary (arising from a retraction of a squamous epithelial lined surface into the target), or secondary (arising from a break in the integrity of the target location). In patients with cholesteatoma of the petrous apex (epidermoid), the clinical and radiologic examination must search for a source outside of the petrous apex, such as the pars flaccida of the middle ear, as in an attic retraction cholesteatoma. This, however, is uncommon. If a source is found, it is usually disproportionately small to the disease within the petrous apex. Cholesteatomas of the petrous apex are therefore most commonly congenital in origin.

Congenital cholesteatomas of the petrous apex may arise from trapped epithelial cells during the time of embryogenesis and subsequent overclosure of the neural tube. Congenital cholesteatomas of the petrous apex may be clinically silent. If they expand to a large enough volume to impinge upon structures within or adjacent to the petrous apex, the clinical manifestations may include hearing loss, aural fullness, facial pain or hypoesthesia, headache, or blurred vision/diplopia. The clinical exam does not necessarily yield a pathological diagnosis, but it may point to the likely site of the lesion.

Effusion

Effusion of the middle ear and mastoid may give the patient a blocked feeling in the ear and cause a conductive hearing loss. This process may extend to the petrous apex. In some cases, the effusion is due to chronic mastoiditis, where the respiratory mucosa of the middle ear and mastoid becomes hypertrophic. In these cases, the mucosa of the middle ear and mastoid will often remain hypertrophic, thus becoming the source of the effusion rather than the result of an active infection. CT will usually reveal a nearly complete middle ear and mastoid effusion without erosion of bony septations or expansion of the apex. The T1-weighted MRI will often be hypointense, whereas the T2-weighted images will be hyperintense. In rare cases, all of the hypertrophic mucosa must be removed with a mastoidectomy and/or a middle ear exploration to allow a new mucosa to replace it. Because the air cell system is contiguous, performing the mastoidectomy will usually provide drainage for the petrous apex.[13]

Mucocele

Rarely, simple obstruction of the regular drainage pathways of the petrous apex may result in a mucocele. The apex expands as mucus continues to collect within it. The CT and MRI characteristics are similar to those of cholesteatomas, with a smooth, expansile appearance. On MRI, mucoceles are hypointense on T1- and hyperintense on T2-weighted images.

The signal on MR may be variable, depending on the protein content of the fluid. Fluid with low protein content is hypointense on T1-weighted images and hyperintense on T2. As time passes, the water content decreases and the protein content increases. This may alter the enhancing characteristics such that both T1- and T2-weighted images become hyperintense.[2,13]

Cerebrospinal Fluid Cysts and Encephaloceles

CSF cephaloceles are meningeal diverticula that may consist of only CSF and dura (meningocele) or both CSF and brain tissue (encephaloceles). Structures that arise from the dura of Meckel's cave are called petrous apex cephaloceles and typically contain only CSF.[14]

Encephalocoeles typically arise from the middle fossa near the mastoid and tegmen tympani and are often associated with chronic ear disease or surgical trauma. CSF cephaloceles may be an incidental finding, or they may present with CSF oto/rhinorrhea, vertigo, hearing loss, diplopia, facial numbness, or meningitis.[15]

Petrous Apicitis/Abscess

In 1904, Gradenigo described an infection of the ear with concomitant paralysis of the abducens

(VI) nerve.[16] Profant[17] first used the term *petrositis* to describe infection of the petrous apex combined with mastoiditis. Inflammation of the leptomeninges around Dorello's canal produces palsy of the VI cranial nerve. Involvement of the adjacent trigeminal ganglion in Meckel's cave (CN V) may lead to periorbital and facial pain. The combination of otorrhea, lateral rectus palsy and pain in the trigeminal distribution constitutes Gradenigo's syndrome in honor of his original description.

Cases of petrous apicitis are almost always found in a setting of acute or subacute otitis media. CT and MRI imaging show air cell opacification with enhancement of the dura over the petrous apex. Complications such as intracranial abscess or venous thrombosis may occur. The cavernous sinus, sigmoid sinus and jugular vein are at risk due to their proximity to the apex. A variety of organisms may cause petrous apicitis. Tuberculosis has been reported to cause this syndrome.[18]

Skull Base Osteomyelitis/ Necrotizing (Malignant) Otitis Externa

Malignant otitis externa, more properly called necrotizing otitis externa (NEO) or skull base osteomyelitis (SBO), does not represent malignancy. The term describes skull base osteomyelitis, usually a result of *Pseudomonas* infection. Toulmouche described a case of progressive osteomyelitis of the temporal bone in 1838 that may have been the first reported case of NEO.[19] Risk factors for this disease include old age, diabetes and any other cause of immunosuppression. The typical complaint is deep-seated, boring pain in the ear with radiation toward the middle of the head. Granulations in the inferior margin of the external canal near the tympanic bone may be seen, though aural discharge is rarely encountered. A conductive hearing loss due to fluid or granulations within the middle ear may be diagnosed. Involvement of cranial nerves indicates more advanced disease. The treatment is initially medical; treating the underlying disorder, such as diabetes, is paramount. Intravenous antibiotic therapy, usually a combination of two different classes of anti-pseudomonal antibiotics, will offer synergy toward the eradication of the offending organism. In extremely rare cases, surgical decompression of a phlegmon or abscess of the skull base may be necessary.[20,21]

Petrous Carotid Aneurysm

A smooth-bordered mass seen within the petrous apex may in fact be an aneurysmal dilatation of the petrous carotid and must always be included in the differential diagnosis. Violation of an aneurysm in this location would lead to catastrophic sequelae for the patient. An easy way to distinguish the lesion from the artery is to include MRA sequences along with the MRI in detailing the soft tissues of the mass. The MRA delineates first and second-order vessels and will be formatted in many different planes. Therefore, if the mass is separate from the vessel in the petrous apex, this will be seen on MRA. If doubt remains after the MRA, a 4-vessel angiogram, with its inherent risks, would be the next step to definitively answer the question.

Asymmetric Pneumatization

This has been discussed above and remains a source of confusion for inexperienced radiologists and clinicians.

Paget's Disease and Fibrous Dysplasia

Paget's disease of bone affects the skull base in sclerotic, lytic and mixed forms. The skull base is rarely involved without simultaneous calvarial disease. In the base of the skull and petrous apex, the lesions are primarily lytic and may thus have an appearance similar to that of metastatic disease. Paget's disease may cause demineralization or erosion of the otic capsule. It often involves the petrous temporal bones in a symmetric fashion.

Fibrous dysplasia has a typical appearance on CT imaging. Areas of bony thickening with a "ground glass" appearance are typical. The medullary region of the lesion may show dense ossification mixed with areas of fibrous tissue. Both T1- and T2-weighted images are of low signal intensity on MR. However, any cystic areas are bright on both sequences. It is rare to find fibrous dysplasia isolated solely to the petrous apex.[2]

These are described in more detail in Chapter 9.

NEOPLASMS OF PETROUS APEX

Primary

Although, primary neoplasms of the petrous apex are rare, they have been reported. These include giant cell tumor, xanthomas, endolymphatic sac tumor, and hemangioma, hemangiopericytoma, chondroma/chondrosarcoma, aneurysmal bone cyst (ABC), plasmacytoma, undifferentiated carcinoma, various sarcomas, and nasopharyngeal carcinoma.

Chondroma/Chondrosarcoma

Chondroma/chondrosarcoma are thought to arise from embryonic rests of cartilage in the region of foramen lacerum.[22] Malignant chondrosarcomas appear more commonly than their benign counterpart. Chondrosarcomas appear as bulky, enhancing, irregular, destructive lesions arising from the midline with "popcorn" calcifications. They are homogeneous on T1-weighted imaging and heterogeneous on T2-weighted imaging and they enhance intensely with contrast.[2] These are described in more detail in Chapter 7.

Sarcomas

Nager describes sarcomas affecting the temporal bone under general categories of rhabdomyosarcoma, extraskeletal Ewing's sarcoma, myxoma, and fibromyxoma (these do not metastasize but spread locally), and osteosarcoma.[23] These malignancies have in common at least one primordial element from supporting, or mesenchymal, tissue. Although all of these cancers are uncommonly seen *solely* in the petrous apex, they may secondarily spread to this site due to their aggressive behavior.

Rhabdomyosarcoma (synonyms include malignant rhabdomyoma, myosarcoma, and rhabdomyoblastoma) is a highly malignant tumor of rhabdomyoblasts more commonly found in children.

Extraskeletal Ewing's sarcoma is a malignant tumor believed to arise from primitive mesenchymal tissue. It is rare in the temporal bone and is included for completeness.

Eosinophilic Granuloma: Langerhans Cell or Histiocytosis X

Langerhans cell histiocytosis may involve the skull base. Any bone may be involved, but the temporal bone is a common site. The clinical history often is that of an ear infection that will not heal despite appropriate aural toilet and antibiotic therapy. The temporal bone may be expanded or destroyed. The bone-lesion interface may be sharp on CT imaging. The internal density of the lesion and the imaging characteristics on MR may be variable. The patient tends to be young, further raising the index of suspicion. Other entities to be considered would be teratoma, neuroma, and giant cell tumor.

Chordoma

These are tumors derived from primitive notochord remnants and are midline masses arising from the clivus that may secondarily spread to the petrous apex. It is possible for notochord remnants to extend laterally toward the petrous apex, thus causing a primary tumor. Chordomas are bulky, lobulated, midline lesions on CT, enhancing with contrast, destructive of bone, and containing calcifications. They appear similar to chondrosarcomas on MR, but tend to arise more in the midline and are less brightly enhancing with gadolinium.

Meningioma

This benign tumor, arising from the meninges, comprises approximately 14% of all intracranial tumors and is the most common solid tumor involving the petrous apex, appearing rarely as a primary tumor but more commonly secondarily invading the apex. They commonly present as broad-based tumors along the posterior petrous wall. They may exhibit calcification within the tumor and enhance with contrast. They may exhibit a characteristic dural "tail." Meningiomas have a predilection for following sites of dural penetration by cranial nerves VII to XII.[24,25]

Paragangliomas

Paragangliomas usually do not arise from within, but may grow into the petrous apex. It would extremely rare to find a glomus tumor primary to the petrous apex in the absence of this lesion elsewhere.

Metastatic Neoplasms

Extratemporal primary cancers may metastasize via hematogenous routes the temporal bone, specifically to the rich marrow spaces of the petrous apex. These include breast, prostate, lung, renal cell CA, and malignant melanoma. The appearance is variable, depending upon the site of the primary. Metastatic cancer to the temporal bone may erode and remodel bone or be less invasive in appearance. A history of known cancer from any of these sites or the presence of additional metastatic disease anywhere raises the index of suspicion.[26]

TREATMENT PARADIGMS

Few lesions of the petrous apex will be solely observed in patients who are in a state of health to allow treatment. Others, such as necrotizing otitis externa or petrous apicitis, will be treated medically with very rare surgical intervention. The majority of lesions of the petrous apex will eventually require surgery to provide either drainage or resection. Many surgical approaches to the petrous apex exist, each tailor-made to the lesion and the extent of disease. One may need the expertise of neurosurgery to manage some processes in this complex area.

Surgical approaches to the petrous apex may be classified according the neighboring anatomy, according to the ability to preserve hearing, or according to the direction of approach. Because the temporal bone is pneumatized by air cell tracts invaginating the mastoid complex around the vestibular and cochlear labyrinths and the facial nerve, a classification scheme is based on hearing preservation/hearing ablation and these named pathways of pneumatization around the otic capsule. All approaches should attempt to preserve and protect the facial nerve.

Flood and Kemink[27] list six requirements which must be fulfilled in approaching tumors of the petrous apex as listed in Table 6–4.

Hearing Preservation Approaches

These surgical approaches aim to reach the petrous apex with the preservation of the otic capsule. These approaches follow established air cell tracts *above*, *below*, or *anterior* to the otic capsule. Many of these approaches were first described in the "preantibiotic era," and were used to exteriorize abscesses of the petrous apex. None of these approaches involves the transposition of the facial nerve or of the petrous carotid artery. The jugular bulb is an inferior anatomic boundary.

Above the Labyrinth

Middle Cranial Fossa Approach. This is an extension of the standard middle cranial fossa approach for decompression of the labyrinthine facial nerve and resection of lesions within the internal auditory canal, as described by William House in 1959 and thereafter.[28] It may be a preferred approach for lesions in which surgical removal and subsequent exenteration is the goal, such as in cholesteatoma. It is difficult to drain lesions to other dependent areas of the temporal bone, although this has been described. The major landmarks to be preserved are the petrous carotid artery, the cochlea, and the facial nerve. This approach affords a "keyhole" window from above, through which a lesion may be more thoroughly exenterated.[29]

Table 6–4. Goals of Surgery in Treatment of Lesions Involving the Petrous Apex

Provide adequate exposure for complete excision or exteriorization.
Preserve useful residual hearing, if possible.
Provide for wound closure without cerebrospinal fluid leak.
Preserve facial nerve and other cranial nerve function when possible.
Preserve the internal carotid artery.
Avoid injury to the brainstem.

Subarcuate Approach. In patients with a well-developed perilabyrinthine air cell tract and a more posterior lesion, this approach may be contemplated following the subarcuate artery. However, the diameter within the SSC is no more than a few millimeters, and thus the vestibular and cochlear labyrinths are both placed at risk with this approach. This approach was developed to drain abscesses of the petrous apex and is mentioned here for historical interest as it is rarely used.

Trans-Attic Approach. This approach is rarely indicated for lesions of the petrous apex with extension above and posterior to the vestibular labyrinth. It may be of value for obtaining a biopsy but would not today itself be considered a definitive approach. It is often combined with other approaches to the petrous apex, especially when the goal is to provide drainage or exteriorization and not definitive resection.

Approach Through the Root of the Zygomatic Arch. This is also mentioned for historical completion only and today would most likely be replaced by or combined with another technique, such as a middle cranial fossa approach.[30]

Below the Labyrinth

Infracochlear (subcochlear) Approach. This approach utilizes the triangular space bordered by the basal turn of the cochlea, the ascending petrous carotid artery, and the jugular bulb. In an anatomical study of 20 preserved temporal bones, Haberkamp[5] found the average window created via this approach to be 9.41 × 7.33 mm. In none of his specimens was this approach impossible. In the living, a well-defined axial and coronal CT with a bone algorithm is needed to approximate the space between the basal turn of the cochlea and the petrous carotid. If the space is greater than approximately 3 to 4 mm, surgical drainage of the petrous apex will likely be possible. This approach is limited by a short distance between these 2 structures or by a high-riding jugular bulb. It is the most common otologic approach in current use and has been described by many authors.[3,5,31,32]

Infralabyrinthine (retrofacial) Approach. This approach is bordered by the posterior semicircular canal, the vertical (descending) facial nerve and the jugular bulb. It is a straightforward approach, an anterior extension of a complete mastoidectomy. A preoperative axial CT with edge enhancement will help in the surgical planning. In an anatomical study of 20 preserved temporal bones, Haberkamp[5] found the average window created via this approach to be 4.99 × 7.23 mm. The major limitation to this approach is a high-riding jugular bulb. In rare cases, the posterior semicircular canal may be blue-lined to allow a few extra millimeters of the operculum of the SSC to be dissected. As in other approaches, the petrous apex is drained to a well-ventilated area, in this case the mastoid, and subsequently to the eustachian tube. In the literature reviewed for this chapter, it is the second most common approach.[5,33,34]

Retrosigmoid (suboccipital) Approach. This is the standard approach toward the posterior cranial fossa for the excision of lesions of the cerebellopontine angle and IAC. It is rarely used alone to approach the petrous apex, but may be combined with another approach when intracranial extension of a petrous apex tumor produces signs of brainstem compression. The surgeon works at a great distance from the petrous apex and the morbidity associated with this technique limits its usefulness as a primary approach to the petrous apex.[22]

Infratemporal Approach. The infratemporal approach to the skull base, with anterior transposition of the facial nerve, as is typically used in the resection of paragangliomas would allow for a combined infracochlear and infralabyrinthine drainage of lesions of the petrous apex with preservation of hearing. Transposition of the facial nerve with attendant facial weakness is the major limiting factor to this approach.[35]

Anterior to Labyrinth

These approaches utilize the triangle formed by the cochlea, the petrous carotid artery and the middle fossa dura. This approach was developed in the pre-antibiotic era and is rarely if ever indicated today.[36,37]

Transsphenoidal Approach. The history of this approach to the pituitary is a veritable history of modern advances in neurotology and neurosurgery. This approach was first popularized in North America by Harvey Cushing, although he claimed no credit for its discovery.[38] It fell into disfavor due to poor anesthesia and limited visibility in an era devoid of the operating microscope. It was revived by Guiot and Jules Hardy with the advent of intraoperative radiofluoroscopy in 1958.[39–41] Although this approach is aimed precisely at lesions of the sella turcica, it may be modified for lesions of the petrous apex. Gray et al[42] have described the transnasal, transsphenoidal marsupialization of a cholesterol granuloma of the petrous apex and sphenoid sinus. This approach may be favored in patients with lesions that expand the far anterior aspect of the petrous apex and in whom the petrous carotid artery has been laterally displaced. Preoperative planning may include an edge enhanced CT of the temporal bone and MRI/MRA to both detail the nature of the lesion and the exact location of the horizontal portion of the petrous carotid artery. An intraoperative navigational system or intraoperative fluoroscopic system is often used to confirm anatomic landmarks. The sphenoid sinus is approached in a trans-nasal fashion. The posterior wall of the sphenoid sinus is thinned with a diamond bur and the anterior face of the petrous apex is opened. Removal of the intrasphenoid septum may facilitate exposure. A drain may be left in place or a posteriorly based flap of septal mucosa may be rotated into the neo-osteum of the petrous apex, as described by Montgomery.[43]

Hearing-Ablation Approaches

These approaches are intended to reach the petrous apex via the cochlear and/or the vestibular labyrinth(s), the most direct pathway, at the expense of the vestibular or cochlear labyrinth(s). None of these approaches intentionally involve the transposition of the facial nerve or of the petrous carotid artery.

Translabyrinthine Approach

In lesions of the petrous apex in which useful hearing is no longer present, the approach through the labyrinth combined with a canal-wall-down mastoidectomy and a sufficient meatoplasty yields a cavity that can be easily visualized and cleaned. The posterior and middle fossa dura may have been thinned by the expansion of the lesion. This allows exteriorization of disease in the petrous apex. It is important that evaluation and cleaning of the cavity in the office be performed under microscopic vision, in an extremely gentle fashion and without the use of sharp instruments in order to avoid a CSF leak.

Transcochlear Approach

This approach has been described by William House and is indicated in the patient with a lesion of the petrous apex in which useful hearing is no longer present.[44] It is important to follow the usual landmarks of the basal turn of the cochlea, the tympanic facial nerve, the eustachian tube orifice, and the petrous carotid artery carefully in order to prevent injury to vital structures. This approach, combined with a canal-wall-down mastoidectomy and a sufficient meatoplasty will yield a cavity that is open and cleanable. This also allows exteriorization of disease in the petrous apex.

Subtotal Petrosectomy

This is a "workhorse" approach, familiar to all skull base surgeons who have studied the work of Professor Fisch.[45] This technique leaves the otic capsule, the facial nerve, the carotid artery, and the jugular bulb as the only remaining anatomic landmarks within the temporal bone. The surgical goal is to exenterate all remaining disease from the external and middle ear clefts and all air cells of the mastoid. All squamous epithelium from the external auditory canal up to and including the tympanic membrane is removed and the canal is overclosed. The ossicular chain, excepting the mobile stapes footplate, is removed. Depending on the pathology, the facial nerve may be decompressed, transposed or grafted, as in the case of trauma. The petrous carotid may be decompressed, according to need. There are many variations of this approach, including leaving the canal open for surveillance.

CLINICAL AND RADIOGRAPHIC FOLLOW-UP

The lesion itself and the ability to preserve the function of the otic capsule in large measure determine the mode of surveillance for patients with lesions involving the petrous apex. If the lesion is being observed, clinical examination and serial audiograms at the 6-month interval or whenever the patient may experience a decrease in hearing would be indicated. If the hearing remains unchanged, a CT or MRI initially at 6 months and thereafter at longer intervals is commonly performed. The patient is instructed to attend to his or her symptoms. If these worsen at any time, new investigations will be ordered.

If the lesion has been medically treated (6- to 12-week intravenous antibiotics for necrotizing or malignant otitis externa involving the petrous apex), the patient should be examined and the hearing tested at shorter and then longer intervals. Many patients will require a full course of treatment only once. A post-treatment gallium scan at three to four months should show significant improvement. It may not, however, become completely clear and must be interpreted according to the clinical state of the patient. In an elderly, diabetic patient, or an immunocompromised patient, the index of suspicion must be raised, especially if deep-seated otitic or base-of-skull pain should return. In this case, in addition to the clinical exam, audiometric and radiographic studies, radionuclide studies may need to be repeated.

If the patient has been treated surgically, the nature of the disease and the surgical approach will dictate the follow-up. If the disease has been exteriorized and can be visualized with a microscope, surveillance radiography may rarely be indicated. If, however, the disease has been drained to an area that is ordinarily not clinically accessible, such as to the mastoid in a canal-wall-up technique or to the hypotympanum, serial CT imaging at the 6- and then 12-month mark would be indicated. Patients who have had subtotal excision of disease processes within the petrous apex with overclosure of the ear must know that lifelong surveillance at appropriate intervals is mandatory. Because there will always be a chance that a residuum of disease may continue to grow, appropriate scanning (CT, MR or other) at appropriate intervals must be organized along with the clinical examination. As long as the patient remains clinically and radiologically stable, the disease may be observed. Radiographic progression of disease, with or without progression of clinical symptoms, must be carefully assessed and a treatment plan outlined. The overall clinical state of the patient with any comorbidities will help determine what is to be done.

CASE ILLUSTRATIONS

P.K., a 56-year-old male has 4-month history of tinnitus and decreased hearing in the right ear. He had no complaints of otitic pain, dizziness/vertigo and did not have facial pain. His ENT examination including cranial nerves II to XII was unremarkable. His clinical tests of balance were normal. He heard the 512-Hz fork midline and A > B bilaterally.

A pretreatment audiogram demonstrated a significant asymmetry of hearing in the right ear at and above 2K Hz (Figure 6–1). His MRI of brain without and with gadolinium demonstrated a 1.7 × 3.1 × 2.5 cm expansile lesion within the right petrous apex, high in signal on both T1 and T2-weighted

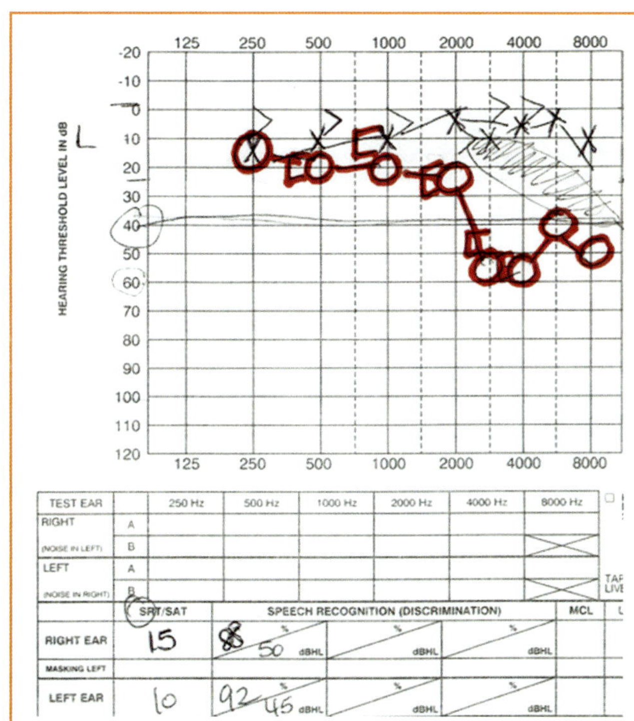

Figure 6–1. Audiogram, pre-op showing asymmetric right hearing loss.

images, with remodeling of bone and expansion in to the CP angle, consistent with cholesterol granulomas (Figure 6–2).

CT of the petrous temporal bone demonstrated thinning and displacement of the posterior horizontal portions of the petrous carotid artery as well as a medial bowing and thinning of the petrous apex. Erosive changes were noted along the lateral margin of the porous acousticus, the clivus and the basisphenoid. A careful review of the coronal images did not favor an infracochlear approach to the petrous apex but did show that a retrofacial (retrolabyrinthine) approach would be possible (Figure 6–3).

The patient elected to have the lesion surgically treated. He underwent a right retrofacial (infralabyrinthine) approach to the petrous apex using the standard landmarks of the posterior semicircular canal, the descending facial nerve, and the jugular bulb. This case was performed with an image navigation system that correlated within approximately 1 mm of the surgical landmarks. The bone over the cystic space was thinned and a 25-gauge needle was used to aspirate dark brown fluid, confirming the cholesterol granuloma. The posterior face of the petrous apex was then opened with graduated diamond burs to a diameter of about 7 mm. This allowed gentle curettage with ringed forceps. Due to the known effacement and displacement of the petrous carotid artery, no attempt was made to strip the lining of the cystic space. A No. 5 Jackson-Pratt drain was placed within the petrous apex and brought out to the mastoid (Figure 6–4). An audiogram performed one month after surgery revealed a slight improvement in hearing at 2, 3, and 4 kHz with 100% speech discrimination (Figure 6–5).

M.A. is a 19-year-old female with right facial weakness, dizziness, hearing loss and fullness in the right ear. She also had pain in the right face for 6 months. Examination revealed a right III/VI facial paresis and bulging in the right epitympanum. No discrete mass was seen. The 512-Hz fork lateralized to the right ear with B > A on the right. The

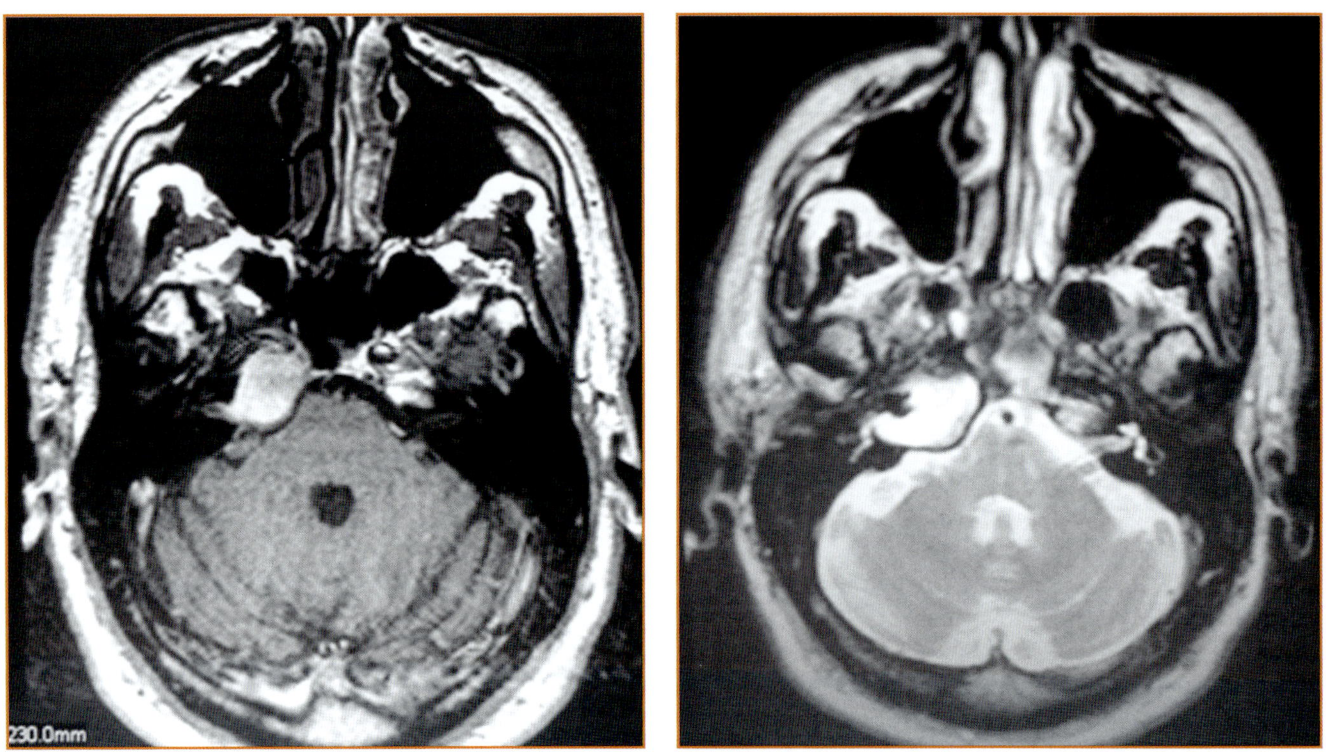

A B

Figure 6–2. MRI of brain. **A.** T1-weighted axial view. **B.** T2-weighted axial view.

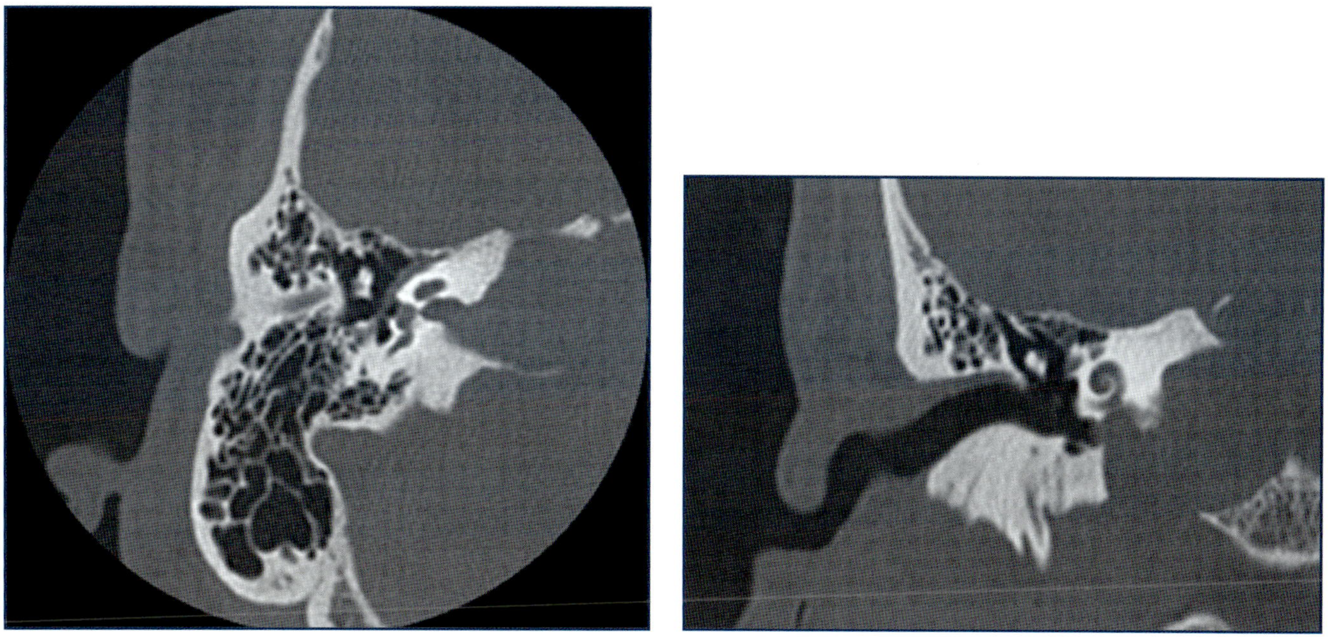

A B

Figure 6–3. CT temporal bone. **A.** Axial views of right. **B.** Coronal views of right. The ascending carotid abuts the cochlea.

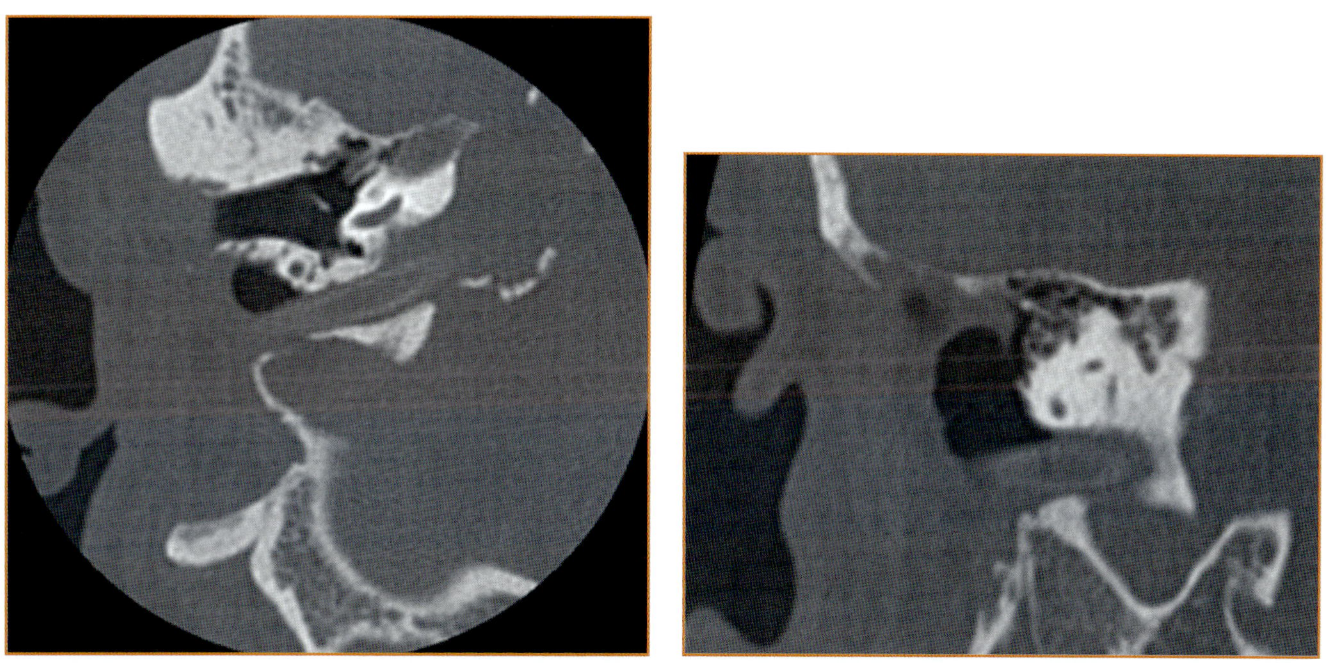

A B

Figure 6–4. Post-op CT. **A.** Axial view. **B.** Coronal view. The Silastic drain may be seen passing underneath the posterior semicircular canal into the petrous apex.

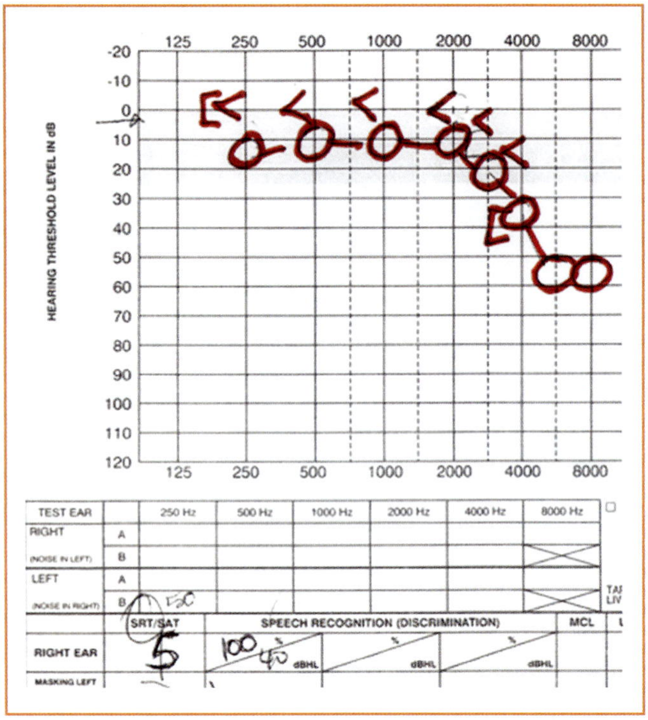

Figure 6–5. Post-op audiogram.

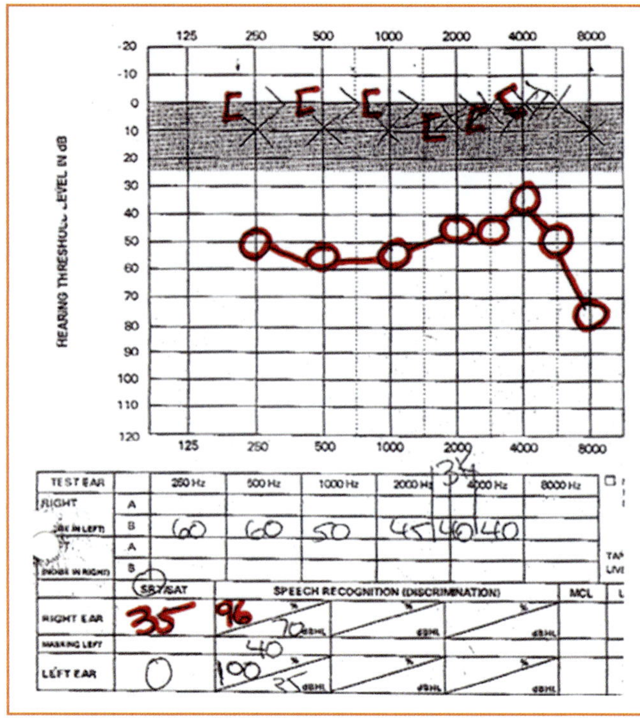

Figure 6–6. Audiogram, pre-op showing right conductive hearing loss.

remainder of the examination was unremarkable. An audiogram revealed a right conductive hearing loss (Figure 6–6).

CT of the temporal bone revealed an expansile lesion in the right petrous apex with extension toward the IAC and labyrinthine portion of the VII nerve, with significant bony erosion (Figure 6–7). An MRI was obtained which showed that the lesion in the right petrous apex was less intense on T1-weighted images and more intense on T2-weighted images, supporting the diagnosis of cholesteatoma of the petrous apex (Figure 6–8).

The patient subsequently moved to Venezuela and was lost to follow-up for about 12 months. When she returned to New York, she complained of worse hearing and worse facial function. On examination, she had complete facial paralysis (VI/VI) on the right side. An ENG was significant for 100% unilateral weakness on the right ear to bithermal caloric irrigation (Figure 6–9). A preoperative ENOG showed 100% degeneration on the right.

The patient was advised that definitive treatment of the mass would be required. She had a right upper lid gold weight inserted and underwent a right infratemporal fossa and transmastoid dissection of the mass. In an effort to preserve hearing, the labyrinth was kept intact. Cholesteatoma was unroofed above the superior semicircular canal and was removed with suction and curettage. The postoperative audiogram showed that little useful hearing remained on the right (Figure 6–10). The patient was followed conservatively with serial debridement and the facial nerve showed signs of slow improvement. She was observed for one year, but the follow-up MRI revealed little change in the overall size of the lesion. Serial debridements under binocular microscopy in the office became increasingly difficult due to stenosis of the meatus. Because the hearing was no longer useful, the patient underwent a right labyrinthectomy, dissection of the cholesteatoma, and meatoplasty. This provided a much wider access to routine debridement of the cholesteatoma. Her right facial nerve function has recovered to a H-B III/VI.

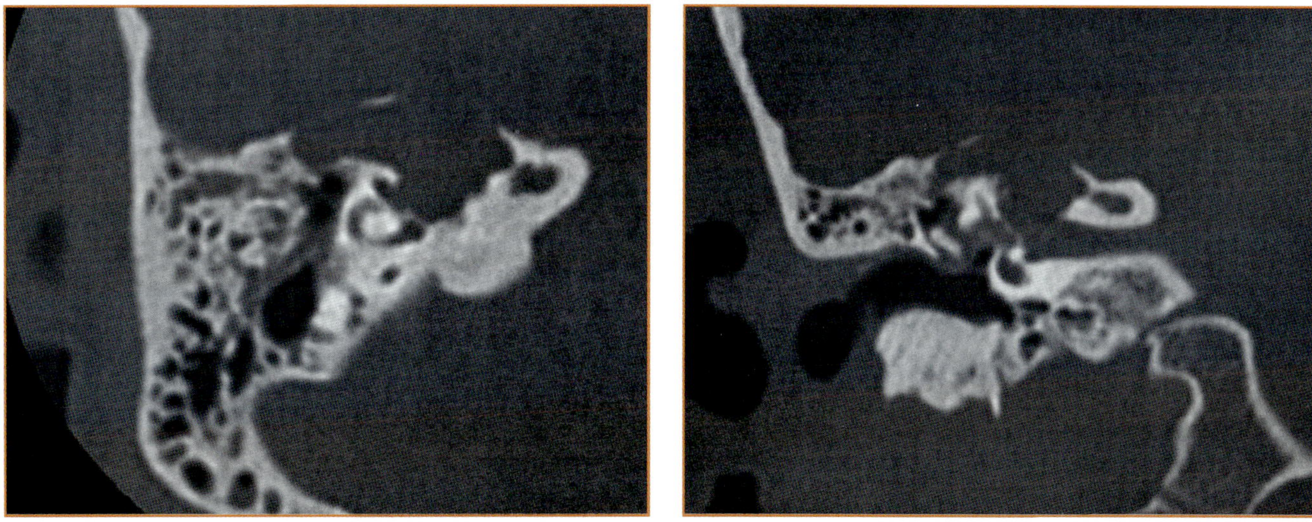

A B

Figure 6–7. CT temporal bones. **A.** Axial view. **B.** Coronal view. Expansile lesion in the right petrous apex with extension toward the IAC and labyrinthine portion of the VII nerve, with significant bony erosion.

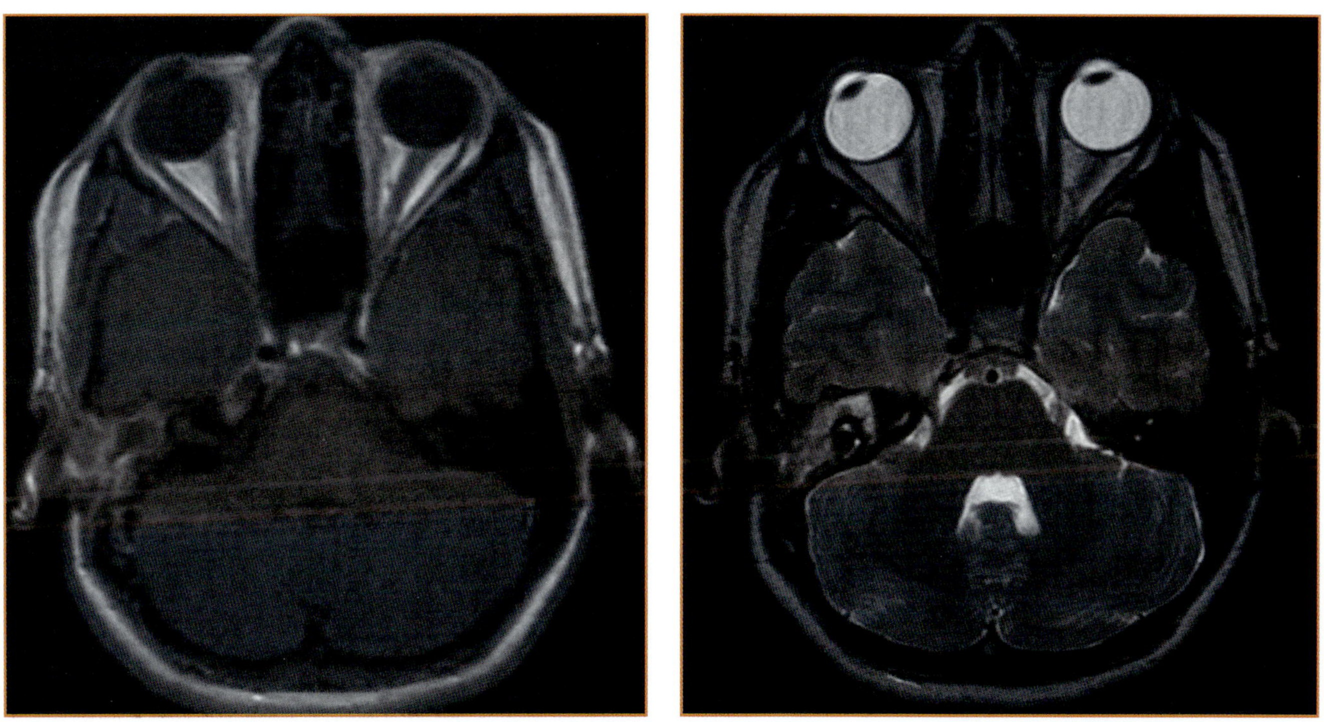

A B

Figure 6–8. MRI brain. **A.** T1-weighted images. **B.** T2-weighted images. The lesion in the right petrous apex was less intense on T1-weighted images and more intense on T2-weighted images, supporting the diagnosis of cholesteatoma.

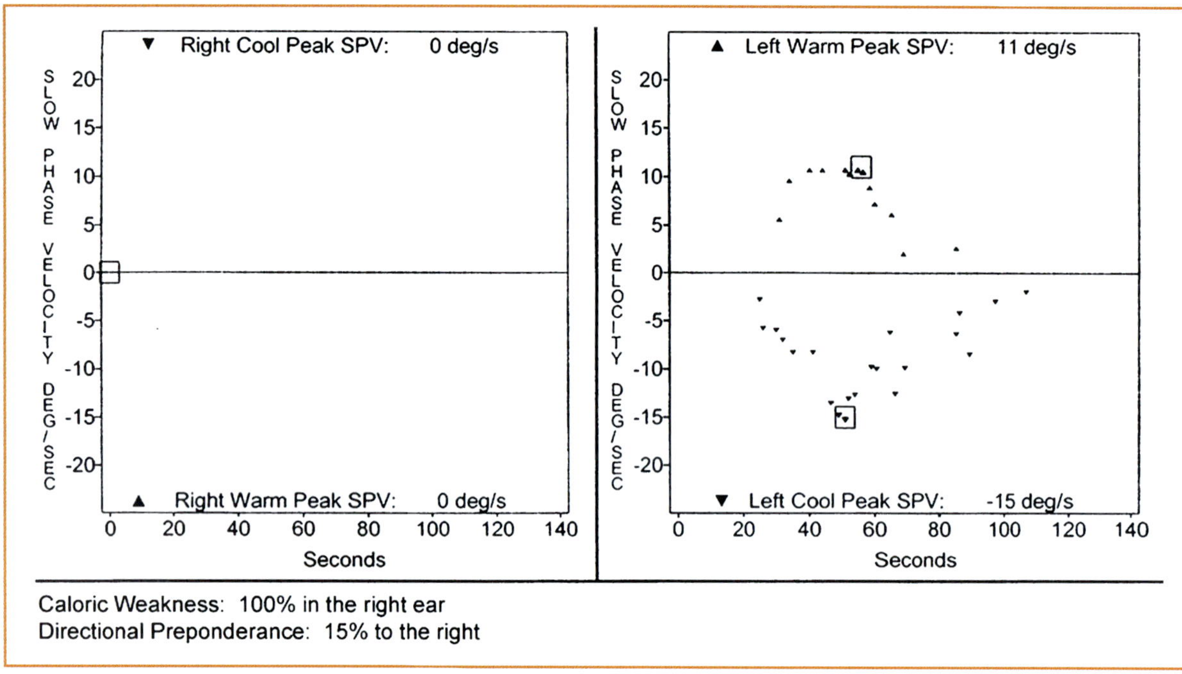

Figure 6–9. ENG shows 100% unilateral weakness on the right ear to bithermal caloric irrigation.

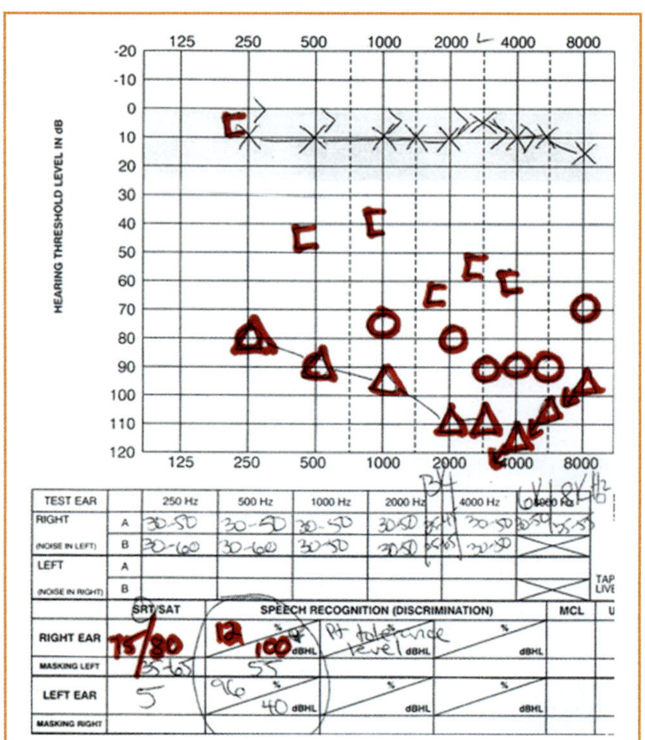

Figure 6–10. The postoperative audiogram showed that little useful hearing remained on the right.

SUMMARY

Though rare in general otolaryngologic practice, lesions of the petrous apex should be recognized and diagnosed. Of the large body of possible lesions presented in the above text, several are by far more common than all of the others combined.

The more common lesions to be distinguished include cholesterol granuloma versus cholesteatoma (epidermoid) versus mucocele (the first entity being 10x and 40x more commonly found than the succeeding two, respectively) versus discrete metastatic disease from several malignancies that favor hematogenous spread to the temporal bone versus an aneurysm of the petrous carotid artery. The first 2 items are by far the major entities that should be distinguished preoperatively.

The history, physical examination, audiometric and radiologic evaluation of the patient presenting with a lesion of the petrous apex has been reviewed. Above all, the co-operation of a skilled neuroradiologist is essential to help clinch the diagnosis prior to surgery.

The rare medical and more commonly performed surgical treatments of lesions of the petrous apex have been described. The surgical approach to lesions of the petrous apex is determined by the nature of the complaint, the age and overall health of the patient, the amount of residual hearing, and the anatomical extent of the lesion. Cystic lesions should be drained to a nearby aerated structure. Solid lesions may be excised or rarely treated with stereotactic radiation. The common surgical approaches to lesions of the petrous apex have been reviewed.

Surveillance for lesions of the petrous apex must be planned according to the age of the patient and the nature of the lesion. It is the rare patient who will be "cured" and in whom follow-up will eventually cease. For the majority of patients, the disease process will be rendered less potentially aggressive, whether by medical care, excision, or drainage, so that clinical and radiographic follow-up at regular intervals will determine the future course of treatment.

REFERENCES

1. Chole RA. Petrous apicitis: surgical anatomy. *Ann Otol Rhinol Laryngol.* 1985;94:251–257.
2. Curtin HD, Som PM. The petrous apex. *Otolaryngol Clin North Am.* 1995;28(3):473–496.
3. Brackmann DE, Toh EH. Surgical management of petrous apex cholesterol granulomas. *Otol Neurotol.* 2002;23:529–533.
4. Isaacson B, Katz W, Roland PS. Lesions of the petrous apex: diagnosis and management. *Otolaryngol Clin North Am.* 2007;40:479–519.
5. Haberkamp TJ. Surgical anatomy of the transtemporal approaches to the petrous apex. *Am J Otol.* 1997;18:501–506.
6. Manasse P. Über Granulationsgeschwulste mit Fremdkörperzellen. *Virch Arch.* 1894;136:245.
7. Miglets AW, Booth JB. Cholesterol granuloma presenting as an isolated middle ear tumor. *Laryngoscope.* 1981;91:410–415.
8. Beaumont GD. Cholesterol granuloma. *J Otol Soc Austral.* 1967;2:28–35.
9. Friedman I. Epidermoid granuloma and cholesterol granuloma. *Ann Otol Rhinol Laryngol.* 1959;58:57–79.
10. Sadé J, Teitz A. Cholesterol and cholesteatoma. *Acta Otolaryngol.* 1983;95:547–553.
11. Jackler RK, Cho M. A new theory to explain the genesis of petrous apex cholesterol granuloma. *Otol Neurotol.* 2003;24:96–106.
12. Pfister MH, Jackler RK, Kunda L. Aggressiveness in cholesterol granuloma of the temporal bone may be determined by the vigor of its blood source. *Otol Neurotol.* 2007;28:232–235.
13. Muckle RP, DelaCruz A, Lo WM. Petrous apex lesions. *Am J Otol.* 1998;19:219–225.
14. Moore KR, Fischbein NJ, Harnsberger HJ, et al. Petrous apex cephaloceles. *Am J Neuro Radiol.* 2001;22:1867–1871.
15. Isaacson B, Cocker NJ, Vrabec JT, Toshor D, Oghalai JS. Invasive cerebrospinal fluid cysts and cephaloceles of the petrous apex. *Otol Neurotol.* 2006;27:1131–1141.
16. Gradenigo G. Sulla leptomeningite circoscritta e sulla paralisi dell' abducente diodigine otica. *Gior Accad Med Torino.* 1904;10:59.
17. Profant HJ. Gradenigo's syndrome. *Arch Otolaryngol.* 1931;13:347–378.
18. Kearns DB, Coker NJ, Pitcock JK, et al. Tuberculous petrous apicitis. *Arch Otolaryngol Head Neck Surg.* 1985;111:406.
19. Toulmouche MA. Observations d'otorhee cérérebrale suivis des reflections. *Gazette Med Paris.* 1838;6:422–426.
20. Chandler JR. Malignant external otitis and osteomyelitis of the base of the skull. *Am J Otol.* 1989;10:108.
21. Linstrom CJ, Lucente FE, Joseph EM. Infections of the external ear. In: *Head and Neck Surgery, Otolaryngology, Vol II.* Byron Bailey, ed. New York, NY: Lippincott Williams & Wilkins; 2001:1711–1724.
22. Gacek RR. Diagnosis and management of primary tumors of the petrous apex. *Ann Otol Rhinol Laryngol.* 1975;84(suppl 18):1–20.
23. Nager GT. *Mesencgymal Neoplastic Processes in Pathology of the Ear and Temporal Bone.* Baltimore, MD: Williams & Wilkins; 1993;448–482.
24. Bataskis JG. *Tumors of the Head and Neck.* Baltimore, MD: Williams & Wilkins; 1979;347–348.
25. Muckle RP, DelaCruz A, Lo WM. Petrous apex lesions. *Am J Otol.* 1998;19:219–225.
26. Jackler RK, Parker DA. Radiographic differential diagnosis of petrous apex lesions. *Am J Otol.* 1992;13:561.
27. Flood L, Kemink J. Surgery in lesions of the petrous apex. *Otol Clin North Am.* 1994;17:565–575.
28. House WF. Surgical exposure of the internal auditory canal and its contents through the middle cranial fossa. *Laryngoscope.* 1961;71:1363–1385.
29. Cristant L, Puchner MA. A keyhole middle fossa approach to large cholesterol granulomas of the petrous apex. *Surg Neurol.* 2000;53:64–71.
30. Mawson SR. Complications of otitis media. In: Ladman H, ed. *Mayson's Diseases of the Ear.* Baltimore, MD: Williams & Wilkins; 1963:347–352.
31. Giddings NA, Brackmann DE, Kwartler JA. Transcanal infracochlear approach to the petrous apex. *Otolaryngol Head Neck Surg.* 1991;104:29–36.
32. Gherini SG, Brackmann DE, Lo WW, et al. Cholesterol granuloma of the petrous apex. *Laryngoscope.* 1985;95:659–664.

33. Graham MD, Kemink JL, Latack JT, Kartush JM. The giant cholesterol cyst of the petrous apex: a distinct clinical entity. *Laryngoscope*. 1985;95:1401–1406.
34. Linstrom CJ, McClure TC, Gamache FW, Saint-Louis LA. Bilateral cholesterol granuloma of the petrous apices: case report and review. *Am J Otol*. 1987;10:393–401.
35. Fisch U. Infratemporal fossa approach to tumors of the temporal bone and base of skull. *J Laryngol Otol*. 1978; 92:949–967.
36. Ramadier J. Exploration de la pointe du rocher par la voie du canal carotidien. *Ann Otolaryngol*. 1933;4:422–444.
37. Lempert J. Complete apicectomy (mastoidotympanoapicectomy). *Arch Otolaryngol Head Neck Surg*. 1937;5:144–147.
38. Cushing H. In: Matson DD, German WJ, eds. *Selected Papers on Neurosurgery*. New Haven, CT: Yale University Press; 1969.
39. Guiot G. *Adénomes hypophysaires*. Paris: Masson: 1958; 165–178.
40. Hardy J. Trans-sphenoidal surgery of the pituitary fossa tumors with televised radiofluoroscopic control. *J Neurosurgery*. 1959;23:612–619.
41. Hardy J. Transphenoidal hypophysectomy. *J Neurosurgery*. 1971;34:582–594.
42. Gray WC, et al. Cholesterol granuloma of the petrous apex and sphenoid sinus: a case report. *Neurosurgery*. 1985;17:67–69.
43. Montgomery WW. Cystic lesions of the petrous apex: transsphenoidal approach. *Ann Otol* 1977;8:429–435.
44. House WF. Surgery of the skull base: transcochlear approach to the petrous apex and clivus. *Otolaryngol*. 1978;86:770–779.
45. Fisch U, Mattox D. *Subtotal Petrosectomy in Microsurgery of the Skull Base*. New York, NY: Thieme; 1988:22–32.

CHAPTER 7

Petroclival Tumors

Wayne Shaia, Sean Wise, and Seilesh Babu

INTRODUCTION

Petroclival tumors can be difficult intracranial tumors to manage clinically and surgically. With the recognized role for conservative management, the accuracy achieved with stereotactic radiosurgery, and the development of new microsurgical approaches, the optimal treatment strategy for petroclival tumors can be challenging for both clinician and patient.

Petroclival tumors are lesions that arise from the upper two-thirds of the clivus, at the petroclival junction, and medial to the trigeminal nerve.[1] Tumors that arise from the lower third of the clivus are more accurately described as foramen magnum lesions, and the approach and management may vary. Similarly, tumors that develop lateral to the trigeminal nerve are best classified as petrosal lesions since their involvement with the clivus is minimal.[2] Petroclival tumors may involve more than one region of the skull base, often extending into both the middle and posterior fossae. Surgical extirpation of such lesions may require combined surgical approaches. These tumors may also displace the brainstem posteriorly. Access to these areas requires the team expertise of both neurotologist and neurosurgeon.

A variety of lesions may originate in the petroclival region, including benign and malignant tumors. Meningiomas are the most common benign tumor of the petroclival region. These are followed by chordomas and schwannomas. Malignancies are rare in the skull base with chondrosarcoma being the most common.[3]

The difficult location of petroclival lesions and the frequency with which they involve both cranial nerves and arterial supply (basilar artery) can create surgical challenges. Mortality rates following resection of petroclival meningiomas approached 50% in some early reports.[4,5] More recently, with advances in microsurgery, endoscopic techniques, and radiation therapy, surgical mortality rates as low as 0 to 2% have been reported.[6,7] The success of surgery in these tumors is dependent on tumor size, their precise location and extent of involvement of the skull base.

Commonly used surgical approaches for these tumors include fronto-orbito-zygomatic, preauricular, subtemporal, retromastoid, retrosigmoid, and suprameatal approaches. Rarely, a translabyrinthine or transcochlear approach is utilized. The optimal approach is most often determined by extension of the tumor into the middle or posterior fossa and cavernous sinus involvement.[8] As previously mentioned, such tumors often require a combined approach.

CLINICAL PRESENTATION

Patients with lesions in the petroclival junction may present with a variety of symptoms. These may include vague symptoms such as headaches, gait disturbances, dizziness, and somatosensory complaints.[9] More specific cranial nerve deficits may occur resulting in visual disturbances, diplopia, and dysphagia. Facial paralysis as a presenting sign was once reported as high as 57%, but now presents in only 10 to 15%.[10] This is most likely due to an improved ability to detect and treat these lesions at an earlier stage. On occasion, tumors in this location may exhibit significant growth prior to the development of symptoms (Figure 7–1).

MENINGIOMAS

Meningiomas are slow growing, benign tumors that can present in the petroclival region. Symptoms typically develop as they become large enough to impinge upon surrounding structures. In a study of the natural history of petroclival meningiomas, Van Havenbergh et al[11] found that symptoms may arise as early as 2 months prior to tumor detection, whereas other tumors may take as long as 10 years to detect and diagnosis. In this series, mean symptom to detection time approached two years.[11] In a review of 21 patients with petroclival meningiomas, 61% exhibited cranial nerve deficits at presentation. These most commonly included deficits in the VIIIth (33%), VIth (28%), Vth (14%), and VIIth (14%) cranial nerves.[12]

Petroclival meningiomas exhibit a female predominance in a ratio of 3:1. Mean presentation occurs between the age of 45 to 53 years old.[13,14] Tumor size at presentation may vary considerably, with tumors less than 2 cm seen in 20%, 2 to 4 cm in 40%, and the remainder presenting at greater than 4 cm.[12,14]

Meningiomas of the clival region are no different from meningiomas that occur in other regions of the skull base. They are benign neoplasms that arise from the dura, and histopathologic findings often include the presence of psammoma bodies (calcifications). Those tumors found in the upper one-third of the clivus are thought to arise from the fusion of the sphenoid and occipital bones (sphenoid-occipital synchondrosis), and tend to grow laterally.[15]

On MRI, these tumors are isointense with brain on T1-weighted imaging, and will enhance brightly following the administration of gadolinium (Figure 7–2). If surgical resection is planned, angiography may be warranted to determine involvement of the cavernous sinus, carotid artery, or basilar artery.

Surgical approaches usually require wide exposure. However, there have been reports of "keyhole" craniotomies to resect these tumors. In one study,

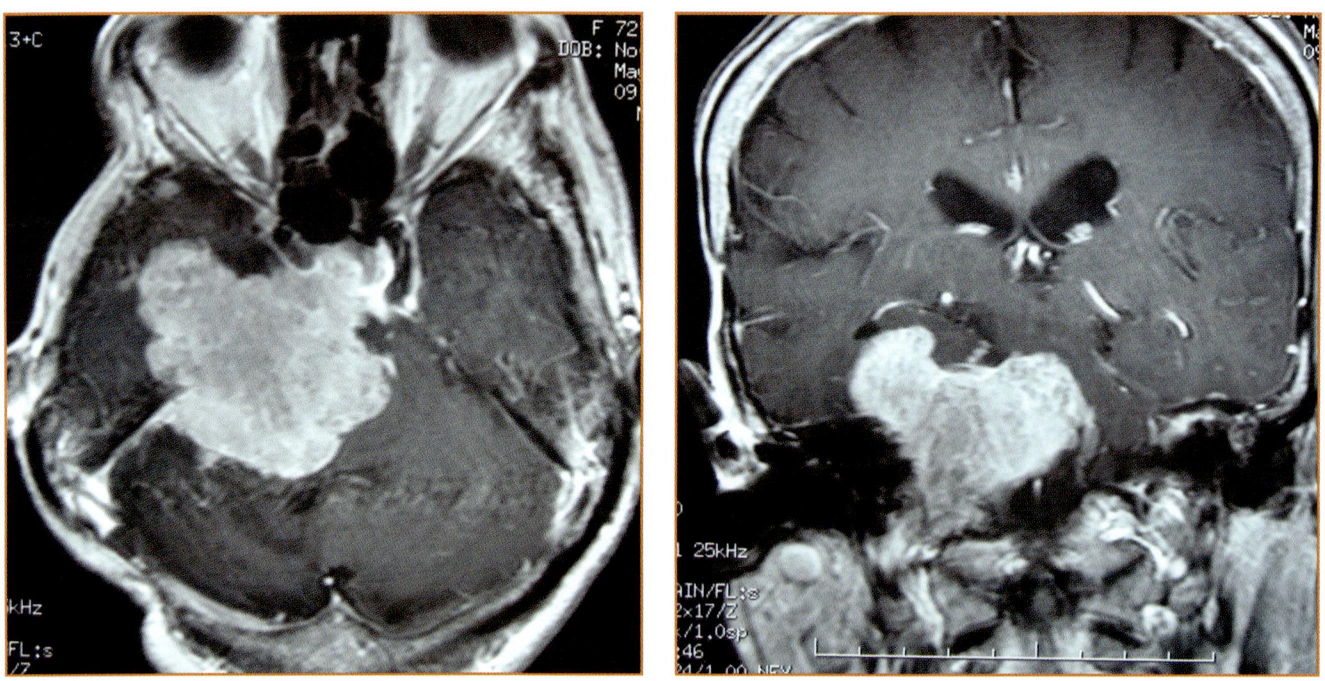

A B

Figure 7–1. A. Axial image of MRI showing a large right petroclival lesion that was not symptomatic until significant in size. **B.** Coronal view of MRI and lesion.

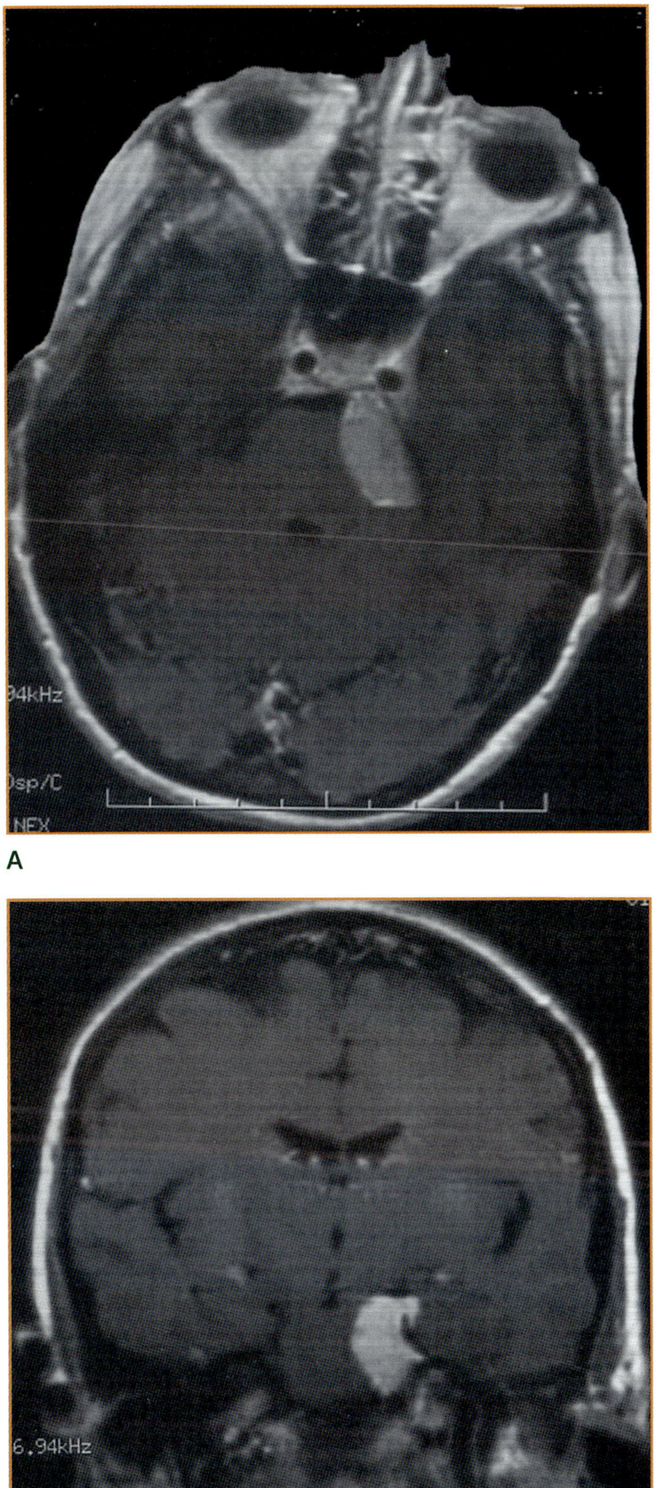

A

B

Figure 7–2. A. Axial image of MRI showing left petroclival meningioma. **B.** Coronal view on MRI.

25 petroclival tumors ranging from 2 to 7 cm were removed using this minimally invasive approach. Almost 60% of patients achieved total resection with minimal cranial nerve deficits.[16] The risk of significant complications, such as disruption of the cavernous sinus, must be weighed against the benefits of such minimally invasive approaches. In addition to the risk of intracranial hemorrhage, other risks to consider with cavernous sinus involvement include the risk of cranial nerve deficits, development of diabetes insipidus (DI), carotid artery injury, as well as an increased risk of incomplete tumor resection. Preoperative tumor size is the most important factor in the determination of morbidity risk. Patients with large tumors are at 13 times greater risk of functional deterioration when compared to patients with small- or medium-sized petroclival tumors.[17] Significant blood supply from the basilar artery is another important factor in the determination of outcome. Patients in this category had a 4.4 times greater risk of permanent functional deterioration following resection.[17]

CHORDOMAS

Chordomas are rare tumors that develop from ectopic notochordal remnants along the neuraxis. As primary intracranial neoplasms, they constitute only 0.2% of all CNS tumors. Chordomas most commonly occur in the sacral region, with the clivus being the next most common location. These tumors, unlike petroclival meningiomas, are twice as prevalent in men. Intracranial chordomas present in a much younger age group than chordomas in other areas of the spinal axis, primarily as a result of their frequent presentation with cranial neuropathies.[18]

With CT imaging, chordomas will typically exhibit multiple areas of decreased attenuation within the clival bone. These tumors possess variable amounts of mucin-containing physaliferous cells, resulting in varying levels of signal intensity on imaging. Chordomas are expansile tumors, and are frequently destructive to the surrounding bone. On MRI, they appear hypointense on T1-weighted images and hyperintense on T2-weighted images, and enhance with the addition of gadolinium.

Chordomas may vary in their histopathologic appearance. The typical chordoma will exhibit the pathognomonic physaliferous cell, or "bubble" cell. These cells contain varying amounts of mucin. Typical chordomas are benign appearing tumors with few mitotic features and pleomorphism. A chondroid type of chordoma contains cartilage and tumor cells in small lacunae. Such changes may be reflected in the radiographic appearance of the tumor, and will commonly prompt additional diagnostic considerations to include entities such as chondrosarcoma, or even ependymoma.[19]

Although they are benign tumors, chordomas are locally aggressive and often behave in a malignant manner. Their recurrence rate is high and survival is low. When compared directly to chondrosarcomas, it has been shown that patients with chondrosarcoma display longer disease free intervals and exhibit better overall survival than equally matched patients with chordomas.[20]

CRANIOPHARYNGIOMA

Craniopharyngiomas can occur in the petroclival region as well. This benign, congenital neoplasm is a derivative of the craniopharyngeal duct (Rathke's pouch). These tumors are benign, but have a malignant behavior, much like chordomas. Craniopharyngiomas present as a single, large cyst or multiple cysts filled with a turbid, proteinaceous material containing cholesterol crystals that appears grossly like "crank-case" oil. Histologically, craniopharyngiomas exhibit palisading epithelial cells that mimic embryonic dental tissue. Calcifications may be seen within the tumor.[21]

Craniopharyngiomas present in a bimodal fashion. They commonly present in children under 15 years of age (40%), with a second increased peak incidence seen in adults in their mid-fifties. Both groups demonstrate an equal male to female ratio. The clinical presentation of patients with craniopharyngiomas is similar to other tumors of the clival region. Presentation with symptoms of increased intracranial pressure is common. Most children present with headache and vomiting that may be accompanied by visual complaints. Endocrine abnormalities may also be present, including diabetes insipidus or hypothyroidism.

MRI is the optimal imaging modality for craniopharyngiomas. On T1-weighted images, the tumor will appear as a hypointense, cystic lesion which enhances with gadolinium. On T2-weighted images, these tumors will be hyperintense.

Total excision is the goal for any surgical extirpation procedure for lesions within the clival region. This holds true for craniopharyngiomas as well. However, associated deficits that occur with aggressive tumor resection may leave significant morbidity that needs to be considered in management decisions as quality of life may be significantly affected.

RADIOTHERAPY

The application of stereotactic radiation in the treatment of petroclival lesions has recently been described with good reported success. At the present time, stereotactic radiosurgery is most commonly employed in the treatment residual or recurrent tumors. In a 1998 study, Subach et al[18] highlighted the utility and limitations of Gamma Knife surgery in 62 residual or recurrent petroclival meningiomas. More details on radiotherapy are covered in Chapter 10.

SURGICAL APPROACHES

The complex anatomy of this region necessitates a thorough and complete knowledge of the vital structures and their relationships. Complete resection may prove difficult because of the location of the tumor anterior to the brainstem, the involvement of cranial nerves, or by the encasement of the vertebral-basilar arteries and their branches. The decision regarding the most optimal surgical approach to facilitate adequate exposure of the tumor and posterior fossa requires careful analysis. Visualization of the lesion and surrounding structures provided by each type of approach must be carefully weighed against the associated potential complications.

Prior to any surgical procedure to access the petroclival region, characterization with interventional radiology is strongly recommended. Angiography can demonstrate vascular relationships that surpass the quality of MRI and CT imaging. Intravascular embolization can also diminish the risk of intraoperative bleeding, decrease surgical time, and may allow for more complete tumor extirpation.

Many approaches to the petroclival region have been described. Unfortunately, the nomenclature is variable depending on the discipline presenting the approach. In addition, strict categorization of the optimal approach has remained elusive.. Numerous attempts have been made to simplify the recognized approaches, and to clearly define their associated risks and benefits. It is generally recommended that the surgical team proceed with the approach that is most familiar to them in order to reduce postoperative morbidity and mortality.

The surgical approaches for petroclival tumors may best be divided into two major categories: anterior midline approaches and lateral approaches, as shown in Table 7–1.

ANTERIOR MIDLINE APPROACHES

Transpalatal Approach

The transpalatal approach is ideal for midline lesions of the middle and lower two-thirds of the clivus. Access as low as the third cervical vertebra (C3) is achievable. With this approach, preoperative antibiotics and tracheostomy are necessary. Mouth guards made from dental impressions are additionally required prior to hard and soft palatal incisions. The mucoperiosteum of the hard palate is reflected and the greater palatine neurovascular bundle is preserved. The hard and soft palate are split and held in place with sutures. The vomer is identified and removed which exposes the basisphenoid area. The posterior median pharyngeal raphe is then identified and sectioned as dissection proceeds through the constrictor muscles and buccopharyngeal fascia. The prevertebral fascia is identified and sectioned, and the longus colli muscles are reflected to expose the caudal half of the basiocciput, or clivus. Dissection then proceeds through the anterior longitudinal and occipital ligaments. A drill is then used to remove any bone overlying the tumor. The dura is opened and the tumor removed. Care must be taken to close the defect in a watertight fashion.

Table 7–1. Approaches to the Petroclival Region

Anterior Midline Approaches
Transpalatal approach
Le Fort I Osteotomy approach
Lateral Approaches
Combined transpetrosal
Retrolabyrinthine, translabyrinthine, or transcochlear approach
Retrosigmoid approach
Extended Middle fossa approach
Cranio-Orbital-Zygomatic (COZ) approach

Le Fort I Approach

If the lesion is midline and more superior, a Le Fort I osteotomy approach may be necessary to achieve surgical exposure. This also allows exposure laterally to the occipital condyles and anteriorly to the pterygoid fossa. Inferiorly, this approach extends down to the C1 level.

A sublabial incision is made and the nasal septum is disarticulated from the maxillary crest. A Le Fort I osteotomy is then made and the hard palate is down fractured. The clivus is now accessible. The osteotomies are reconstructed with titanium plates, and normal eating may resume on the first postoperative day. Disadvantages of this approach include possible malocclusion and trigeminal (V2) numbness. Cosmesis is preserved and postoperative pain is minimal.

LATERAL APPROACHES

Lateral approaches are more frequently utilized as masses in the clival region commonly exhibit lateral extension from the midline. Terminology differs slightly in the neurosurgical and neurotologic literature, so some clarification is necessary. Petrosectomy, or transpetrosal approaches imply that some degree of the petrous portion of the temporal bone is resected. Anterior and posterior petrosectomy are described, and are based on the relationship to the internal auditory canal. Such bone removal allows maximal surgical exposure while minimizing brain retraction. The posterior petrosectomy includes the retrolabyrinthine, translabyrinthine, and transcochlear approaches, and provides access to the posterior cranial fossa. When combined with a far-lateral or subtemporal approach, the entire cranial base from the foramen magnum to the clivus may be visualized. The anterior petrosectomy includes dissection in Kawase's triangle to allow access from the middle cranial fossa when combined with a subtemporal craniotomy.

Before selection of the approach is made, careful examination of the preoperative MR imaging and audiometric evaluation is required. Small petroclival lesions can generally be resected via the anterior petrosal approach (or middle cranial fossa approach). Larger tumors that extend below the internal auditory canal will require a posterior petrosal approach. Tumors extending across the midline of the clivus, or into the anterior cavernous sinus, will most commonly require a combined petrosal approach. Patients with large tumors and profound hearing loss may benefit from the extended exposure provided by a complete petrosectomy (transcochlear approach).

Combined Petrosal Approach

The combined transpetrosal approach is the workhorse for tumors of the clival region. It combines the advantages of a transtemporal (transmastoid) approach with a subtemporal craniotomy. The combination of approaches can further extend the exposure, taking advantage of the benefits of each individual approach. Without the middle fossa approach, access to the petroclival area is limited by the tentorium and petrous apex. Without the posterior approach, the posterior fossa and inferior clival exposure is limited by the petrous bone. With the combined petrosal approach, superior petroclival exposure is obtained from the extended middle fossa approach, while the more inferior clival and posterior fossa exposure is obtained from one of the various posterior approaches. The posterior petrosal approaches additionally allow for minimal cerebellar retraction for tumor exposure.

The degree of anterior extension of the lesion will determine how much of the temporal bone needs to be removed to provide adequate exposure. This determination generally dictates whether the retrolabyrithine, translabyrinthine, or transcochlear approach is most appropriate. Each approach carries different implications with respect to expected deficits of hearing and risk of facial nerve injury. The retrolabyrinthine approach allows limited access to the clivus, whereas the transcochlear approach allows the surgeon to access areas of the mid- and upper clivus while requiring mobilization of the facial nerve.

Surgical Technique

The patient is placed in a supine position with a shoulder roll to allow rotation of their head towards the opposite shoulder with the zygomatic arch elevated. Extreme rotation and flexion can cause venous congestion and engorgement, and must be avoided. Facial, acoustic, and somatosensory evoked potential monitoring is performed.

A large postauricular incision is made approximately 6 cm behind the ear on the affected side (Figure 7–3). The superficial temporal artery is preserved on the muscle layer. The skin is reflected anteriorly along with the temporal fascia to preserve the frontal branch of the facial nerve. The zygomatic arch is cut anteriorly and posteriorly, and the temporalis muscle is reflected inferiorly to allow for the subtemporal craniotomy (middle cranial fossa craniotomy). The bone flap is made along the floor of the middle fossa and crosses the sphenoid wing. A mastoidectomy is performed. Depending on the location of the tumor and the need for anterior exposure, the inner ear structures may need to be sacrificed. If the labyrinth needs removal, this is performed in a similar fashion to translabyrinthine acoustic neuroma resection. If a transcochlear approach is necessary, the facial nerve is identified and its bony covering carefully removed to allow mobilization of the nerve. This approach does allow greater visibility of the clival region, and may be necessary for complete resection

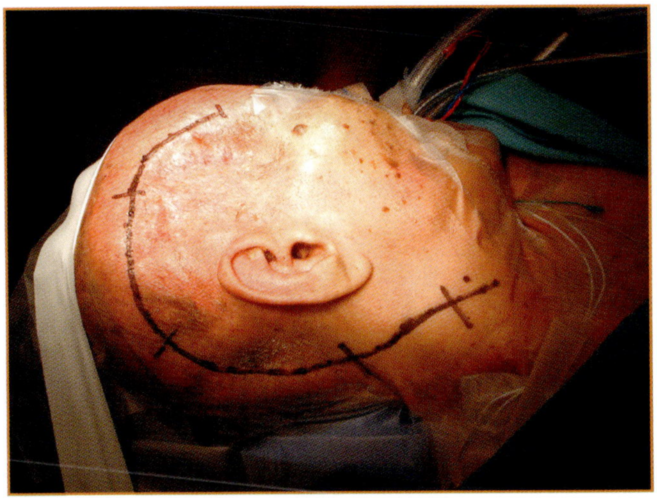

Figure 7–3. Intraoperative photograph of right head and neck prepped for transpetrosal combined approach. Incision is marked as a large C in order to gain complete access to the petroclival region.

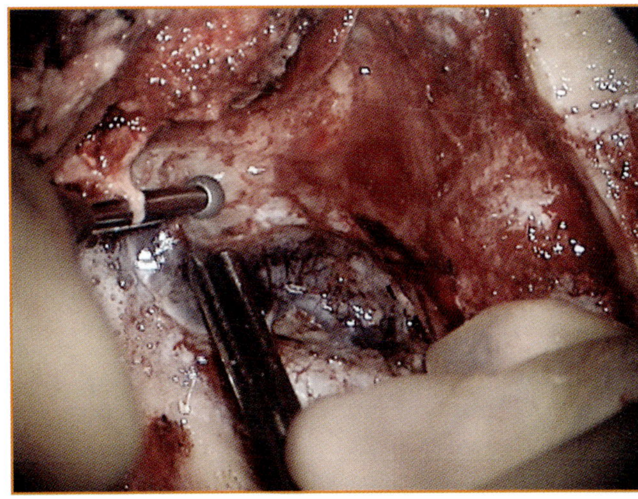

Figure 7–4. Intraoperative photograph of left combined approach with sigmoid sinus being decompressed from the inferior jugular bulb (*left side of picture*) and the superior transverse sinus (*right side of picture*).

of clival lesions. With such an approach, the external auditory canal is oversewn and watertight closure is performed.

The sigmoid sinus is widely decompressed from the transverse sinus to the jugular bulb to allow unimpeded posterior retraction (Figure 7–4). The sigmoid sinus is tethered at the tentorium and the superior petrosal sinus, which need to be carefully transected. A retrosigmoid craniotomy may be added to allow greater decompression of the sigmoid sinus. Transection of the sigmoid sinus has been described to allow sufficient exposure for resection of petroclival meningiomas, but this is usually not necessary and risks the possibility of venous outflow issues. The anatomy of the vein of Labbé plays a critical role in the posterior petrosal approach. Anatomical variations of the vein exist which include its potential insertion into the superior petrosal sinus in the tentorium before the transverse-sigmoid sinus junction. During dural opening, the insertion of the vein must be inspected to ensure that the incision across the tentorium is made anterior to this insertion.

The dura mater incision is extended anteriorly along the floor of the middle fossa. The tentorium is incised anteriorly to the incisura, posterior to the trochlear nerve insertion, and is connected with a tentorial cut paralleling the superior petrosal sinus. With this exposure, the tumor can be approached through the petrous bone anterior and posterior to the labyrinth and middle ear apparatus (Figure 7–5).

The combined petrosal approach is optimal for patients with large petroclival tumors who have serviceable hearing (utilizing the retrolabyrinthine approach). This exposure takes advantage of the benefits of both anterior and posterior petrosal approaches, while preserving hearing.

Retrosigmoid Approach

The retrosigmoid approach is a limited approach when used solely for the purpose of gaining access to the clival region. This approach works well when the tumor lies infratentorially and laterally. Such an approach will typically allow biopsy, diagnosis, and surgical debulking. Its advantages include shorter operative time and a lower risk of postoperative cerebrospinal fluid leak. The disadvantages are the small opening and limited view of the clivus, the lack of supratentorial exposure, and an increased risk to

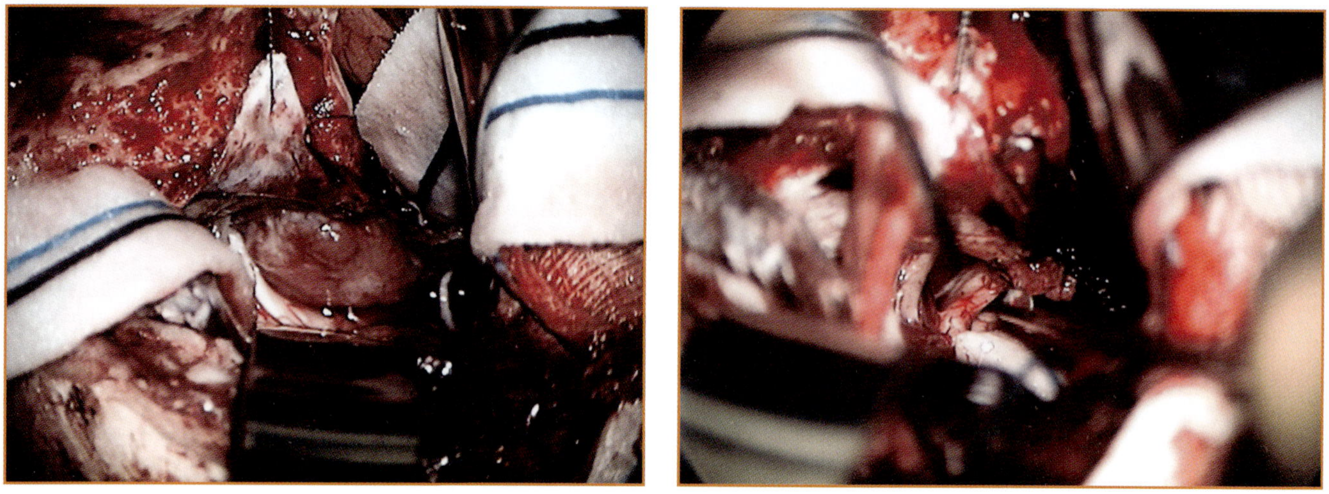

A B

Figure 7–5. Intraoperative photograph of left combined approach with tentorial incisions made and connecting posterior and middle fossa. **A.** Tumor is seen in the center of the picture. **B.** Tumor has been removed and the trigeminal nerve is seen free of disease.

the trochlear nerve (CN IV) when supratentorial extension is required. The retrosigmoid approach can be enhanced with removal of the occipital condyle to improve exposure anterior to the brainstem. The mid-clivus can also be exposed by this approach by drilling a presigmoid extension. Alternatively, the sigmoid sinus may be isolated and sectioned.[14]

Extended Middle Fossa Approaches (Anterior Petrosectomy)

The middle fossa approach is commonly utilized for hearing preservation surgery for acoustic neuromas. The anterior petrosectomy is a middle cranial fossa approach that was initially described as a technique for exposing the cerebellopontine angle and visualizing the brainstem by cutting the tentorium and drilling the petrous apex. It is limited in its ability to expose tumors deeper in the posterior fossa, and requires more manipulation of the trigeminal nerve. With this approach, the fifth cranial nerve is exposed and remains in the center of the surgical field.

This approach can be extended anteriorly to allow access to the ventral pons and the anterior cerebellopontine angle. It can be justified as the correct approach in the removal of medium-sized tumors originating above the internal auditory canal in the anterior petroclival region.

Surgical Technique

The patient is positioned supine with a shoulder roll placed under the ipsilateral shoulder. The head is turned to the contralateral side. A curvilinear incision is made beginning anterior to the tragus at the level of the zygomatic arch, and is continued behind the hairline to the midline, approximately 8 cm in length. The superficial and deep layers of the temporal fascia are elevated with the skin flap to protect the frontal branch of the facial nerve. The zygomatic arch is cut anteriorly and posteriorly, and the temporalis muscle is elevated and retracted inferiorly. A craniotomy is made along the floor of the middle fossa with two-thirds of the bone plate anterior to the external auditory canal. The dura mater is elevated from the floor of the middle fossa until the middle meningeal artery is encountered at the foramen spinosum. This is coagulated and cut. The greater superficial petrosal nerve is dissected in a posterior to anterior direction to prevent injury to the facial nerve.

Bone is then removed in Kawase's triangle medial to the carotid, exposing the posterior fossa dura anterior to the internal auditory canal down to the inferior petrosal sinus. The petrous apex is drilled away from the internal auditory canal anteriorly to the petroclival junction, taking care to prevent injury to the cochlea. If necessary, bone can be removed off the horizontal carotid canal creating less need for temporal lobe retraction.

Once the bone removal has been completed, the dura is opened and the tentorium is divided. When dividing the tentorium, the superior petrosal sinus is initially encountered and is ligated. The tentorium is then divided to the incisura just posterior to the dural entrance of the trochlear nerve. Care is taken to identify the trochlear nerve at the tentorial edge as it enters the dura. Dural incisions are then made along the internal auditory canal and continued along the bony edge of the petrous apex. The dura of the middle fossa above the superior aspect of the petrosal bone and the tentorium, and over the trigeminal nerve, is resected. This exposes the site of the anterior petrosectomy and the trigeminal nerve. The cavernous sinus can be identified as well, depending on extent of the tumor. The dura is further elevated, and the mandibular division of the trigeminal nerve (V3) is identified in the foramen ovale. Meckel's cave and the gasserian ganglion are identified. Tumor may then be carefully dissected away from these structures, towards the petrous apex and the petroclival junction. Tumor debulking may be undertaken once the adjacent cranial nerves have been identified and protected.

Disadvantages of this approach include extended operative time, limited exposure of posterior fossa contents, risk to the abducens nerve in Dorello's canal, and risks associated with significant temporal lobe retraction. Advantages include the potential for hearing preservation, lack of a need for facial nerve re-routing, and no brainstem retraction.

CRANIO-ORBITAL-ZYGOMATIC (COZ) APPROACH

The cranio-orbito-zygomatic (COZ) approach has become popular over the past several decades as a neurosurgical procedure of choice to gain access to a wide range of tumors. The approach maximizes the surgeon's operative advantage by providing wide tumor exposure with multiple angles of view. Less brain retraction is necessary than with other approaches described, thereby decreasing the potential for associated morbidity. Further details of this approach can be found in the neurosurgical literature.

SUMMARY

Petroclival lesions are uncommon. Treatment for patients with mild symptoms may sometimes include simple observation. Radiosurgery may be considered if adequate decompression cannot be accomplished, or for regrowth following subtotal resection. Surgery is generally indicated in patients with worsening symptoms of brainstem dysfunction, and in younger patients with cranial nerve deficits.

Surgical treatment of these lesions requires expertise in the fields of otology and neurosurgery to ensure adequate resection while minimizing injury to critical structures. Access to petroclival tumors may require lateral skull base approaches with petrous temporal bone resection for improved exposure. The extent of temporal bone resection required for adequate exposure depends on many factors. Anterior, posterior, and combined petrous bone resections must be tailored to the individual clinical scenario. Appropriate surgical treatment of these lesions requires that the surgeon be comfortable with all of the possible skull base approaches.

REFERENCES

1. Al Mefty O, Smith R. Clival and petroclival meningioma. In: Al Mefty O, ed. *Meningioma*. New York, NY: Raven Press; 1991: 517–538.
2. Couldwell WT, Fukushima T, Giannotta SL, Weiss MH. Petroclival meningiomas: surgical experience in 109 cases. *J Neurosurg*. 1996;84:20–28.
3. Goel A. Chordoma and chondrosarcoma: relationship to the internal carotid artery. *Acta Neurochir (Wien)*. 1995; 133:30–35.
4. Goel A. Extended lateral subtemporal approach for petroclival meningiomas: report of experience with 24 cases. *Br J Neurosurg*. 1999;13:270–275.

5. Hakuba A, Nishimura S, Jang BJ. A combined retroauricular and preauricular transpetrosal-transtentorial approach to clivus meningiomas. *Surg Neurol.* 1988;30: 108–116.
6. Kawase T, Shiobara R, Ohira T, Toya S. Developmental patterns and characteristic symptoms of petroclival meningiomas. *Neurol Med Chir (Tokyo).* 1996;36:1–6.
7. Kawase T, Shiobara R, Toya S. Anterior transpetrosal-transtentorial approach for sphenopetroclival meningiomas: surgical method and results in 10 patients. *Neurosurgery.* 1991;28:869–875; discussion 875–866.
8. Malis L. Surgical resection of tumors of the skull-base. In: Wilkins RH, Rengachary S, eds. *Neurosurgery. Vol 1.* New York, NY: McGraw-Hill; 1985:1011–1021.
9. Mayberg MR, Symon L. Meningiomas of the clivus and apical petrous bone. Report of 35 cases. *J Neurosurg.* 1986;65:160–167.
10. Petty AM, Kun LE, Meyer GA. Radiation therapy for incompletely resected meningiomas. *J Neurosurg.* 1985; 62:502–507.
11. Van Havenbergh T, Carvalho G, Tatagiba M, Plets C, Samii M. Natural history of petroclival meningiomas. *Neurosurgery.* 2003;52(1):55–62.
12. Pomeranz S, Umansky F, Elidan J, Ashkenazi E, Valarezo A, Shalit M. Giant cranial base tumours. *Acta Neurochir (Wien).* 1994;129:121–126.
13. Samii M, Ammirati M, Mahran A, Bini W, Sepehrnia A. Surgery of petroclival meningiomas: report of 24 cases. *Neurosurgery.* 1989;24:12–17.
14. Samii M, Tatagiba M, Carvalho GA. Retrosigmoid intradural suprameatal approach to Meckel's cave and the middle fossa: surgical technique and outcome. *J Neurosurg.* 2000;92:235–241.
15. Sekhar LN, Jannetta PJ, Burkhart LE, Janosky JE. Meningiomas involving the clivus: a six-year experience with 41 patients. *Neurosurgery.* 1990;27:764–781; discussion 781.
16. Sekhar LN, Schramm VL, Jr., Jones NF, et al. Operative exposure and management of the petrous and upper cervical internal carotid artery. *Neurosurgery.* 1986;19:967–982.
17. Spetzler RF, Daspit CP, Pappas CT. The combined supra- and infratentorial approach for lesions of the petrous and clival regions: experience with 46 cases. *J Neurosurg.* 1992;76:588–599.
18. Subach BR, Lunsford LD, Kondziolka D, Maitz AH, Flickinger JC. Management of petroclival meningiomas by stereotactic radiosurgery. *Neurosurgery.* 1998;42:437–443; discussion 443–435.
19. Taylor BW Jr, Marcus RB Jr, Friedman WA, Ballinger WE Jr, Million RR. The meningioma controversy: postoperative radiation therapy. *Int J Radiat Oncol Biol Phys.* 1988;15:299–304.
20. Weber AL, Liebsch NJ, Sanchez R, Sweriduk ST Jr. Chordomas of the skull base. Radiologic and clinical evaluation. *Neuroimaging Clin North Am.* 1994;4:515–527.
21. Yasargil M, Moratra R, Curcic M. Meningiomas of basal posterior fossa. In: H K, ed. *Advances and Technical Standard in Neurosurgery. Vol 7.* New York, NY (Wien): Springer-Verlag; 1980:115.

CHAPTER 8

Temporal Bone Malignancy

John Zappia, Matthew Kircher, and Seilesh Babu

INTRODUCTION

Fortunately, malignancies of the temporal bone are rare. These tumors are mostly of epithelial origin, arising from the external auditory canal and middle ear. Tumors of nonepithelial origin, tumors extending from adjacent areas and metastatic lesions also occur. Temporal bone malignancies tend to be aggressive, difficult to diagnose, and sometimes difficult to treat. These factors, along with the frequent delay in diagnosis and the complex temporal bone anatomy, generally result in a poor prognosis. These unusual tumors and their treatment options are discussed in this chapter.

TUMOR TYPES

Most tumors involving the temporal bone are of epithelial origin with squamous cell carcinoma representing over 80% of the total and basal cell carcinoma being much less prevalent.[1] Adenocarcinoma and adenoid cystic carcinoma occur significantly less frequently. Although relatively rare, rhabdomyosarcoma is the most common malignancy of the temporal bone in children. Overall, about 10% of all rhabdomyosarcomas involve the temporal bone. Additional tumors arising in this area include chondrosarcoma, melanoma, Ewing's tumor, fibroxanthoma, and verrucous carcinoma. Tumors such as meningiomas, chordomas, parotid malignancies, and nasopharyngeal carcinomas may spread to the temporal bone from contiguous sites. Metastatic carcinoma to the temporal bone presents similarly to primary tumors and, although rare, must be considered. Primary sites include breast, lung, kidney and prostate. Squamous cell carcinoma treatment will be discussed in detail as it is the most common lesion and the treatment considerations are representative of most of the other tumors in this region.

ETIOLOGY

Although the true cause of primary temporal bone malignancies is unknown, chronic irritation may play a role. Squamous cell carcinoma appears to be associated with chronic otitis externa and chronic suppurative otitis media. The resultant chronic inflammation may lead to squamous metaplasia and thus predispose some to temporal bone malignancy. Human papillomavirus (HPV) has been implicated in squamous cell carcinomas of the middle ear.[2] Radiation exposure after treatment of other nearby sites (ie, nasopharynx) has been implicated in temporal bone cancer and carries a poor prognosis for these patients.[3]

ANATOMY OF TEMPORAL BONE

Several relevant points regarding the anatomy deserve review in considering malignancies of the temporal bone and its treatment. The fissures of Santorini are small defects in the anterior cartilaginous external auditory canal (EAC) wall adjacent to the parotid region. Within the bony portion of the inferior EAC is the foramen of Huschke, which is a defect of the tympanic ring. The critical vascular structures within or adjacent to the temporal bone include the internal carotid artery, jugular bulb, sigmoid sinus, and cavernous sinus. Important neural structures in assessing these lesions include the cochleovestibular, facial, trigeminal, and chorda tympani nerves. The lymphatic drainage of the EAC is to the postauricular nodes posteriorly, the internal jugular and upper cervical nodes inferiorly, and the parotid and preauricular nodes anteriorly. The middle ear and mastoid tend to drain deep into the retropharyngeal and deep upper jugular lymph nodes.

TUMOR SPREAD

Direct extension is common and problematic in and around the temporal bone with its close population of important structures. Although these generally aggressive tumors can grow in any direction, there are some patterns that are important. The fissures of Santorini predispose to spread anterior to the EAC into the parotid region. Spread outside the inferior EAC is facilitated by the foramen of Huschke. The bony-cartilaginous junction is a weak barrier and a source of direct access to the area around the parotid gland. There are few barriers to a lesion in the lateral EAC. Most commonly the cancer will extend anteriorly from the EAC to the parotid gland and less likely to the temporomandibular joint. Tumor may spread from the EAC medially through the tympanic membrane to the middle ear, otic capsule, carotid canal, or petrous apex. Posteriorly, it may extend into the mastoid bone and involve the facial nerve or sigmoid sinus. Superiorly, the tumor may spread into the middle fossa and inferiorly into the jugular foramen.[4] Squamous cell carcinoma has a strong predisposition for perineural spread. As a result of its intimate position in the temporal bone, the facial nerve is most commonly involved.[5]

Spread to the lymph nodes is uncommon but tends to follow the routes defined by the anatomy above. The first nodes that tend to become involved, however, are in the periparotid area. Hematogenous spread from the temporal bone to distant sites is rare. Mortality is most often due to locoregional disease/recurrence.

CLINICAL PRESENTATION

Signs and symptoms of temporal bone malignancy can mimic other disease processes and require a keen sense of suspicion to make the diagnosis. Patients are usually elderly with symptoms of chronic otalgia and bloody otorrhea that have been present for some time, usually years. Patients with otalgia may require further evaluations such as imaging and nasopharyngoscopy in order to diagnose occult disease including malignancey. Patients may have a conductive hearing loss as well. Failed treatment with topical and systemic antibiotics with continued complaints usually occurs. Presentation with facial or other cranial nerve weakness is an ominous sign.[6]

Physical examination usually reveals a bleeding mass in the ear canal with a conductive hearing loss. A periparotid or neck mass may also be palpable, which raises the suspicion as well. A thorough head and neck exam, including all cranial nerves should be performed.

DIAGNOSIS

The most accurate way to determine the type of lesion is with a biopsy. Open biopsy of the primary lesion can usually be done in the office. If the diagnosis continues to be uncertain, then a deeper biopsy needs to be performed in the operating room for patient comfort. Needle biopsy can be performed for any possible neck mass or parotid lesion.

Computed tomography (CT) of the temporal bones and neck should be obtained to evaluate for involvement or erosion of the adjacent bony structures. Magnetic resonance imaging (MRI), which is particularly good for looking at soft tissue, will show spread along soft tissue planes and involvement of neurovascular structures. Preoperative planning may include angiography to assess carotid artery involvement.

For advanced lesions where carotid sacrifice may be a consideration, some have advocated preoperative carotid balloon occlusion testing for evaluation of the flow through the vertebrobasilar and contralateral carotid artery systems. Carotid sacrifice can result in significant morbidity and may not affect survival; therefore some no longer perform arteriography with balloon occlusions especially because this investigation in itself is not without risk.[7] Consultation with a neurosurgeon may be necessary if involvement of the dura is suspected.

Metastatic work up should be done with CBC, liver profile, chest x-ray, and CT of chest, abdomen, and/or pelvis if warranted. Preoperative audiogram should be done to assess the hearing of the contralateral ear.

STAGING

There is no standard staging system for cancers of the temporal bone. Squamous cell carcinoma may be staged by a system proposed by the University of Pittsburgh has been shown useful and has gained support in the literature.[8,9] This staging system is shown in Table 8–1.

Table 8–1. Staging System Proposed by University of Pittsburgh for Tumors of Temporal Bone

T1	Tumor limited to the EAC without bony erosion or evidence of soft tissue involvement
T2	Tumor with limited EAC bone erosion (not full thickness) with limited (<0.5 cm) soft tissue involvement
T3	Tumor eroding the osseous EAC (full thickness) with limited (<0.5 cm) soft tissue involvement or tumor involving the middle ear, mastoid, or both
T4	Tumor eroding the cochlea, petrous apex, medial wall of the middle ear, carotid canal, or jugular foramen of dura; or with extensive soft tissue involvement (>0.5 cm), such as involvement of the temporomandibular joint or stylomastoid foramen; or with evidence of facial paresis
Nodal involvement and stage can be classified as it is for other cancers of the head and neck:	
• N1—Single ipsilateral lymph node, size less than 3 cm • N2—Single ipsilateral node, size 3–6 cm • N2b—Multiple ipsilateral nodes, all less than 6 cm • N2c—Bilateral or contralateral nodes, all less than 6 cm • N3—Nodes involved greater than 6 cm	
Cancer is staged as follows:	
• Stage 0—Tis N0 M0 • Stage I—T1 N0 M0 • Stage II—T2 N0 M0 • Stage III—T3 N0 M0, T1 N1 M0, T2 N1 M0, T3 N1 M0 • Stage IV—T4 N0 M0, T4 N1 M0, any T N2 M0, any T N3 M0, any T any N M1	

MANAGEMENT OF TEMPORAL BONE CARCINOMA

Medical Therapy

Radiotherapy as a sole modality has not been shown to be effective for this disease process. Surgery with postoperative radiation is indicated in stage T3, T4, and some aggressive T2 lesions.[10] The temporal bone and neck should be treated with 50 to 60 Gy for tumors staged T3 and T4.[11] Good coverage with vascularized tissue in the surgical defect is required if postoperative radiation is planned in order to reduce the risk of osteoradionecrosis.

Chemotherapy may be indicated in patients with residual disease, T4 tumors, and in metastatic disease. A combination of cisplatin with 5-fluorouricil may be the best chemotherapeutic treatment. One report showed that use of 5-fluorouricil after tumor resection improved 5-year survival rate to 74%. Some of these were extensive lesions, but many of these tumors were T1 and T2 lesions.[12]

Surgical Therapy

Surgical intervention is the treatment of choice for patients who are medically stable and who have tumors that are felt to be resectable. The goal of surgery is complete eradication of the cancer with negative margins and preservation of neurovascular structures as this provides the greatest chance of cure. When this is not possible, surgery may still have a role in palliation and quality of life but will not likely affect survival. Options for surgery include sleeve resection, lateral temporal bone resection, subtotal temporal bone resection, and total temporal bone resection. Usually a parotidectomy and selective neck dissection are indicated as well. Advanced tumors with intracranial invasion have a grave prognosis, and aggressive resection does not seem to improve survival.

Surgical Procedures: Management of the Primary Site

Lateral Temporal Bone Resection

The lateral temporal bone resection (LTBR) is a procedure that can be performed for direct therapeutic effect in resecting tumors of the external auditory canal. Depending on the size, location, invasion, and nature of tumor, the lateral temporal bone resection can be combined with partial or total auriculectomy, parotidectomy, and/or neck dissections to provide appropriate complete surgical extirpation of neoplastic disease. This resection is performed when the tumor involves the external auditory canal and extends to, but not beyond, the tympanic membrane. The lateral margin depends on the extent of spread. The otic capsule and facial nerve are preserved. The LTBR is appropriate for T1 and T2 tumors.[13] In cases where the tumor has extended beyond the bony confines of the external auditory canal or through the tympanic membrane and involving the mesotympanum or mastoid air cells, a subtotal or total temporal bone resection is indicated.

A postauricular incision is made and carried forward to transect the external auditory meatus. In cases in which partial or total auriculectomy are to be performed, the corresponding degrees of auricular resection are included within the incision. If a meatus is to be preserved, the meatal skin is everted and oversewn in two layers to create a blind meatal pouch. Care must be taken to remove all of the epithelium in order to prevent cholesteatoma formation medial to a closed-off meatus.

A wide mastoidectomy is performed and the sigmoid sinus skeletonized. The posterior wall of the external auditory canal is thinned in preparation for later resection. The incus is identified within the fossa incudis. An extended facial recess is performed, from the fossa incudis downward, transecting the iter chordae posterius and into the tympanic ring inferiorly. The incudostapedial joint is carefully separated to minimize vibrational trauma to the intact stapes, and the incus is removed.

The inferior tympanic ring is resected anterior to the fallopian canal and followed forward to the anterior canal wall. Dissection in this area is performed slowly and only using diamond burs, as the caroticojugular spine and great vessels are directly medial to the dissection plane along the inferior tympanic ring. The dissection plane along the inferior tympanic ring must be maintained medial to the tympanic membrane to provide complete resection of the external auditory canal.

The superior limit of the mastoidectomy is extended anteriorly to resect the root of the zygomatic arch, and the superior cortex and air cells are extirpated to fully expose the epitympanic space. The cog (bone that separates the anterior epitympanic recess from the attic proper) is resected and supratubal air cell exposed. The dissection is carried forward from the supratubal air cell until the glenoid fossa is entered. The anterosuperior canal bone is completely separated from the root of the zygoma along the plane of the glenoid fossa. Care should be taken during drilling of the superior cuts, as the petrous carotid artery lies medial to the supratubal air cell and eustachian tube.

Once the superior and inferior cuts are accomplished, the external auditory canal is attached to the temporal bone medially only by the anterior bony annulus. This thin bony attachment is readily fractured by placing firm digital pressure in an anterior direction on the posterior surface of the external auditory canal, which has now been essentially circumferentially skeletonized. After the canal is freed of all bony attachments, the soft tissue attachments anteriorly along the glenoid fossa and parotidomasseteric fascia are carefully incised and the external auditory canal removed en bloc. The extratemporal facial nerve should be identified prior to these soft tissue incisions to prevent injury.

If a superficial or total parotidectomy is to be performed as well, the external auditory canal can be kept attached to the parotidomasseteric fascia, with the parotidectomy performed en bloc with the lateral temporal bone resection.

The external auditory meatus is overclosed. A temporalis muscle flap or other local subcutaneous rotation flap can be used to fill in the bony defect, followed by closure of the postauricular incision in standard fashion.

Subtotal Temporal Bone Resection

The medial limit of dissection in a lateral temporal bone resection is the incudostapedial joint, lateral to which all tissues are resected. When tumor has extended into the middle ear cleft, a subtotal temporal bone dissection is warranted. However, recurrence rates and long-term mortality are significantly increased when tumors have breached this plane and entered the medial temporal bone.

The subtotal temporal bone dissection encompasses all the components of the lateral temporal bone resection with further resection of the bony otic capsule. The remaining anterior petrous apex is preserved. As the lateral temporal bone resection is removed separately from bony extirpation of the otic capsule, the subtotal temporal bone resection is, by necessity, a form of piecemeal oncologic resection. The margins of resection are the sigmoid sinus and posterior fossa dura posteriorly, middle fossa dura superiorly, internal carotid artery anteriorly, jugular bulb inferiorly, and petrous apex medially. Based on the extent of tumor spread, dissection may include the condyle of the mandible, the facial nerve, dura, sigmoid sinus, and contents of the intratemporal fossa. The morbidity of resection of critical structures must be weighed against benefit in terms of improving survival.

Total Temporal Bone Resection

When neoplastic disease has invaded the medial temporal bone and resection beyond the otic capsule is necessary to achieve total tumor resection, a total temporal bone resection is performed. Despite the aggressive nature of the procedure, long-term and disease-free survival following this resection is dismally poor.

The total temporal bone resection involves exactly its namesake: the entire temporal bone is resected. An oncologically sound resection is attempted, but the nature of the temporal bone anatomy makes piecemeal resection the standard. Intratemporal neural and vascular structures are resected when oncologically indicated, often including the facial nerve, cochleovestibular nerve, and lateral sinus/jugular bulb. When the petrous carotid artery is resected, the procedure is sometimes termed a radical temporal bone resection. Involvement of the intrapetrous carotid artery by neoplastic disease portends dismal short term survival and reports prove that resection may cause more morbidity than cure.[14]

Management of Parotid and Neck

Tumors of the EAC and middle ear will spread to the parotid lymph nodes initially as this is the first echelon of nodes draining this region. A superficial parotidectomy should be performed en bloc with the temporal bone for T1 and T2 lesions. If facial nerve involvement is present, a total parotidectomy including the facial nerve may need to be performed.

Neck metastasis is uncommon, but selective neck dissection may be performed as identification and control of the great vessels is usually necessary. However, the presence of metastasis is associated with a poor prognosis, and neck dissection does not improve survival.[15]

Reconstruction of Defect

Large resections will result in soft tissue defects, as well as increase the risk for osteoradionecrosis during radiation therapy. Pedicled muscle flaps or free flaps can be used to reconstruct these defects. The temporalis muscle flap may work for smaller defects. For larger ones, a trapezius or pectoralis flap may be used. The rectus abdominus free flap and radial forearm flap have been used successfully as well.[16] A watertight dural closure is warranted if the dura has been violated.

COMPLICATIONS

Cranial Nerve Injury

Facial nerve paralysis may be present as a result of tumor involvement or may be related to surgery either inadvertently or intentionally depending on the tumor extent and exact procedure performed. In those with facial paralysis, corneal protection is essential and may require a gold weight insertion or tarsorrhaphy. Re-anastamosis or hypoglossal-facial nerve grafting may be considered, but usually not performed in the face of malignancy.

The lower cranial nerves may become involved as well and result in subsequent morbidity. This may result in dysphagia, aspiration, and voice difficulties. This may require feeding assistance (nasogastric tube, percutaneous gastrostomy tube) and procedures to improve the voice and decrease aspiration risk (thyroid medialization).

Cerebrospinal Fluid Leak

Cerebrospinal fluid leak is a potential complication of any skull base procedure when the dura is breached. Good watertight dural closure and postoperative lumbar drain insertion help prevent such occurrence. Antibiotics may become necessary, but prophylaxis does not reduce the risk of developing meningitis.

PROGNOSIS

Prognosis for cancers of the temporal bone is related to the primary site, the histologic type, and the treatment that is initiated.[17] Early stage tumors do well with 90% survival rate.[18] As tumors become more advanced, the survival drops to 50 to 75% despite surgery and radiation therapy[18,19] Larger tumors with cranial nerve, carotid, or intracranial involvement have an even worse survival of 0 to 30%.[20] Positive margins at the time of resection, involvement of neck lymphadenopathy, and dural involvement are associated with poorer prognosis.[21,22]

Prasad et al[23] concluded that limited lesions could be treated with LTBR and additional radiotherapy did not improve survival. Lesions involving the middle ear treated with STBR and radiotherapy did better than either treatment alone. They also noted that involvement of the petrous apex, dura, carotid artery, and brain tissue did not respond do aggressive surgical resection and had a poor prognosis.

SUMMARY

Temporal bone malignancy is rare, and usually presents with minimal symptoms until advanced disease has occurred. Early diagnosis is needed for successful therapy so the clinician needs to have a keen suspicion of this diagnosis. The treatment involves surgical resection, but debate continues regarding optimal treatment for advanced disease. The morbidity of aggressive surgical resection may lead to poorer quality of life without improving ultimate survival.[24] The surgeon needs to understand this and educate the patient as to the limits of surgical resection. Appropriate selection of patients with the most appropriate choice of surgical resection and postoperative radiotherapy may achieve an adequate quality of life with better survival rate. Resection of involved dura mater, involved brain parenchyma, or internal carotid artery is of limited or no clinical improvement.

REFERENCES

1. Morton RP, Stell PH, Derrick PPO. Epidemiology of cancer of the middle ear cleft. *Cancer.* 1984;53:1612–1617.
2. Jin YT, Tsai ST, Li C, et al. Prevalence of human papillomavirus in middle ear carcinoma associated with chronic otitis media. *Am J Pathol.* 1997;150(4):1327–1333.
3. Lustig LR, Jackler RK, Lanser MJ. Radiation-induced tumors of the temporal bone. *Am J Otol.* 1997;18:230–235.
4. Leonetti JP, Smith PG, Kletzker GR, Izquierdo R. Invasion patterns of advanced temporal bone malignancies. *Am J Otol.* 1996;17(3):438–442.
5. Hirsch BE, Chang CYJ. Carcinoma of the temporal bone. In: Myers EN, ed. *Operative Otolaryngology-Head and Neck Surgery.* Philadelphia, PA: WB Saunders; 1997:1434–1458.

6. Arriaga M, Hirsch BE, Kamerer DB, Myers EN. Squamous cell carcinoma of the external auditory meatus (canal). *Otolaryngol Head Neck Surg*. 1989;101(3): 330–337.
7. Gillespie MB, Francis HW, Chee N, Eisele DW. Squamous cell carcinoma of the temporal bone: a radiographic-pathologic correlation. *Arch Otolaryngol Head Neck Surg*. 2001;127(7):803–807.
8. Arriaga M, Curtin HD, Takahashi H, Kamerer DB. The role of preoperative CT scans in staging external auditory meatus carcinoma: radiologic-pathologic correlation study. *Otolaryngol Head Neck Surg*. 1991;105(1):6–11.
9. Hirsch BE. Staging system revision. *Arch Otolaryngol Head Neck Surg*. 2002;128:93–94.
10. Spector JG. Management of temporal bone carcinomas: a therapeutic analysis of two groups of patients and long-term follow-up. *Otolaryngol Head Neck Surg*. 1991; 104(1):58–66.
11. Pemberton LS, Swindell R, Sykes AJ. Primary radical radiotherapy for squamous cell carcinoma of the middle ear and external auditory cana—an historical series. *Clin Oncol (R Coll Radiol)*. 2006;18(5):390–394.
12. Knegt PP, Ah-See KW, Meeuwis CA, et al. Squamous carcinoma of the external auditory canal: a different approach. *Clin Otolaryngol*. 2002;27:183–187.
13. Medina JE, Park AO, Neely JG, Britton BH. Lateral temporal bone resections. *Am J Surg*. 1990;160(4):427–433.
14. Pensak ML, Gleich LL, Gluckman JL, Shumrick KA. Temporal bone carcinoma: contemporary perspectives in the skull base surgical era. *Laryngoscope*. 1996;106: 1234–1237.
15. Moffat DA, Wagstaff SA, Hardy DG. The outcome of radical surgery and postoperative radiotherapy for squamous carcinoma of the temporal bone. *Laryngoscope*. 2005;155(2):341–347.
16. Manolidis S, Pappas D Jr, Von Doersten P, Jackson CG, Glasscock ME 3rd. Temporal bone and lateral skull base malignancy: experience and results with 81 patients. *Am J Otol*. 1998;19(6 suppl):S1–15.
17. Stell PM, McCormick MS. Carcinoma of the external auditory meatus and middle ear. Prognostic factors and a suggested staging system. *J Laryngol Otol*. 1985;99(9):847–850.
18. Kunst H, Lavieille JP, Marres H. Squamous cell carcinoma of the temporal bone: results and management. *Otol Neurotol*. 2008;29(4):549–552.
19. Kuhel WI, Hume CR, Selesnick SH. Cancer of the external auditory canal and temporal bone. *Otolaryngol Clin North Am*. 1996;29:827–852.
20. Nyrop M, Grontved A. Cancer of the external auditory canal. *Arch Otolaryngol Head Neck Surg*. 2002;128:834–837.
21. Moffat DA, Grey P, Ballagh RH, et al. Extended temporal bone resection for squamous cell carcinoma. *Otolaryngol Head Neck Surg*. 1997;116(pt 1):617–623.
22. Austin JR, Stewart KL, Fawzi N: Therapeutic prognosis based on a proposed staging system. *Arch Otolaryngol Head Neck Surg*. 1994;120:1228–1232.
23. Prasad S, Janecka IP. Efficacy of surgical treatments for squamous cell carcinoma of the temporal bone: a literature review. *Otolaryngol Head Neck Surg*. 1994;110(3):270–280.
24. Kwok HC, Morton RP, Chaplin JM, et al. Quality of life after parotid and temporal bone surgery for cancer. *Laryngoscope*. 2002;112:820–823.

CHAPTER 9

Diffuse Osseous Lesions of Temporal Bone

Michael Hoa and Seilesh Babu

INTRODUCTION

Diffuse osseous lesions of the temporal bone are a heterogeneous group of disorders that can represent manifestations of either systemic disease or a focal disease process. The usual clinical presentation of this diverse group of diseases includes hearing loss, progressive stenosis of the external auditory canal (EAC), and cranial nerve dysfunction that occurs as a result of progressive narrowing of skull base foramina and changes to the lateral skull base surface.

SUGGESTED DIAGNOSTIC WORKUP

Although these disease entities are histologically distinct, clinical presentation and conventional radiologic examination often fail to distinguish between them. However, the use of high-resolution computed tomography (HRCT) has enhanced diagnostic differentiation of these clinically similar but histologically diverse groups of diseases.[1] HRCT should be employed with special attention to the external auditory canal, middle ear space, otic capsule, facial nerve, and internal auditory canal.

FIBROUS DYSPLASIA

Fibrous dysplasia (FD) is characterized by progressive replacement of normal bone marrow by a mixture of fibrous tissue and disordered bony trabeculae. Histologically, FD consists of bony trabeculae consisting of immature woven bone with varying amounts of fibrous stroma. Fibrous dysplasia has been classified into three distinct subtypes: monostotic, polyostotic, and McCune-Albright syndrome. Monostotic FD, which accounts for 70% of all cases and is the mildest subtype, manifests as an isolated bony lesion and is typically diagnosed between ages 20 and 30 years.[2] The skull and face are involved in 25% of the cases in monostotic FD.[3] Polyostotic FD, which accounts for approximately 25% of all cases, has an earlier onset, typically in childhood, and more severe skeletal and craniofacial involvement. The skull and face are involved in 50% of the cases in polyostotic FD. McCune-Albright syndrome, which accounts for approximately 5% of cases, is more common among females and is associated with endocrine abnormalities and pigmented cutaneous lesions. In addition, short stature is common due to premature closure of epiphyses. This last type is thought to be a subtype of polyostotic FD, but appears earlier and affects more bones more severely.

In general, there is a female predominance (3:1). Clinical presentation of temporal bone involvement often consists of bulging of the temporal area, EAC stenosis, and hearing loss (conductive, sensorineural or mixed). Prognosis is generally excellent for the monostotic subtype with a poorer prognosis for the polyostotic subtype (although not generally life threatening). Poorer prognosis is noted for McCune-Albright syndrome. Most lesions spontaneously "burn out" or cease to grow by age 20 to 25. Differential diagnosis may include Paget's disease, osteomyelitis of the temporal bone, ossifying fibroma, and giant cell tumors.

With respect to imaging, the best diagnostic clue to this disorder is the appearance of increased bone volume with "ground glass" appearance. Manifestations can be localized or diffuse and lesions themselves may reach many centimeters in size. On HRCT, these lesions can have one of 3 appearances (which relate to relative content of fibrous versus osseous tissues). Pagetoid FD (50%) consists of mixed osseous and fibrous components and appearance on CT may be one of either "ground glass" or mixed sclerotic-cystic appearance (Figure 9–1). Sclerotic FD (25%) consists of predominantly osseous components and density approaches that of cortical bone. Finally, cystic FD (25%) consists of predominantly fibrous components and has a hypodense appearance on CT. This variant is somewhat problematic as malignancy cannot be excluded and biopsy by mastoidectomy is recommended. With respect to disease activity, cystic, pagetoid, and sclerotid FD may represent most active to least active, respectively. In general, middle ear, otic capsule and internal auditory canal stenosis are rare in fibrous dysplasia. Appearance on MRI is often low signal or hypointense on both T1 and T2 images with some occasional patches of high signal on T1 and enhancement with gadolinium which may correlate with areas of increased activity. However, MRI generally should be reserved for unusual cases and not for standard evaluation.

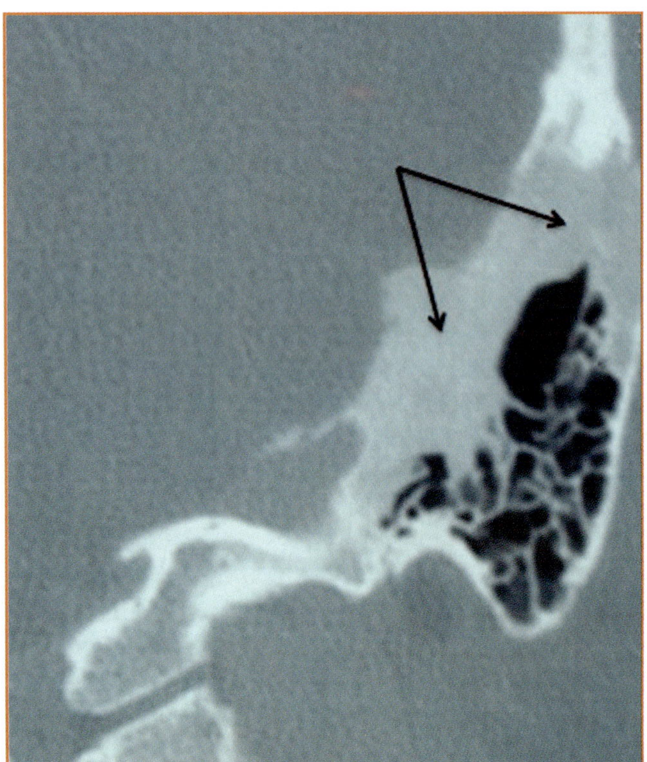

Figure 9–1. Coronal CT image of left temporal bone shows expansile "ground glass" fibrous dysplasia lesions (*arrows*) involving mastoid.

No specific medical therapy exists for fibrous dysplasia. Regular clinical monitoring is essential to assess for progressive external auditory canal stenosis and cranial neuropathy. Treatment is generally targeted towards maintenance of external auditory canal patency to stabilize hearing and prevent complications from entrapped cholesteatoma. Aggressive surgical management is not recommended in most cases and nondisabling surgical interventions are utilized when safe. Radiation therapy is contraindicated due to the risk of malignant degeneration.

OSTEOPETROSIS

Osteopetroses are a group of inheritable metabolic bone disorders characterized by diffuse dense sclerosis and faulty bony remodeling. Histologically, osteopetrotic bone is immature, thick, dense and brittle lending to the names chalk, or marble bone, disease. Classically, two types have been described, autosomal recessive osteopetrosis (AROP) or osteopetrosis congenita and autosomal dominant osteopetrosis (ADOP). AROP is the childhood form that is almost uniformly lethal with death occurring early in the disease process secondary to hemorrhage, anemia, or overwhelming infection. Hepatosplenomegaly and mental retardation usually accompany the autosomal recessive form. ADOP is the adult form and consists of less severe osteopetrosis with two types. The most common type is Type II, otherwise known as Albers-Schönberg disease, which results from a genetic mutation in a chloride channel gene that is highly expressed in osteoclasts and enables acidification of the extracellular environment required for bone breakdown.

Clinically, these patients may be asymptomatic. Some patients with temporal bone involvement may present with conductive hearing loss, which is more common than sensorineural hearing loss, and progressive bilateral hearing loss. Cranial nerves may become involved as compression occurs from the abnormal bony growth causes narrowing. Facial nerve involvement generally presents with acute and recurrent episodes of facial palsy that result in progressive worsening of facial nerve function. With respect to HRCT findings, AROP is notable for generalized density of the entire skull base, sclerotic otic capsule beyond normal bony labyrinth margins, enlarged subarcuate fossa, and a short and trumpet shaped or flared internal auditory canal (Figure 9–2).

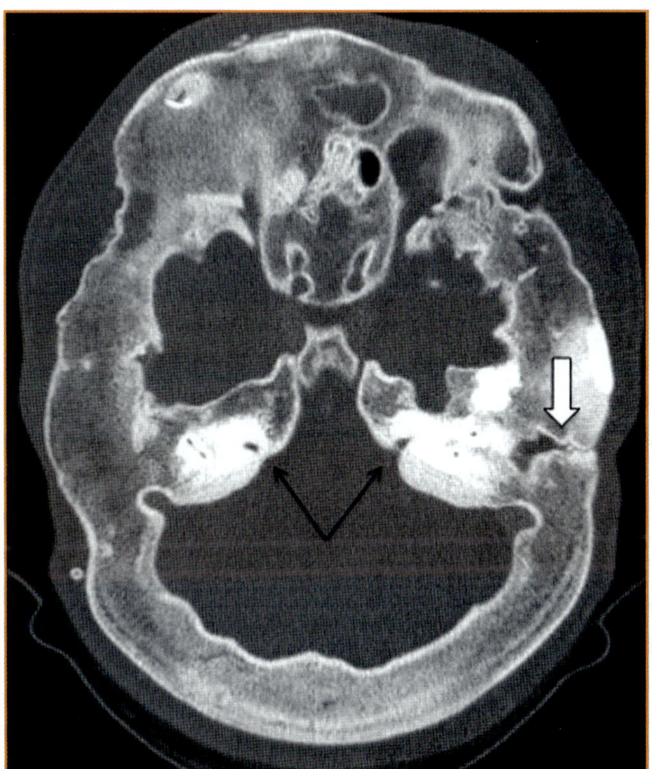

Figure 9–2. Axial CT of skull demonstrating diffuse and extensive sclerosis and thickening of entire skull including the temporal bone. Left external auditory canal is completely obstructed by the thickened bone (*white arrow*). Internal auditory canals are being compressed as well (*black arrows*).

MRA in AROP may reveal petrous internal carotid artery (ICA) compromise. In general, involvement of the EAC, middle ear, otic capsule, and internal auditory canal (IAC) are common. On HRCT, ADOP is manifest by dense sclerosis of the skull base and calvarium in type I and dense sclerosis of the skull base that spares the calvarium in type II.

No effective medical therapy exists and thus, intervention is largely surgical. Interventions may be aimed toward recontouring the external canal to facilitate fitting of amplification devices. Improvement of conductive hearing loss by ossiculoplasty may be technically difficult due to dense middle ear bony disease and footplate abnormalities. Amplification should be considered in these patients. Bone anchored hearing aids may be a consideration, as well. Surgical therapy, particularly facial nerve decompression, appears to be beneficial for facial paralysis in osteopetroses.[4,5] The surgery itself can be technically challenging due to the abnormally thickened bone of the skull and around the facial nerve (Figure 9–3).

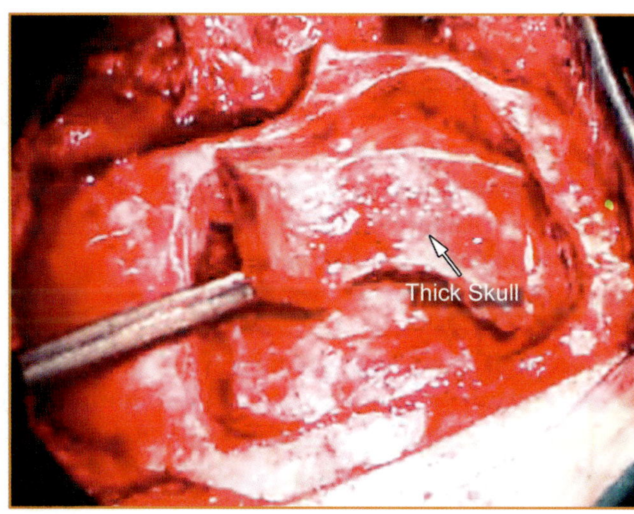

Figure 9–3. Intraoperative picture of patient with osteopetrosis with facial paralysis. Patient underwent total facial nerve decompression. The bone flap was exceedingly thick, as was the bone surrounding the facial nerve. Decompression of the internal auditory canal was performed with significant recovery of facial nerve function.

PAGET'S DISEASE

Paget's disease is a bony dysplasia characterized by excessive remodeling of bone primarily of the axial skeleton. The inheritance pattern is mostly sporadic, yet an autosomal dominance pattern is noted in 15% of cases. The disease tends to occur after the fifth decade. The cause is thought to be viral as suggested by an immune-regulatory defect in chromosome 6 associated with viral inclusions in osteoclasts.

Histologically, alternating waves of osteoclastic and osteoblastic activity result in disorganized bony resorption followed by deposition of structurally weakened, demineralized cancellous bone. Three phases are typically seen. In the early phase, bone resorption predominates, manifesting as lytic lesions. Subsequently, repeated mixed osteoclastic-osteoblastic activity results in the marrow space being filled with fibrovascular tissue. Finally, the sclerotic phase is marked by mosaic pattern of coarse fibers composed of disorganized layers of bone. Monostotic and polyostotic varieties exist. However, primary monostotic involvement of the temporal bone is rare and bilateral temporal bone involvement is common.

These patients most commonly present with bilateral mixed hearing loss (30 to 50%), tinnitus and vertigo (20%). The conductive component is most marked in the lower frequencies, whereas the sensorineural component is most pronounced in the higher frequencies.

The best diagnostic radiologic clues include diffuse thickening of the calvarium and cranial base with "cotton-wool" appearance (demonstrative of the coexistence of osteolysis and sclerosis) and "ground glass" bony changes with thinning of the otic capsule on temporal bone CT (Figure 9–4). Other temporal bone findings on CT include tortuous EAC, middle ear cleft constriction, pagetoid changes to the ossicular chain with increased mass loading, and otic capsule demineralization.

The treatment of symptomatic Paget's disease (bone pain, neuropathies, and cardiovascular stress) with calcitonin and bisphosphonates has been shown to induce biochemical and clinical improvement.[6] Clinical improvement is seen in association with decreasing levels of alkaline phosphatase and urinary hydroxyproline. Alendronate (Fosamax) and pamidronate (Aredia) are used most frequently and will cause an approximately 70% decrease in biochemical markers in one-half of patients.[6] Other bisphosphonates currently approved for treatment of Paget's disease include tiludronate (Skelid), risedronate (Actonel), and etidronate (Didronel). Calcitonin-salmon is available in injectable and nasal-spray forms, but only the injectable form is approved for treatment of Paget's disease by the FDA. Table 9–1 shows FDA approved medications and recommended dosages.[7] Compared to bisphosphonates, calcitonin is not as potent and does not suppress disease activity for as long after cessation. Patients should also receive adequate doses of calcium (1,000 to 1,500 mg per day) and vitamin D (400 IU per day).[7] In general, surgical therapy in Paget's disease should be considered as a last resort when medical therapy has failed. Amplification should strongly be considered as an alternative to middle ear exploration. Persistent symptomatic IAC stenosis with sensorineural hearing loss and facial nerve dysfunction may be an indication for surgical decompression. Importantly, because surgical landmarks can be distorted by the dysplastic process, surgical intervention is quite hazardous, and should be performed with facial nerve monitoring.

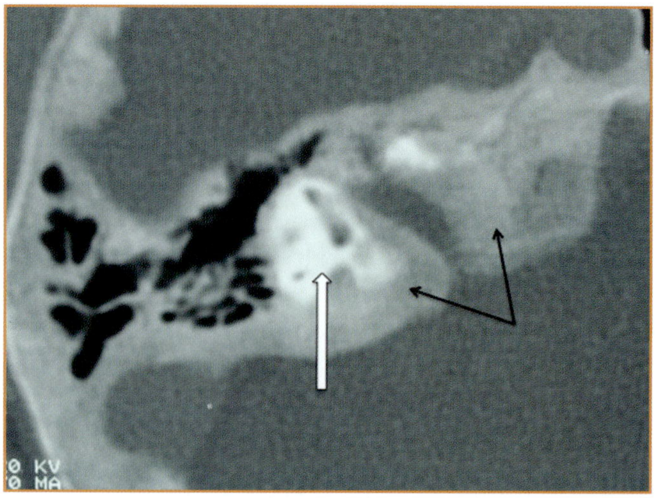

Figure 9–4. Axial CT right temporal bone shows "ground glass" appearance of petrous bone (*black arrows*). Otic capsule demineralization (*white arrow*) also noted.

Table 9–1. List of Approved Medications for the Treatment of Paget's Disease (recommended treatment regimens and dosages are listed)

Medications	Dosage
Alendronate (Fosamax)	40 mg PO once a day for 6 months; may reinstate treatment after 6 months if necessary
Pamidronate (Aredia)	30 mg IV over 4 hours on 3 consecutive days; 60 mg IV over 2 to 4-hour period for 2 or more consecutive or nonconsecutive days
Tiludronate (Skelid)	400 mg PO once a day for 3 months; may reinstate treatment after 3 months if necessary
Risedronate (Actonel)	30 mg PO once a day for 2 months; may reinstate treatment after 2 months if necessary
Etidronate (Didronel)	5 mg per kg per day (if ineffective, then 11 to 20 mg per kg per day for a maximum of 6 months); may reinstate treatment after 3 months if necessary
Calcitonin-salmon	200 U per mL; 100 U subcutaneously or intramuscularly once daily for 6 to 18 months.

LANGERHANS CELL HISTIOCYTOSIS

Langerhans cell histiocytosis (LCH), previously known as histiocytosis X, is a poorly understood non-neoplastic disease that consists of proliferation of Langerhans type histiocytes with variable bone and soft tissue involvement. LCH has been classified into three forms. Unifocal LCH or eosinophilic granuloma is the mildest form which manifests as unifocal osseous lesions of the long bones, skull base and temporal bones often seen in children over 5 years. Hand-Schuller-Christian disease, which has an earlier onset and more severe presentation, consists of the common triad of diabetes insipidus, proptosis, and skeletal involvement. Finally, Letterer-Siwe disease, which has the worst prognosis of the three forms, presents with fulminant disseminated multiorgan disease including liver, spleen, lymphatic, lung, and bone involvement. Common clinical presentation is that of a young male with otalgia, otorrhea, and a postauricular mass.

Histopathology shows histiocyte-like cells with folded nuclei, known as Langerhans cells, which release osteoclastic activating factor and result in eosinophilic infiltration. Characteristic histologic finding are Birbeck granules which represent rod shaped cytoplasmic organelles with striated appearance and a central linear density. Typical temporal bone findings on HRCT include a lytic mastoid bone with "punched out" borders, ossicular and otic capsule destruction.

Typical treatment is surgical curettage or mastoidectomy for localized mastoid-middle ear disease. Low-dose radiotherapy is reserved for larger destructive lesions and systemic disease is treated with chemotherapy in combination with radiation therapy.

SUMMARY

Although diffuse osseous lesions of the temporal bone can have similar presentations, this heterogeneous group of disorders can often be distinguished by recognition of certain imaging features on HRCT along with a thorough history. The accurate differentiation of these diseases allows for appropriate treatment and referrals. In this heterogeneous group of diseases, treatment is generally based on patient symptomatologyo. In summary, accurate and efficient diagnosis of these disorders is essential and close medical follow-up is important for monitoring of disease progression.

REFERENCES

1. Cheung SW, Munck K, Jackler RK. Diffuse osseous lesions of the temporal bone. In: Brackmann DE, Jackler RK, eds. *Neurotology.* 2nd ed. Philadelphia, PA: Mosby; 2005:1125–1133.
2. Lustig LR, Holliday MJ, McCarthy EF, Nager GT. Fibrous dysplasia involving the skull base and temporal bone. *Arch Otolaryngol Head Neck Surg.* 2001;127(10):1239–1247.
3. Schwartz JD. Fibrous Dysplasia, T-Bone. In: Harnsberger R, Hudgins P, Wiggins R, Davidson C, eds. *Diagnostic Imaging: Head and Neck.* Philadelphia, PA: Elsevier; 2005: 202–215.
4. Hamersma H. Osteopetrosis (marble bone disease) of the temporal bone. *Laryngoscope.* 1970;80:1518–1539.
5. Miyamoto RT, House WF, Brackmann DE. Neurotologic manifestations of the osteopetroses. *Arch Otolaryngol.* 1980;106:210–214.
6. Hullar TE, Lustig LR. Paget's disease and fibrous dysplasia. *Otolaryngol Clin North Am.* 2003;36(4):707–732.
7. Delmas PD, Meunier PJ. The management of Paget's disease of the bone. *N Engl J Med.* 1997;336:558–566.

CHAPTER 10

Stereotactic Radiotherapy for Skull Base Lesions

Yoav Hahn, Brent J. Benscoter, and Dennis Bojrab

INTRODUCTION

Stereotactic radiation has become both an alternative and adjunctive treatment to surgery for the management of skull base tumors, including schwannomas, meningiomas, and paragangliomas. Considerable improvements in computer technology and delivery devices have made use of radiation for skull base tumors more common, though the exact understanding of its efficacy is continually evolving. Skilled teams including neurotologists, neurosurgeons, radiation oncologists, and medical physicists work together to accumulate data on techniques and results in order to improve patient outcomes. Long-term results and rates of tumor control in the literature are very favorable for this treatment modality.

HISTORY

The initial radiosurgical concept occurred in 1951. Since then, many studies have assessed the effects of various radiation doses on normal brain tissue. The first patient treated with Gamma Knife radiation was in 1967 for a craniopharyngioma, and thus the era of tumor radiosurgery began. Lars Leksell described the indications and technique of acoustic tumor radiosurgery, as first performed in a patient in 1969.[1] Due to the high morbidity associated with acoustic neuroma surgery at the time, Leksell believed that stereotactic radiosurgery offered a new, safer approach to treatment of these tumors.

Initial treatment planning was based on air or contrast encephalography. The acoustic tumor in each of three patients was originally irradiated with 179 Cobalt-60 radiation beams focused to a single point.[1] Soon thereafter, computed tomography (CT) scanning, metrizamide cisternography, and in some cases, pneumoencephalography were utilized for pre-treatment planning replacing older techniques. In the early days of radiosurgery, many questions were raised regarding the accuracy of targeting with such crude imaging and calculations performed without computers.[2] When radiosurgery was planned with relatively poor quality imaging, developing a radiosurgical plan that fit the tumor margin precisely was difficult to achieve. In addition, early nonsurgical treatment of acoustic neuromas utilized high doses of radiation, with doses at the tumor margin of up to 45 gray.[3]

In the early 1990s, significant improvements in imaging technology led to the evolution of the specialty. The advent of high-resolution stereotactic magnetic resonance imaging (MRI) improved the targeting of acoustic neuroma tumors.[4,5] In addition, the use of multiple isocenters to achieve conformality was now possible because of advances in imaging techniques and treatment planning programs.[6] Finally, improvements in stereotactic imaging, dose planning, and computer technology enhanced stereotactic radiation as a legitimate option in the treatment of skull base tumors.

CONVENTIONAL RADIOTHERAPY

Currently, conventional external beam radiation therapy is seldomly used for tumors of the skull base. Conventional radiation is delivered via a photon beam at 1.5 to 2 gray for 5 days per week over a course of 4 to 6 weeks with a cumulative dose of 40 to 50 gray.[7] Because the radiation preferentially affects dividing cells, a long course of therapy affords the opportunity to affect more cells in the mitotic stage. However, acoustic neuromas have a very low index of mitoses and thus, a small number of cells will enter the mitotic stage during treatment. Several studies have shown that conventional radiation therapy results are clearly poorer than those of surgical excision and stereotactic radiation.[7,8]

Adverse effects associated with treatment often complicate conventional radiotherapy. Conformality is difficult to achieve in this modality, and injury to adjacent healthy tissues is a particular concern. In addition, because of dose limitations of the surrounding or adjacent tissues, some tumors cannot be treated effectively. This is especially true with external beam radiation therapy at the skull base as the brainstem and surrounding neurovascular structures limit dosing and carry increased risk.

STEREOTACTIC RADIATION THERAPY

Stereotactic radiation therapy is the term used to define the method of delivery of a precise dose of high-energy radiation through stereotactically directed narrow beams.[9] Beam shaping and intensity modulation provide flexibility and optimal tumor dosing. Whereas conventional radiotherapy is delivered over weeks, stereotactic radiation is designed to induce necrosis in the irradiated tissue. This occurs in a large dose delivered during a single session (stereotactic radiosurgery) or a few fractions delivered within a short period of time (fractionated stereotactic radiotherapy).

Stereotactic radiation treatment delivers a precise, conformal dose of radiation with isodose lines tailored to the margins of the tumor. Various delivery devices and types of radiation are used including: gamma radiation from a fixed-array of multiple Cobalt-60 sources in a treatment unit, high energy photon radiation from linear accelerators (LINAC) systems which also use wavelike radiation, and heavy particle radiation such as proton beam therapy.

Proton beams provide the best control of penetration depth compared with x-ray or gamma radiation. LINAC systems achieve radiation targeting and rapid dose falloff by rotating the patient and the treatment unit gantry simultaneously. Conversely, Gamma Knife units have 201 fixed Cobalt-60 sources aimed precisely at the focus of the unit. Collimators are used to conform the radiation to the shape of the tumor. Both the Gamma Knife and LINAC systems have been shown to have targeting accuracy in the sub millimeter range.[10] Neither system has consistently shown superior accuracy in targeting lesions, and dose distributions with sharp falloff can be expected for both devices.

Both Gamma Knife and LINAC radiation systems require immobilization of the head during treatment (Table 10–1). To perform accurate fractionated stereotactic radiotherapy, positioning of the patient with respect to the treatment space must be reproducible.[11] Repositioning accuracy within 1 mm is of utmost importance. Head fixation methods include those that are minimally invasive through the use of pins that penetrate the scalp and rest on the skull, and those that are completely noninvasive such as the thermoplastic face mask (Figures 10–1 and 10–2). Invasive frames have been used for stereotactic radiosurgery where accurate reapplication is not necessary. However, fractionated stereotactic treatment plans require a comfortable, noninvasive, precisely relocatable frame.

Based on the limited initial Swedish experience in the 1980s, with some uncertainties in the dosimetry of their early treatment plans, it was believed that minimum tumor doses of 16 to 20 gray were necessary to control acoustic neuromas.[12] Secondary to early postradiation complications in these patients, the marginal dosages of 20 gray have been lowered to approximately 12.5 gray, which is currently administered at most centers. Multiple centers are now collecting important information about hearing, tinnitus, balance, and facial nerve results,

Table 10–1. Characteristics of Gamma Knife and LINAC

	Gamma Knife	LINAC
Sites Treated	Intracranial only	Intracranial and Extracranial
Imaging in System	Not necessary to perform treatment	Yes, in some models only
Immobilization	Frame	Frame and Frameless
SRS Time	30–60 minutes	3–4 hours
SRS	Intracranial	Intracranial and Extracranial
Fractionated Therapy	Yes, in certain circumstances	Yes
Machine Purpose	Intracranial SRS only	Stereotactic Radiosurgery, (SRS), Stereotactic Radiotherapy (SRT)

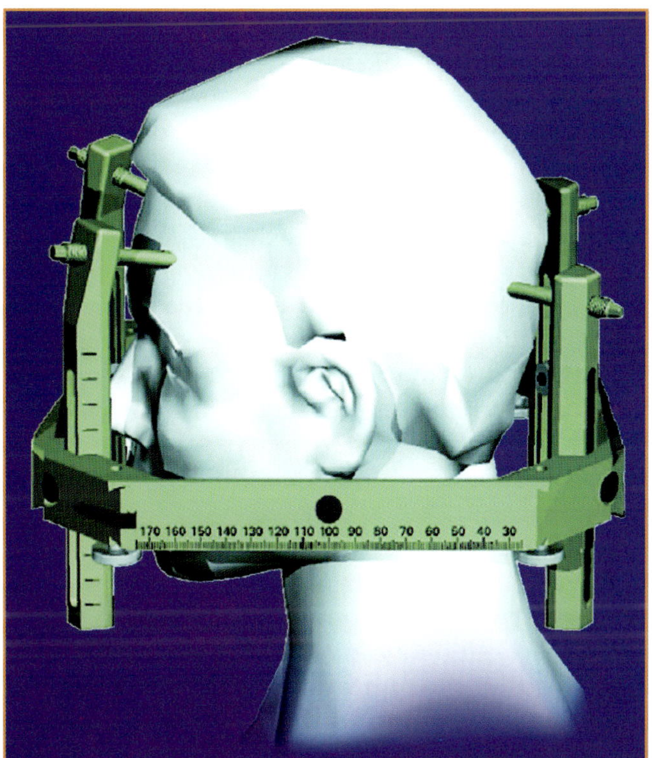

Figure 10–1. Head fixation held in place with pins that penetrate the scalp and rest on the skull.

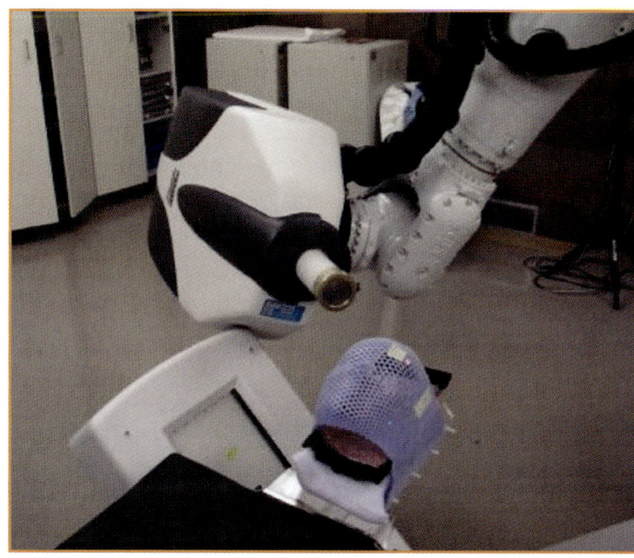

Figure 10–2. Head fixation device that is noninvasive using a thermoplastic face mask.

along with intracranial complication rates. Follow-up data will be necessary for 10 to 20 years to assess control rates with these lower treatment levels.

Fractionated Stereotactic Radiation

Stereotactic radiotherapy uses beams of radiation generated by a linear accelerator aimed directly at a target where a higher radiation dose is administered. This is usually accomplished by designing arcs of radiation that intersect at the target region which has a larger volume than that volume considered ideal for stereotactic radiosurgery. This also has a significant impact upon the volume of normal tissue that is irradiated. Higher total doses can be delivered to the tumor with fractionated therapy because of increased tolerance of the surrounding healthy tissues to each fractionated dose.

Fractionated stereotactic radiotherapy allows the treatment radiation to specifically target a lesion, minimizing the effects to the surrounding healthy tissues. Because noninvasive fixation devices are now available, single-treatment delivery of stereotactic radiation is no longer mandatory. The total dose can be delivered in a fractionated fashion and thus be increased from typical nonfractionated treatment protocols. For acoustic neuromas, 5 to 30 fractionated treatments are typically administered. The main advantage of fractionation is that it allows higher total doses to be delivered to the tumor because of increased tolerance of the surrounding healthy tissues to each individual, smaller fractionated dose.

Fractionated stereotactic radiotherapy techniques developed when several centers using linear accelerator irradiation technology were dissatisfied with the accuracy and results after single fraction stereotactic radiosurgery. To decrease morbidity and potentially improve results, they began delivering radiation over several sessions (fractionation). The goal of this approach is to weaken the effect of each radiation administration and maintain brain or nerve function. Unfortunately, this also weakens the effect of the radiation on the tumor.[13]

The noninvasive fixation options often used for stereotactic radiation include frameless technology utilizing implanted 2-mm gold fiducial markers around the head to provide a coordinate system, and a mask system using mesh. In the frameless systems, the implanted markers are used as a reference frame for localization prior to each radiation treatment, and the computer uses these references to update the treatment plan. Mask systems use a mesh material to create an individual mask molded for each patient that may be held in place with vacuum-attached markers. In assessing reproducible positioning, there is variability noted between treatments using the mask system of up to 2 mm in an uncooperative patient. While this is a small value, vital structures including the labyrinth, facial nerve, and brainstem are within 1 to 2 mm of tumor margins.[14]

Stereotactic Radiosurgery

Stereotactic radiosurgery, not to be confused with stereotactic radiotherapy, is a technique utilizing small beams of radiation accurately directed at a precise, three-dimensionally located target of small volume. This radiation is delivered with a single treatment. The treatment usually involves a high dose of radiation delivered in one fraction from a specially equipped linear accelerator or a specialized unit using multiple Cobalt-60 sources. The method by which the linear accelerator delivers the radiation is either a series of arcs or collimated ports or nodes. This technique limits the radiation dose to the surrounding normal tissue and structures. Thus, much higher doses can be delivered accurately to the tumor, yielding improved control rates and decreased complications. As shown in Table 10–2, there are a variety of devices and associated software used for stereotactic radiosurgery.

Stereotactic radiosurgery is used to treat a variety of malignant and benign conditions for which the endpoints are different. The Gamma Knife (AB Elekta, Stockholm, Sweden) was the first unit designed primarily for the treatment of functional disorders in the early 1950s. The applications were expanded to pituitary tumors and arteriovenous malformations, and evolved to the treatment of acoustic tumors, glomus jugulare tumors, meningiomas, metastases, trigeminal neuralgia, epilepsy, parkinsonism, essential tremor, and other conditions, benign and malignant.

The differential diagnosis for base of skull tumors and cerebellopontine angle tumors includes meningiomas, acoustic neuromas, cranial nerve sheath tumors, and glomus jugulare tumors. Depending on the volume of the tumor, the critical structures surrounding the tumor, and the extent of the damage done by the tumor and/or the surgery, there may be a choice among the options of stereotactic radiosurgery, stereotactic radiotherapy or standard radiation therapy. Tumors or residual tumors, if being considered for stereotactic radiosurgery, should be less than 4 centimeters in any linear dimension. Tumors that are long and thin but constitute a small total volume are not required to fall into the same size guideline. Edema after stereotactic treatment in patients with larger tumors can be significant with inherent

Table 10–2. Devices and Software Used for Stereotactic Radiosurgery

Manufacturer	Radiation Source	Trade Name	Energy Type	Localization Device	Software
Varian	LINAC	NovalisTx RapidArc	X Rays	Frame or Mask	iPlan Eclipse
Siemens	LINAC	Oncor	X Rays	Mask	Oncor
Accuray	LINAC	CyberKnife	X Rays	Laser X Ray	Multiplan
Elekta	LINAC	Axesse	X Rays	X Ray Mask	Pinnacle
Elekta	Co-60	Gamma Knife Perfexion	Photons	Stereotactic Frame	Leksell Gamma Plan
American Radiosurgery	Co-60	RGSVertx360	Photons	Frame	Explorer4D

increased risk. In addition, functional preservation will not be as great in larger tumors undergoing stereotactic radiation.

THE RADIOSURGICAL PROCEDURE

Stereotactic radiosurgery is predominantly performed as a minimally invasive, same day surgical procedure. The decision to perform stereotactic radiosurgery is made based on preoperative images, symptoms, patient options, and patient desires. On the day of the procedure, the patient is brought to the Gamma Knife suite, given a mild sedative, and the Leksell frame is applied using a local anesthetic for the insertion of the pins that fix the frame to the outer table of the skull, as shown in Figure 10–1. Placement of the head frame establishes both a reference frame with a coordinate system for target determination and a means of precise patient positioning. The patient is imaged with CT and/or magnetic resonance imaging (MRI) and rests while the images are imported into the treatment-planning computer.

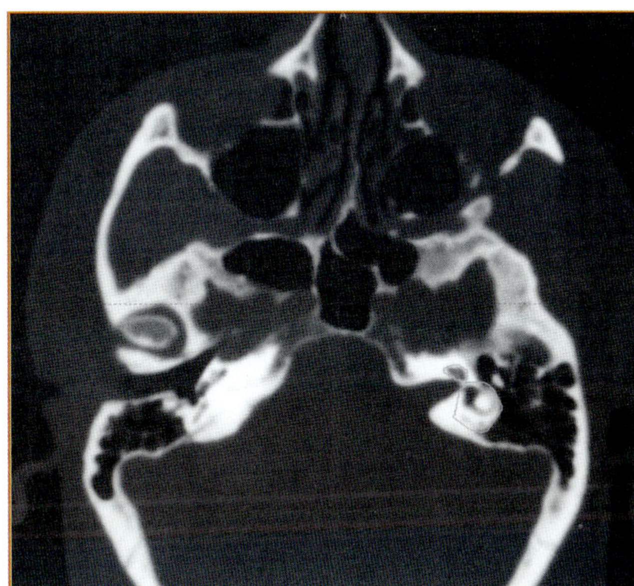

Figure 10–3. CT with areas to be protected from radiotherapy are carefully outlined at the workstation computer. The cochlea and vestibular system are carefully outlined here.

The physician carefully outlines the cochlea and vestibular system on the computer workstation utilizing the CT images attained (Figure 10–3). The tumor area is then plotted on the MRI images to effectively treat the tumor while minimizing injury to nearby structures (Figure 10–4). Final verification is performed on the target positions and a trial run performed. Then, the patient's head frame is secured

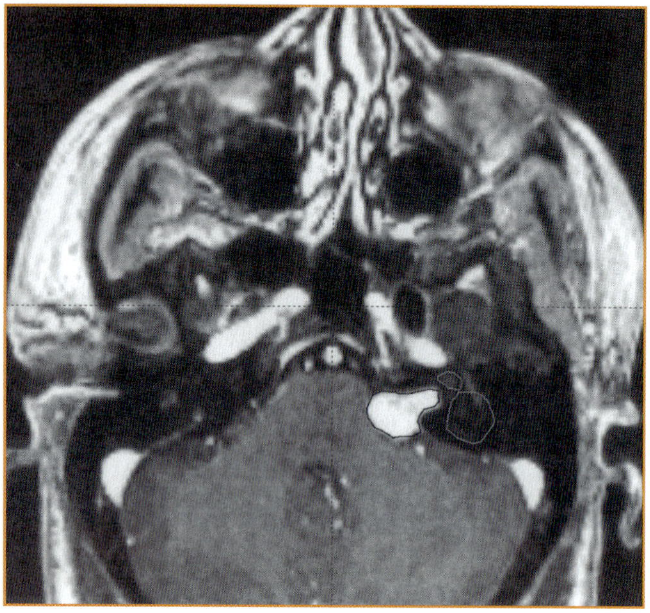

Figure 10–4. MRI scan with tumor area marked in order to effectively treat it while minimizing injury to vital structures nearby.

into position and radiation treatment is administered (Figure 10–5). After the treatment is completed, the frame is removed and the patient recovers for a short period of time, usually one to two hours, and is then discharged home.

Treatment Planning

When designing the treatment plan in stereotactic radiosurgery, the keys lie in conformality, protection of critical areas, and the decision of a radiation dose that is biologically effective. In order to create an optimal treatment plan, it requires the expertise of several disciplines: a neurotologist or neurosurgeon, a radiation oncologist, a neuroradiologist, and a medical physicist.

Specifically in Gamma Knife radiosurgery, the dose falloff is quite steep. While not a rigid rule, historically the convention has been to prescribe to the 50% isodose level. The term "isodose level"

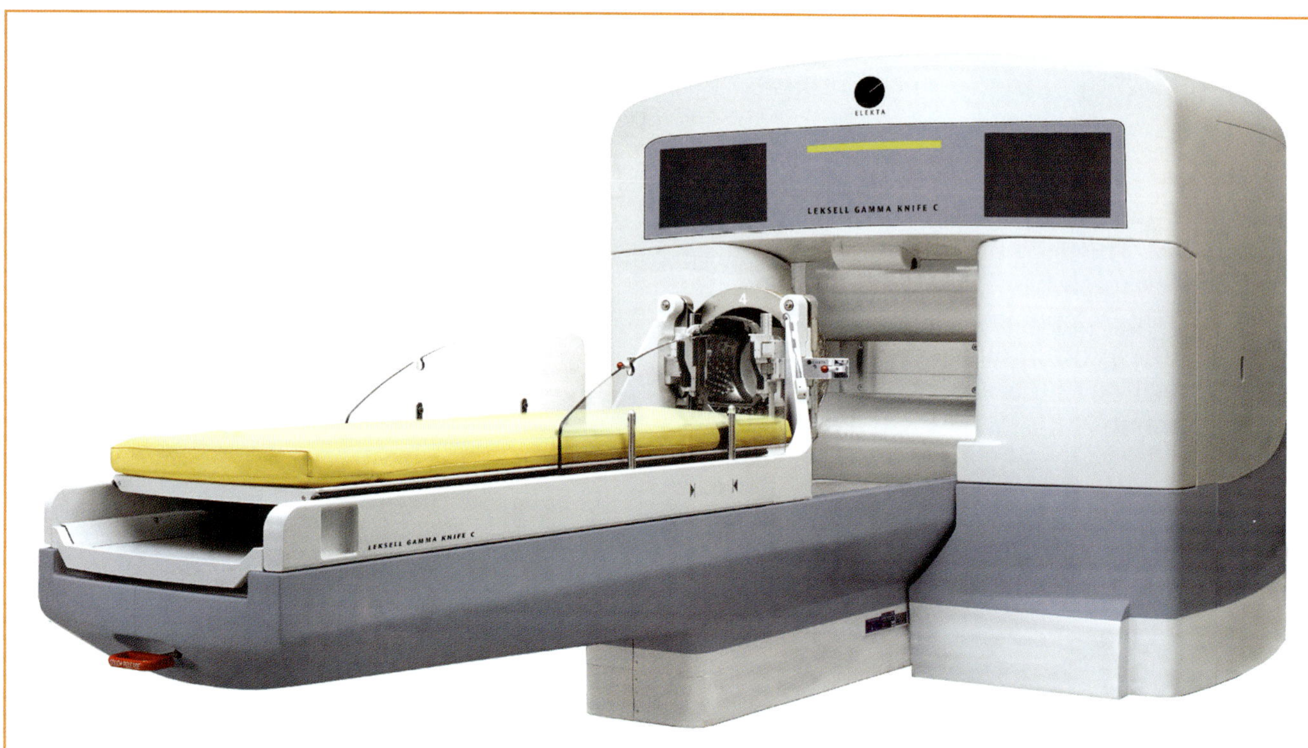

Figure 10–5. Leksell Gamma Knife machine.

is often referred to in the radiation therapy arena to mean the percentages of the maximum dose to be delivered to the target volume. A 50% isodose level means that the marginal dose to the tumor is that which is considered to be biologically effective to achieve the desired endpoint, and the area outlined to be the tumor will receive 50% or more of the maximum dose prescribed.

Conformality has been somewhat controversial since it relies on the human perception of tumors on images. An interesting concept for the advancement of neuroradiology is to develop specific markers for specific tumor cells, since relying on imaging has disadvantages when compared with microscopy and generic enhancing agents. As seen in Figure 10–4, the dose delivered to this acoustic tumor quite closely conforms to the outline of the tumor. In order for this to be truly useful, the tumor must be outlined prior to the development of the treatment plan for the tumor. Theoretically, fewer complications are expected the closer the treatment dose conforms to the outline of the tumor. It is quite challenging, especially after surgical resection, to differentiate between residual or recurrent tumor and normal postoperative changes. Critical structures must also be outlined so that accurate dose assessments can be made and structure tolerances can be considered. For example, in acoustic tumors the critical structures of the cochlea and labyrinth are protected, as well as the brainstem in compressive tumors.

As the field of stereotactic radiosurgery has progressed from its infancy, the marginal dose considered to be effective in tumor control has been decreased and the mean dose to the cochlea and labyrinth is currently being assessed for toxicity. The original marginal doses for acoustic tumors ranged from 15 to 18 gray, and are currently around 12 to 13 gray. In other cerebellopontine angle tumors, additional cranial nerve toxicity is being evaluated.

The tolerance doses for the optic apparatus and brainstem have been further identified related to findings from standard radiation therapy in terms of maximum dose, which may be volume or track length dependent. These doses were discovered by various methods including: (1) overdosing and following the effects; (2) animal studies; and (3) underdosing and observing tumor progression. Studies were all performed with fractionated therapy for pituitary tumors, cavernous sinus tumors, brainstem tumors and spinal cord tumors. Extrapolation from fractionated dose treatments to single dose delivery continues to be studied as long-term responses of tumors irradiated with a single high dose are evaluated.

Smaller lesions without brainstem compression are ideal for primary stereotactic radiosurgery. Stereotactic radiosurgery is also used in conjunction with surgery as a method of treating the residual tumor in critical or difficult locations unreachable by the surgeon. Finally, elderly, patients refusing surgery, and medically high-risk patients who are unable to undergo open surgical procedures are excellent candidates for stereotactic radiosurgery. It is also important to note that in the event of radiosurgical failure, surgery may remain an option.

There has been some controversy regarding the ease of surgery after radiosurgery. A recent study of microsurgery after failed Gamma Knife radiosurgery evaluated 12 patients.[15] These tumors were found to be severely adherent to the brainstem. In addition, there was considerable difficulty identifying the facial nerve intraoperatively and dense adhesions of tumor to the facial nerve led to the inability to dissect tumor free from the nerve. Deterioration of facial function after the surgery was seen in 25% of the patients. Another recent study showed that the quality of microsurgical tumor resection and of facial nerve preservation was impaired after Gamma Knife radiosurgery in 10 of 20 cases requiring surgical resection after radiosurgery.[16]

An additional retrospective review assessed 38 patients with microsurgical salvage after failed stereotactic radiosurgery compared to a matched random sample of 38 patients with primary surgery.[17] Tumor adherence to the facial nerve, facial nerve grade, and complications were reviewed. The mean time from radiation to surgical salvage was 3.3 years. Mean tumor size was 2.6 cm in each group. The irradiated group had more adherence of tumor than the controls and a lower rate of good facial function postoperatively if surgery was required. Thus, surgical salvage was found to have poorer outcomes and was more difficult when compared to those patients with no prior irradiation.

Radiobiologic Rationale

The desired endpoints of the different conditions treated with radiotherapy vary. The goals of performing stereotactic radiation are to achieve the highest probability of local tumor control with the lowest achievable incidence of adverse effects, to prolong the life of the patient, and to provide the best quality of life with as few anatomic and physiologic defects as possible.

Various treatment endpoints exist regarding radiosurgery. At a minimum, the goals of radiosurgery include stopping the growth of the tumor in hopes that it will eventually recede and relieve the patient's symptoms. Another endpoint is to protect the pre-procedure function of nerves, such as hearing and vision, pituitary gland function, and optic apparatus function. For secreting pituitary tumors, a single high dose of appropriately directed radiation can curtail the secretions and preserve what vision is unaffected. The ultimate endpoint for trigeminal neuralgia is to eradicate the pain without causing anesthesia dolorosa, thus eliminating the need for medication. The desired effect for arteriovenous malformations is obliteration of the nidus by the thickening of the lumen of the involved vessels. Timeframe to reach the anticipated endpoint varies. Whereas arteriovenous malformation effects are generally seen after two to three years, other condition endpoints may be observed over weeks to months.

After radiation treatment of an acoustic neuroma, little change in tumor characteristics or tumor volume is detected over the first 6 months. Some swelling of the tumor is often noted within the first 18 months after treatment, but typically this process declines with time. Occasionally, these patients may be treated with steroids or even ventriculoperitoneal (VP) shunt. Partial involution of the tumor typically occurs by 2 years, and residual enhancing tumor may be noted on MRI imaging examination for long periods. This is thought to be tumor that is locally controlled. Post radiation MRI scanning should be continued for years to ensure stabilization of tumor and no evidence of further growth.

Control of acoustic neuroma tumor growth with radiation is thought to occur via two mechanisms: direct cellular injury and vascular fibrosis. In the higher dose central region, tumor histopathology has revealed necrosis, decreased tumor cell population, and fibrosis. In the lower dose peripheral region, vascular occlusion, macrophage infiltration, fibrin deposits, and thrombus formation have been identified. In general, apoptosis is the mechanism of cellular death and direct tumor control.

CONSIDERATIONS OF STEREOTACTIC RADIOSURGERY FOR ACOUSTIC NEUROMA

Acoustic neuromas are the most common tumor of the posterior fossa. The three options for the management of acoustic neuromas are observation, surgical excision, or stereotactic radiosurgery. In a select group of patients with large or giant tumors, a planned subtotal resection with follow-up MRI scanning and stereotactic radiosurgery for growth of the remaining tumor is indicated. Each treatment option has its advantages and disadvantages. Individualized decisions are made considering tumor size, hearing status, balance signs and symptoms, age and comorbidities, and experience of the treating physician.

Results with Stereotactic Radiosurgery

Approximately 35 to 50% of untreated acoustic neuroma tumors show no growth when monitored over time.[18–21] In most studies assessing results of stereotactic radiation for treatment of acoustic neuromas, treatment is delivered even if no proof of growth is identified. It is important to realize that any stereotactic radiation treatment results are somewhat biased since most acoustic neuromas treated with radiosurgery are neither followed until growth occurs, nor determined to be a growing tumor prior to treatment.

The number of publications assessing results using stereotactic radiosurgery has increased substantially in the past several years. A recent report summarizes outcomes for 829 patients treated between 1989 and 2002 with a mean follow-up of 10 years.[22]

Marginal dose was 13 gray with a mean tumor volume of 2.5 mL. With this treatment protocol, tumor control rate remained 97% during that period, while hearing level, graded with the Gardner-Robertson scale, was preserved in 50% of these patients.

Hasegawa and colleagues in Japan reported outcomes on a similarly large cohort of patients with long follow-up.[23] Their group followed 317 patients treated with a marginal dose of 13 gray at the 50% isodose line, with a mean follow-up period of 7.8 years. Hearing preservation was 68% in those treated with marginal doses of 13 gray or less at the 50% isodose line, while it was only 13% in those receiving greater than 13 gray at the 50% isodose line. They reported that 91% of the patients demonstrated tumor control, defined as stable or smaller tumor volume at last imaging. Of note, only 2 patients had complete remission of tumor volume. Of the 26 that failed, 4 died of tumor progression or radiation-induced edema and intracerebral complications, 6 underwent second radiosurgery treatment (3 of whom later required craniotomy), and 21 developed hydrocephalus requiring ventriculoperitoneal shunting. In addition, one patient had malignant transformation at 51 months and succumbed to progression of malignant acoustic tumor.

A follow-up study by the Hasegawa group reported on 71 patients with a mean follow-up of 135 months.[24] In this group, 62 had stable or smaller tumor volumes, while 9 had either progression of tumor or uncontrolled tumor edema causing intracranial complications and requiring craniotomy and resection.

A recent series of 216 acoustic neuroma patients treated with radiosurgery between 12 to 13 gray revealed the actuarial 10-year clinical tumor control rate at 98.3%.[25] This study was performed on patients regardless of progression of symptoms or increase in tumor size. Facial nerve preservation was 100% and normal trigeminal nerve function was preserved in 94.9% of patients. The 10-year actuarial preservation rate of serviceable or useful hearing (GR Class 1–2) was 44.5%. This study showed continued hearing loss beyond 6 years after radiosurgery.

Treatment results of stereotactic radiosurgery versus observation of acoustic tumors is an important topic. To date, no randomized controlled studies have been completed evaluating patient outcomes with acoustic tumors in the two treatment options. Long-term data from early studies that used higher marginal dose levels showed that there were higher cranial nerve complication rates but the results were favorable for better tumor control.[26] Most centers now use lower dosing paradigms, but long-term follow-up is necessary.

Reporting hearing preservation outcomes has multiple challenges. Post radiation hearing must be followed and documented for years after treatment, and timing reported in various studies is inconsistent. One classification system has not been universally used in the literature to document hearing before and after treatment. Grading systems for hearing outcomes include the AAO-HNS and Gardner Robertson Classification Systems (Figures 10–6 and 10–7). Reports of hearing outcomes should be standardized across one classification system and reported only when there is useful hearing prior to treatment. Reports of preservation of hearing when there is no pre-radiosurgery useful hearing skew the results and are difficult to interpret as clinically relevant. For example, many reports show a high percentage (90%) of radiosurgery patients do not demonstrate any change in their classification. This conclusion, though, does not imply that there has been sparing of serviceable hearing. Standardizing the hearing preservation results in the literature would aid in the understanding of the true benefit of radiosurgery over traditional surgical resection.

A recent review study reported that 40% of 219 patients had pre-radiosurgery serviceable hearing (GR I–II).[27] Of the patients with serviceable hearing before treatment, 44% retained useful hearing after radiosurgery. This compared favorably to microsurgery, which included 42% of 599 patients with serviceable hearing preoperatively. Of these patients, 44% retained useful hearing postoperatively. Average follow-up in this pooled population was 24 months.

Advantages of Stereotactic Radiosurgery

Advantages of stereotactic radiosurgery over surgical treatment include decreased hospital stay,

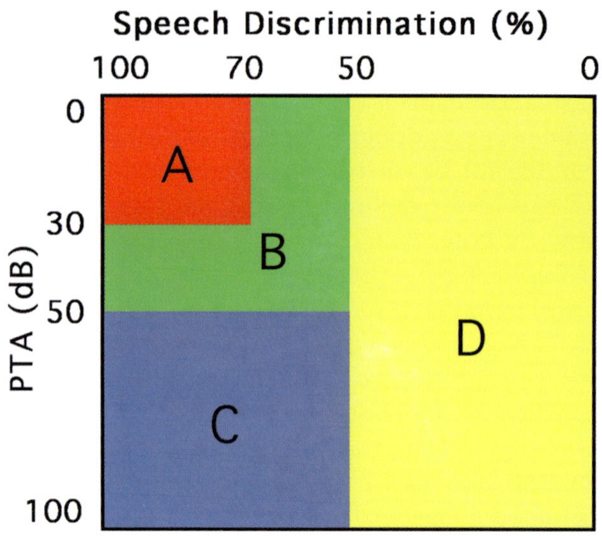

Figure 10–6. AAO-HNS grading system for hearing outcome. PTA (Pure Tone Average).

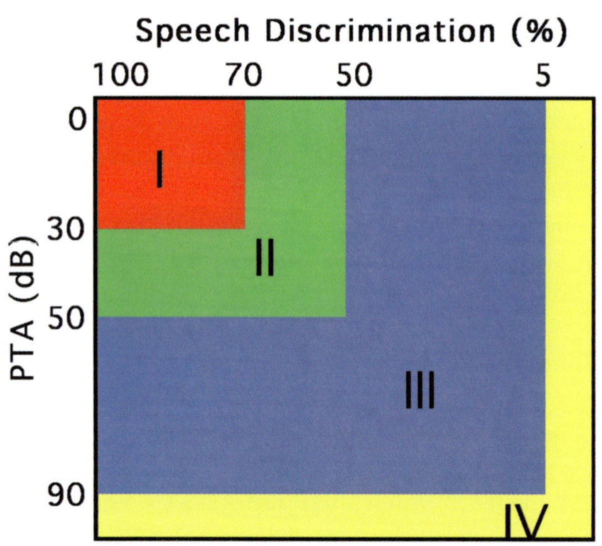

Figure 10–7. Gardner-Robertson Classification Systems for grading hearing outcome. PTA (Pure Tone Average).

a quicker return to work, and lower cost in treatment. This may be a particularly appealing option for elderly or medically infirm patients with documented tumor growth. Tumor recurrence after surgical resection may also be an indication for radiosurgery in a select group of patients. The surgical complications of cerebral spinal fluid leak, infection, and other inherent risks are obviated with radiosurgery. The results of hearing preservation and facial nerve function are quite similar with either radiosurgery or surgical resection.

Disadvantages of Stereotactic Radiosurgery

Stereotactic radiosurgery is not without risks and side effects. Patients may experience headache, nausea, and dizziness after stereotactic radiosurgery.[28] Approximately one-third of patients undergoing stereotactic radiosurgery exhibited one of these immediate side effects after treatment. In patients with significant disequilibrium or recurrent vertigo prior to radiation, symptoms may remain or actually worsen with stereotactic radiation. Balance and dizziness outcomes need further investigation with long-term follow-up.

Stereotactic radiosurgery has the potential to cause sudden hearing loss, likely owing to swelling that occurs soon after treatment. Additional decline in cranial nerve function may occur over several years following radiation, but this phenomenon has also been observed in surgical patients as well. Long-term follow-up with documentation in a large series of patients must be completed for more accurate results.

A potential complication of stereotactic radiosurgery is radiation-induced hydrocephalus. Its occurrence is associated directly with tumor size, though it has been reported after treatment of tumors as small as 18 mm.[29] Radiation-induced hydrocephalus was more common in early reports, but thankfully its occurrence has been reduced recently to a range of 1.4 to 9.2% with modern dosing and protocols.[30] Some studies have reported great difficulty preserving facial nerve function in the surgical salvage of schwannomas that have failed radiation.[31,32]

The risk of a previously benign schwannoma undergoing malignant degeneration is a concern, especially in the younger patients. Of 8,000 vestibular schwannomas treated with stereotactic radiation since 1969 worldwide, Noren[33] reports an estimated 0.1% rate of malignant change. All patients whose tumors underwent malignant transformation died despite microsurgical excision. Histopathologic analysis revealed a malignant spindle cell neoplasm with numerous mitotic figures.[34–37] While the incidence of malignant transformation is low, the majority of studies have relatively short follow-up. Finally, it should be recognized that malignant schwannomas might occur spontaneously in nonradiated patients. Because stereotactic radiosurgery is often performed without tissue pathology, it is unknown if the "malignant transformation" was definitively radiation induced, the original tumor pathology, or a normal sequelae for that tumor.

A distinct advantage of stereotactic radiosurgery versus stereotactic radiotherapy is the application of a head frame to the outer table of the skull, thus allowing the three-dimensional localization to be fixed from the imaging segment of the procedure through the treatment. Still, similar to all treatments using stereotaxy for localization, the procedure's limitation relies on the quality and method of imaging. Sources of imprecision in treatment protocols can include mechanical inaccuracy of the treatment delivery unit, contributing to potential procedural imprecision. The mechanical accuracy is assessed at the time of acceptance testing, radiation unit commissioning, and at least annually thereafter. Some units are required by law to be tested more frequently.

Controversies of Stereotactic Radiosurgery

Controversies surrounding stereotactic radiosurgery of acoustic neuroma are abundant in the literature, mainly surrounding the definitions of outcomes. This includes the definition of tumor control, inherent risks of radiation, and potential increased of salvage surgery after radiation.

In many studies tumor control is poorly defined. Some studies use as an outcome measure "no additional treatment needed" which does not define tumor outcomes. Other reports state that unchanged tumor size was considered evidence of tumor control. The degree of success, however, is not necessarily correct when considering that the control rate also includes patients whose tumors were stable prior to radiation. Quite simply, the natural history of acoustic neuroma tumors is that 35 to 50% of them will show no growth over time, thus skewing the results towards success, In a different study looking at the natural history of 53 patients with acoustic neuromas, up to 60% had no demonstrable tumor growth within the first 2 to 3 years of conservative management and observation.[38] One must interpret study results with caution as they may grossly overstate the actual improvement in control rate from stereotactic radiosurgery.

As a primary treatment, stereotactic radiotherapy has lower risks of treatment complications when compared to microsurgery in the acute setting. Thus, stereotactic radiotherapy is advantageous as a treatment modality in patients who are older, medically infirm, require anticoagulant therapy, or who are otherwise poorer surgical or anesthetic candidates. If surgical salvage is necessary, then issues of surgical results must also be included in the decision tree as outcomes are fraught with increased potential complications such as facial nerve paralysis, loss of opportunity for hearing conservation surgery, incomplete tumor removal, and cerebrospinal fluid leak. Finally, the consideration of malignant transformation with radiation must be discussed openly as a potential risk, especially in the younger patient who will have a longer life expectancy.

Stereotactic radiotherapy displays an advantage over microsurgery in the setting of treatment of only-hearing ears in the acute setting. However, the initial advantages of stereotactic radiotherapy, whether fractionated, hypofractionated, or single-dose, are offset by the long-term rates of cranial neuropathy and hearing loss that eventually occurs. While these tend to be comparable to those seen following microsurgical resection, the long-term hearing outcome must still be part of the outcomes discussion.

NEUROFIBROMATOSIS II

Neurofibromatosis Type 2 (NF2) is an autosomal dominant genetic disorder caused by mutations on chromosome 22.[39] The disease process represents a special challenge with the hallmark of bilateral acoustic neuromas. Traditionally, these tumors have been treated with microsurgical resection after documented growth, though all treatment options are fraught with drawbacks. In patients with NF2, the acoustic tumors often engulf the cochlear nerve, making hearing preservation surgery very difficult. In addition to the high risk of complete deafness, multiple cranial neuropathies including the facial and trigeminal nerves can be associated with microsurgical resection of NF2 tumors. In recent years, stereotactic radiosurgery has emerged as a potential first-line treatment for tumors associated with NF2.[23,40]

In a recent study, stereotactic radiosurgery was used to treat 74 schwannomas in 62 patients with NF2.[41] To better define the tumor control rate and long-term functional outcome, the authors reviewed their experience in treating these lesions. The median follow-up period was 53 months, and two patients were lost to follow-up. Actuarial local control rates were 85, 81, and 81% at 5, 10, and 15 years, respectively. Tumor volume was significant as a predictor of local control. The actuarial serviceable hearing preservation rate was 73% at 1 year, 59% at 2 years, and 48% at 5 years after radiosurgery. Facial neuropathy occurred in 8% of tumors, trigeminal neuropathy occurred in 4%, and vestibular dysfunction occurred in 4%. Radiation dose and tumor volume were predictive of development of new deficits.

Based on this study, the results of radiosurgery for tumors associated with NF2 are clearly worse when compared with sporadic tumors. The short follow-up period (<5 years) is a considerable weakness of this study. In addition, the patients with the longest follow-up were treated with much higher doses of radiation. It is not known if patients treated with lower doses in an attempt to decrease side effects will have worse long-term control rates. Patients undergoing stereotactic radiosurgery may experience growth of their tumors many years after treatment, and one patient in this series had tumor progression 7 years after treatment.

Balasubramaniam and colleagues reviewed all reported cases of secondary neoplasms following stereotactic radiotherapy.[42] Including their institution's one case as of 2007, 20 cases of secondary tumors associated with prior stereotactic radiotherapy were reported. Of these 20, half (10) were de novo tumors, and eight were malignant. Accelerated growth of primary benign acoustic neuromas and subsequent resection with histopathologic confirmation of malignant transformation was found in 6 patients, all who had NF-2. Although extremely low, the risk of malignant transformation and/or de novo secondary malignancy must be discussed with patients, particularly NF-2 patients and those with high neoplastic potential. Finally, there are reports of an increased relative risk of new tumors (18.8 relative risk for new schwannomas) and a real risk of malignant transformation of treated schwannomas.[43]

The tumors most amenable to stereotactic radiation are smaller in size and associated with better hearing. Unfortunately, these tumors are also the best cases for microsurgical resection and hearing preservation. The management decisions of NF2 patients with bilateral acoustic neuromas are extremely challenging, fraught with many increased risks and drawbacks. Radiosurgery should be an important therapeutic option for NF2 patients.

GLOMUS TUMORS

Definition

Glomus tumors are the most common benign tumors of the temporal bone. They demonstrate considerable biologic variability in their clinical behavior. Glomus tumors may be discovered as small, easily removed middle ear tumors with minimal symptoms and no sequelae, or as large, destructive tumors with intracranial extension and multiple cranial neuropathies.

Glomus tumors are paragangliomas or chemodectomas. Glomus tympanicum and jugulare arise from paraganglionic tissue intimately related to Jacobson's nerve along the promontory and the adventitia of the jugular bulb. Histologically, the tumors are benign lesions despite their clinically destructive course. Eighty percent of paragangliomas are sporadic, and the remainder are inherited as an autosomal dominant trait. Inherited forms tend to be multicentric, bilateral, and with an earlier onset of symptoms.[44,45] Malignant forms are rare with an incidence ranging from less than 1% for glomus jugulare tumors, to 6.4% for carotid body tumors, and up to 17% for glomus intravagale.[46,47]

All glomus tumors have the potential to secrete catecholamines, although only 1 to 3% so resulting in symptoms such as headache, sweating, palpitations, and hypertension. Counterintuitively, chronic norepinephrine intoxication may manifest orthostatic syncope because of chronic intravascular volume depletion and must be investigated further.

Treatment Options

As with all benign neurotologic tumors, therapeutic options aim to improve local control while minimizing resultant morbidity. Decisions are made individually with specific patient presentation of tumor size, cranial nerve or posterior fossa signs and symptoms, age and comorbidities, and experience of the physician team in treating these benign tumors.

Traditionally if the patient is a surgical candidate, surgical resection is thought to be the main treatment modality. With larger tumors that encroach on cranial nerves, involve the carotid artery, or invade into the posterior fossa, other options of treatment must be considered. Though there are no long-term treatment studies available for guidance, we typically recommend preoperative embolization, safe surgical resection preserving cranial nerves, with staged radiosurgery following if necessary. Radiosurgery is an intriguing theoretical option because of the effects on the vasculature of the tumor. If cranial nerve injury occurs after radiosurgery, it would theoretically be better tolerated because of the slow progression of the neuropathy and increased time for compensation.

Conventional fractionated, external beam radiotherapy has been used most commonly in the past to treat residual tumors with varying degrees of success. Various studies have published success rates ranging from a maximum of 61 to 71%. Side effects of radiation include osteoradionecrosis of the temporal bone, radiation necrosis of the temporal lobe, mastoiditis and secondary malignancies.[48–51] Although the glomus cells are thought to be radioresistant, radiotherapy helps halt tumor growth by inducing fibrosis around the supplying vessels. Stereotactic radiosurgery, with the ability to deliver precise, high-dose radiation to a small, localized field, increases the chance of obliterative endarteritis while reducing complications by sparing adjacent normal structures.

No randomized, controlled clinical trial have objectively assessed the long-term outcomes of treatment options of observation, surgery, radiosurgery, or a combined approach of surgery with postoperative radiosurgery. There are several studies assessing tumor control and growth after stereotactic radiation with short follow-up periods.[52–54] A recent study of 17 patients with glomus jugulare tumors who underwent Gamma Knife radiosurgery showed improvement in clinical symptoms in eight patients (47.1%), worsening of clinical symptoms in two patients (11.8%), and unchanged symptoms in the remainder of patients.[52] The median radiosurgical dose to the tumor margin was 15 gray. No patients experienced new lower cranial nerve palsies. Tumor volume on latest MRI scan showed an increase in the size of the tumor in four patients. Median follow-up was 48 months.

In another study, 42 patients with glomus jugulare tumors underwent stereotactic radiosurgery with Gamma Knife.[55] Nineteen patients (45%) underwent stereotactic radiosurgery as their primary tumor management. The mean number of isocenters used was 8.3 with a mean tumor margin dose of 14.9 gray. The mean follow-up duration after radiosurgery was 44 months (range 6 to 149 months). One tumor (2%) enlarged after radiosurgery. This enlargement in tumor size was noted 99 months after radiosurgery. Hearing preservation was attained in 81% of the patients after 4 years.

Glomus tumors are slow-growing benign tumors, thus, long-term follow-up of at least 10 years is required to accurately assess control and success of stereotactic radiosurgery. The glomus cells are radioresistant and may behave unpredictably with time. Quality of life is critical to consider, especially when dealing with a disease that is benign. Preliminary studies examining quality of life after microsurgery and radiosurgery clearly show an improved quality of life with radiosurgery as the treatment modality.

When considering treatment options in patients with glomus tumors, the natural history of the disease must be considered. There are no long-term results of stereotactic radiosurgery for glomus tumors. The potential benefit of control of the disease with preservation of cranial nerve function and lack of operative complications makes this treatment worth studying in long-term follow-up studies. As with radiosurgery for acoustic tumors, we must know growth, not "control," of the residual glomus tumor with a time frame of 10 to 15 years. The results must be documented by strict cranial nerve examination of function, not symptoms as currently used. The benefit over surgery is exciting if in fact we are able to limit possible surgical risks and preserve cranial nerve function with long-term stagnation of tumor growth.

CONCLUSION

Stereotactic radiosurgery has undergone significant advances since first introduced for skull base tumors. This treatment minimizes acute risks in tumor treatment associated with craniotomy and microsurgical procedures. The ability to treat these difficult tumors on an outpatient basis with minimal acute morbidity is exciting. However, patients should be counseled that their exposure to radiation puts them at higher risk of acute, long-term, or latent complications that microsurgery and definitive resection avoid.

Radiosurgery dosage has been reduced over the years, decreasing the incidence of cranial nerve injury and other complications after treatment. Long-term studies need to assess success of these new lower dose treatment protocols. In addition, long-term post-radiosurgery tumor growth needs to be documented.

Acknowledgment

Thank you to Roger Gonda, MD, for his help with the images used in this chapter.

REFERENCES

1. Leksell L. A note on the treatment of acoustic tumours. *Acta Chir Scand.* 1971;137(8):763–765.
2. Kondziolka D, Lunsford LD, Flickinger JC. Acoustic neuroma radiosurgery. Origins, contemporary use and future expectations. *Neurochirurgie.* 2004;50(2–3 pt 2):427–435.
3. Noren G, Arndt J, Hindmarsh T. Stereotactic radiosurgery in cases of acoustic neurinoma: further experiences. *Neurosurgery.* 1983;13(1):12–22.
4. Forster DM, Kemeny AA, Pathak A, Walton L. Radiosurgery: a minimally interventional alternative to microsurgery in the management of acoustic neuroma. *Br J Neurosurg.* 1996;10(2):169–174.
5. Kondziolka D, Dempsey PK, Lunsford LD, et al. A comparison between magnetic resonance imaging and computed tomography for stereotactic coordinate determination. *Neurosurgery.* 1992;30(3):402–406; discussion 406–407.
6. Flickinger JC, Kondziolka D, Pollock BE, Lunsford LD. Evolution in technique for vestibular schwannoma radiosurgery and effect on outcome. *Int J Radiat Oncol Biol Phys.* 1996;36(2):275–280.
7. Wallner KE, Sheline GE, Pitts LH, Wara WM, Davis RL, Boldrey EB. Efficacy of irradiation for incompletely excised acoustic neurilemomas. *J Neurosurg.* 1987;67(6): 858–863.
8. Darrouzet V, Maire, J., Guerin J., Bebear JP. Fractionated radiation therapy in the treatment of stage III and IV cerebellopontine angle tumors: preliminary results in 20 cases. In: Tos M, Thomsen, J, eds. *Proceeding of the First International Conference on Acoustic Neuroma.* Amsterdam: Kugler; 1992:305–307.
9. Diaz R, Brodie, HA, Schwaber, MK. Fractionated stereotactic radiation for acoustic neuroma. *eMedicine.* October 6, 2008.
10. Solberg TD, Goetsch SJ, Selch MT, Melega W, Lacan G, DeSalles AA. Functional stereotactic radiosurgery involving a dedicated linear accelerator and gamma unit: a comparison study. *J Neurosurg.* 2004;101(suppl 3):373–380.
11. Shoshan Y, Suh, JH, Barnett, GH. *Fractionated Stereotactic Radiosurgery. Vol 1.* AANS; 2000.
12. Leksell L. Stereotactic radiosurgery. *J Neurol Neurosurg Psychiatry.*1983;46(9):797–803.
13. Kondziolka D, Lunsford LD, Flickinger JC. Acoustic tumors: operation versus radiation—making sense of opposing viewpoints. Part II. Acoustic neuromas: sorting out management options. *Clin Neurosurg.* 2003;50: 313–328.
14. Hoogeman MS, Nuyttens JJ, Levendag PC, Heijmen BJ. Time dependence of intrafraction patient motion assessed by repeat stereoscopic imaging. *Int J Radiat Oncol Biol Phys.* 2008;70(2):609–618.
15. Shuto T, Inomori S, Matsunaga S, Fujino H. Microsurgery for vestibular schwannoma after gamma knife radiosurgery. *Acta Neurochir (Wien).* 2008;150(3):229–234; discussion 234.
16. Roche PH, Khalil M, Thomassin JM, Delsanti C, Regis J. Surgical removal of vestibular schwannoma after failed gamma knife radiosurgery. *Prog Neurol Surg.* 2008;21: 152–157.
17. Friedman RA, Brackmann DE, Hitselberger WE, Schwartz MS, Iqbal Z, Berliner KI. Surgical salvage after failed irradiation for vestibular schwannoma. *Laryngoscope.* 2005;115(10):1827–1832.
18. Shin YJ, Fraysse B, Cognard C, et al. Effectiveness of conservative management of acoustic neuromas. *Am J Otol.* 2000;21(6):857–862.

19. Rosenberg SI. Natural history of acoustic neuromas. *Laryngoscope.* 2000;110(4):497–508.
20. Flint D, Fagan P, Panarese A. Conservative management of sporadic unilateral acoustic neuromas. *J Laryngol Otol.* 2005;119(6):424–428.
21. Smouha EE, Yoo M, Mohr K, Davis RP. Conservative management of acoustic neuroma: a meta-analysis and proposed treatment algorithm. *Laryngoscope.* 2005;115(3):450–454.
22. Lunsford LD, Niranjan A, Flickinger JC, Maitz A, Kondziolka D. Radiosurgery of vestibular schwannomas: summary of experience in 829 cases. *J Neurosurg.* 2005;102 suppl:195–199.
23. Hasegawa T, Fujitani S, Katsumata S, Kida Y, Yoshimoto M, Koike J. Stereotactic radiosurgery for vestibular schwannomas: analysis of 317 patients followed more than 5 years. *Neurosurgery.* 2005;57(2):257–265; discussion 257–265.
24. Hasegawa T, Kida Y, Kobayashi T, Yoshimoto M, Mori Y, Yoshida J. Long-term outcomes in patients with vestibular schwannomas treated using gamma knife surgery: 10-year follow-up. *J Neurosurg.* 2005;102(1):10–16.
25. Chopra R, Kondziolka D, Niranjan A, Lunsford LD, Flickinger JC. Long-term follow-up of acoustic schwannoma radiosurgery with marginal tumor doses of 12 to 13 Gy. *Int J Radiat Oncol Biol Phys.* 2007;68(3):845–851.
26. Hoistad DL, Melnik G, Mamikoglu B, Battista R, O'Connor CA, Wiet RJ. Update on conservative management of acoustic neuroma. *Otol Neurotol.* 2001;22(5):682–685.
27. Kaylie DM, McMenomey SO. Microsurgery vs gamma knife radiosurgery for the treatment of vestibular schwannomas. *Arch Otolaryngol Head Neck Surg.* 2003; 129(8):903–906.
28. Werner-Wasik M, Rudoler S, Preston PE, et al. Immediate side effects of stereotactic radiotherapy and radiosurgery. *Int J Radiat Oncol Biol Phys.* 1999;43(2):299–304.
29. Thomsen J, Tos M, Borgesen SE. Gamma knife: hydrocephalus as a complication of stereotactic radiosurgical treatment of an acoustic neuroma. *Am J Otol.* 1990;11(5): 330–333.
30. Martens F, Verbeke L, Piessens M, Van Vyve M. Stereotactic radiosurgery of vestibular schwannomas with a linear accelerator. *Acta Neurochir Suppl.* 1994;62:88–92.
31. Slattery WH, 3rd, Brackmann DE. Results of surgery following stereotactic irradiation for acoustic neuromas. *Am J Otol.* 1995;16(3):315–319; discussion 319–321.
32. Ito K, Kurita H, Sugasawa K, Mizuno M, Sasaki T. Analyses of neuro-otological complications after radiosurgery for acoustic neurinomas. *Int J Radiat Oncol Biol Phys.* 1997;39(5):983–988.
33. Noren G. Long-term complications following gamma knife radiosurgery of vestibular schwannomas. *Stereotact Funct Neurosurg.* 1998;70(suppl 1):65–73.
34. Bonetti B, Panzeri L, Carner M, Zamboni G, Rizzuto N, Moretto G. Human neoplastic Schwann cells: changes in the expression of neurotrophins and their low-affinity receptor p75. *Neuropathol Appl Neurobiol.* 1997;23(5):380–386.
35. Comey CH, McLaughlin MR, Jho HD, Martinez AJ, Lunsford LD. Death from a malignant cerebellopontine angle triton tumor despite stereotactic radiosurgery. Case report. *J Neurosurg.* 1998;89(4):653–658.
36. Thomsen J, Mirz F, Wetke R, Astrup J, Bojsen-Moller M, Nielsen E. Intracranial sarcoma in a patient with neurofibromatosis type 2 treated with gamma knife radiosurgery for vestibular shwannoma. *Am J Otol.* 2000;21(3): 364–370.
37. Sangueza OP, Requena L. Neoplasms with neural differentiation: a review. Part II: malignant neoplasms. *Am J Dermatopathol.* 1998;20(1):89–102.
38. Wiet RJ, Zappia JJ, Hecht CS, O'Connor CA. Conservative management of patients with small acoustic tumors. *Laryngoscope.* 1995;105(8 pt 1):795–800.
39. Evans DG, Huson SM, Donnai D, et al. A genetic study of type 2 neurofibromatosis in the United Kingdom. I. Prevalence, mutation rate, fitness, and confirmation of maternal transmission effect on severity. *J Med Genet.* 1992;29(12):841–846.
40. Kondziolka D, Lunsford LD, McLaughlin MR, Flickinger JC. Long-term outcomes after radiosurgery for acoustic neuromas. *N Engl J Med.* 1998;339(20):1426–1433.
41. Mathieu D, Kondziolka D, Flickinger JC, et al. Stereotactic radiosurgery for vestibular schwannomas in patients with neurofibromatosis type 2: an analysis of tumor control, complications, and hearing preservation rates. *Neurosurgery.* 2007;60(3):460–468; discussion 468–470.
42. Balasubramaniam A, Shannon P, Hodaie M, Laperriere N, Michaels H, Guha A. Glioblastoma multiforme after stereotactic radiotherapy for acoustic neuroma: case report and review of the literature. *Neuro Oncol.* 2007;9(4): 447–453.
43. Evans DG, Birch JM, Ramsden RT, Sharif S, Baser ME. Malignant transformation and new primary tumours after therapeutic radiation for benign disease: substantial risks in certain tumour prone syndromes. *J Med Genet.* 2006;43(4):289–294.
44. van der Mey AG, Frijns JH, Cornelisse CJ, et al. Does intervention improve the natural course of glomus tumors? A series of 108 patients seen in a 32-year period. *Ann Otol Rhinol Laryngol.* 1992;101(8):635–642.
45. Hu K, Persky MS. Multidisciplinary management of paragangliomas of the head and neck, Part 1. *Oncology (Williston Park).* 2003;17(7):983–993.
46. Sniezek JC, Netterville JL, Sabri AN. Vagal paragangliomas. *Otolaryngol Clin North Am.* 2001;34(5):925–939, vi.
47. Shamblin WR, ReMine WH, Sheps SG, Harrison EG Jr. Carotid body tumor (chemodectoma). Clinicopathologic analysis of ninety cases. *Am J Surg.* 1971;122(6):732–739.
48. Cole JM, Beiler D. Long-term results of treatment for glomus jugulare and glomus vagale tumors with radiotherapy. *Laryngoscope.* 1994;104(12):1461–1465.
49. Larner JM, Hahn SS, Spaulding CA, Constable WC. Glomus jugulare tumors. Long-term control by radiation therapy. *Cancer.* 1992;69(7):1813–1817.

50. Schild SE, Foote RL, Buskirk SJ, et al. Results of radiotherapy for chemodectomas. *Mayo Clin Proc.* 1992;67(6): 537–540.
51. Jordan JA, Roland PS, McManus C, Weiner RL, Giller CA. Stereotastic radiosurgery for glomus jugulare tumors. *Laryngoscope.* 2000;110(1):35–38.
52. Varma A, Nathoo N, Neyman G, et al. Gamma knife radiosurgery for glomus jugulare tumors: volumetric analysis in 17 patients. *Neurosurgery.* 2006;59(5):1030–1036; discussion 1036.
53. Eustacchio S, Trummer M, Unger F, Schrottner O, Sutter B, Pendl G. The role of gamma knife radiosurgery in the management of glomus jugulare tumours. *Acta Neurochir Suppl.* 2002;84:91–97.
54. Sharma MS, Gupta A, Kale SS, Agrawal D, Mahapatra AK, Sharma BS. Gamma knife radiosurgery for glomus jugulare tumors: Therapeutic advantages of minimalism in the skull base. *Neurol India.* 2008;56(1):57–61.
55. Pollock BE. Stereotactic radiosurgery in patients with glomus jugulare tumors. *Neurosurg Focus.* 2004;17(2):E10.

CHAPTER 11

Intraoperative Cranial Nerve Monitoring

Jack M. Kartush and Alice Lee

INTRODUCTION

The increasing availability and sophistication of intraoperative cranial nerve monitoring (IOM) within the last few decades has opened a new era in the pursuit of functional neural preservation during microsurgery. The use of intraoperative electromyographic (EMG) facial nerve monitoring has been a standard of care for the resection of acoustic neuromas and other cerebellopontine angle tumors for over a decade.[1] Parallel applications are now routinely being used to monitor cranial nerves during other otolaryngology procedures involving the parotid gland, thyroid, neck, middle ear, and mastoid. Although monitoring is becoming more commonly used for these procedures, polls suggest that there is currently no consensus on the role of IOM as being a standard of care in these settings. Nonetheless, it is interesting to note that, although litigation 20 years ago for iatrogenic facial palsy focused on whether or not monitoring was used, litigation today focuses on whether or not it was used *correctly*. Thus, a key objective of this chapter is to examine common pitfalls in intraoperative monitoring because "poor monitoring is worse than no monitoring."

HISTORY

The concept of intraoperative nerve monitoring has been in existence for over a century. Early forms of intraoperative facial nerve monitoring consisted of visual confirmation of facial motion or tactile confirmation by an assistant's hand. As early as 1898, Krauze described galvanic stimulation of the facial nerve during an acoustic neurectomy, with visual confirmation of the response.[2] In the 1940s, Olivecrona[3] made a concerted attempt to routinely preserve the facial nerve during acoustic tumor resections using a facial nerve stimulator and a nurse whose responsibility was to observe the patient for facial contractions. At times, the surgery was performed under a local anesthetic to allow the patient to move their face upon demand. During the mid-1960s, Parsons, Jako, and Hilger independently reported on dedicated facial nerve monitors that were intended for use during otologic and parotid surgery.[4–6] Jako's device was distinguished by a mechanical transducer placed along the patient's cheek that detected facial contractions. Delgado et al[7] were the first to report on intraoperative electromyographic (EMG) facial nerve monitoring during cerebellopontine angle (CPA) surgery. Using surface electrodes, they reviewed a printout of the EMG tracings. Sugita and Kobayashi[8] modified this technique by using accelerometers to transduce facial motion into electrical energy, but commented on one false-positive error due to inadvertent stimulation of the motor portion of the trigeminal nerve. More importantly, they used a loudspeaker to provide acoustic feedback that allows the surgeon to interpret the evoked responses in context to ongoing surgical events. Prass and Luders[9] subsequently correlated specific patterns of EMG activity to surgical manipulations. Silverstein et al[10] enhanced Jako's motion-detector device (WR Electronics, St Paul, MN) and recommended its use for many otologic procedures. Kartush and Prass[11] developed the "Nerve Integrity Monitor" (NIM) with Nicolet Company (Madison, WI) in 1984 that was subsequently purchased by Xomed (Medtronic) and has become the most commonly used device in the United States.[11] Many other companies now produce "multimodality" monitoring devices that can monitor up to 32 channels of responses not only of EMG but also EEG making them ideal for complex spine and brain monitoring. Their sophisticated multimodality features, however, add a high degree of complexity and, therefore, are typically only used by specially trained technologists. Many devices are available that are acceptable for cranial nerve monitoring. This chapter uses the NIM for many examples simply because of the senior author's 25 years of experience with it: including its strengths and weaknesses. A few other dedicated devices for cranial EMG monitoring include the Magstim Neurosign, the WR Electronics Silverstein, WR Electronics Brackmann and the IOM Solutions Nerveana (Figure 11–1).

NEUROMONITORING BASICS

Goals of Monitoring

The goals of intraoperative neural monitoring have been well established. First and foremost is to assist in identifying the nerve of interest. Second, information gleaned from responses during monitoring assists in the detection of injury to the nerve during dissection. Third, stimulation proximal to the manipulated nerve post dissection can provide a predictive assessment of nerve function.

Responsibility of Monitoring

There are two aspects of monitoring. One is the technical component, which consists of using and setting up the monitoring equipment correctly and

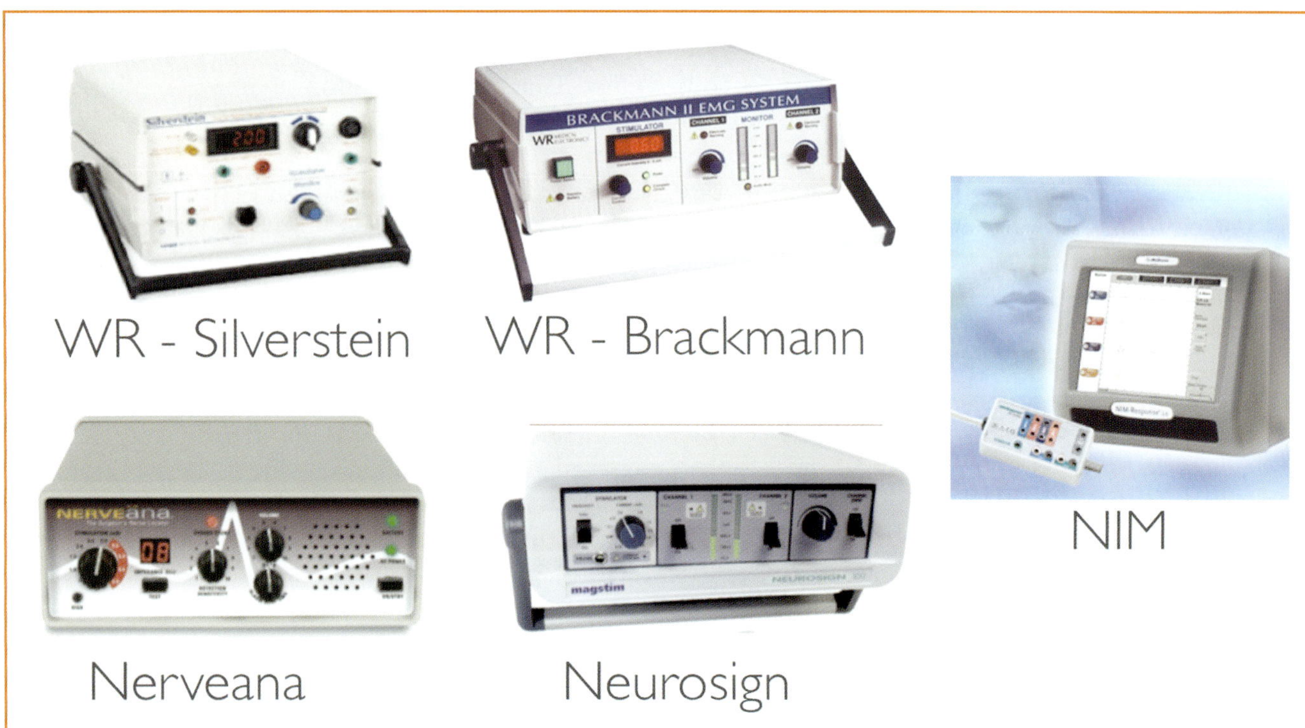

Figure 11–1. Numerous dedicated EMG nerve monitors are commercially available. (Reprinted with permission, courtesy of Jack M. Kartush, MD)

understanding the inherent properties of the system to avoid an erroneous setup (eg, no muscle relaxation, correct electrode placement, low impedance, etc). The other aspect is the interpretive component. Is the person performing the monitoring able to distinguish between a true response versus an artifactual one? When problems occur, can they perform appropriate troubleshooting to identify and correct the issue at hand? With something relatively simple, such as facial nerve monitoring, it is often possible for the surgeon to perform both components, assuming that he or she has undergone the proper training to do so. Many features of the NIM were specifically designed to allow for surgeon interpretation such as auditory representation of the EMG through both raw EMG and intelligently designed alarms that alert the surgeon to significant responses as well as potential problems such as electrode displacement or high impedance. Another important feature is confirming current flow during stimulation with both visual and auditory displays. In fact, a surgeon trained in monitoring is unequivocally the ideal person to interpret the responses as he or she can immediately correlate them to the surgical events. Even the best trained technologist, neurophysiologist, or neurologist will have difficulty separating true responses from artifact without the benefit of seeing and understanding the surgical events in real time.

In contrast, complex types of monitoring that require the averaging of small potentials such as auditory brainstem recording (ABR) and somatosensory evoked potentials (SSEP) typically require too much time and effort for the surgeon, which could distract from the operation. Furthermore, many surgeons simply are not trained in performing the technical or interpretive aspects of these more complex monitoring. Thus, either the surgeon has undergone sufficient training to manage both the technical and interpretive aspects of nerve monitoring or a well-trained technician, neurophysiologist, or neurologist should assist in monitoring. Unfortunately, poor reimbursement in this country has made it prohibitive for neurologists to spend hours or an entire day in one operating room. Thus, with a trained technologist in the operating room, professional interpretation is increasingly being performed by remotely located neurophysiologists and neurologists, who receive real-time information through the internet. While there is little need for such remote monitoring for basic EMG modalities if the surgeon is well trained, complex procedures (EEG for carotidectomy, transcranial motor evoked potentials [MEP] for scoliosis surgery) benefit greatly from a well-trained team of local technologist and remote neurologist/neurophysiologist. Today, most hospitals seek monitoring service companies who specialize in these complex procedures and have the requisite information technology (IT) resources to ensure appropriate hardware, software, and systems management to optimize connectivity from the OR to the remote monitoring professional.

Monitoring Pitfalls

Monitoring is an adjunct, not a replacement for anatomical knowledge and surgical skill. When neurophysiologic responses appear to conflict with anatomy and surgical findings, one must either troubleshoot for a solution or disregard the monitor. As the senior author (JMK) has stated for decades, "Poor monitoring is worse than no monitoring." Monitoring can be likened to going into a minefield with a minesweeper that is malfunctioning. Under this circumstance, it is better to disregard the minesweeper rather than to depend on something that is unreliable. There are many possible pitfalls even for relatively simple monitoring modalities such as facial nerve recording. Just as physicians learn to generate a differential diagnosis for medical disorders, so must the well-trained surgeon develop consistent protocols and a differential diagnosis for intraoperative monitoring problems if they are to perform both technical and interpretive components without a technologist or neurophysiologist. As the use of monitoring has become increasingly routine in otolaryngology, neurosurgery, and spine surgery, surgical residency programs should begin to include monitoring courses in their core curriculum, and test for competency in this area just as they do in other critical areas. General surgeons are just beginning to adopt monitoring for thyroidectomy and, without any prior experience in monitoring, it is critical that they actively pursue IOM training. A great deal of effort has gone into the training of IOM technologists and reading professionals over the last 20 years. Organizations such as the American Society of Neurophysiologic Monitoring (ASNM) provide training courses for surgeon, technologists, neurophysiologists, and neurologists as well as a means to certify levels of monitoring interpretative competence (eg, American Board of Neurophysiologic Monitoring [ABNM]). In contrast, the American Board of Registration of Electroencephalographic and Evoked Potential Technologists (ABRET) has focused on a certification exam for technologists, Certification for Intraoperative Monitoring (CNIM). Thus, surgeons who choose to perform technical and/or interpretive aspects of monitoring should take advantage of these educational resources.

There are numerous technical and interpretive pitfalls that can lead to false-positive and false-negative errors. A false-positive error occurs when a signal is interpreted as being a true response from the nerve of interest when in fact it was generated by artifact or another neuromuscular generator. Examples include (a) mistaking a response from a pharyngeal constrictor while seeking a vocal fold response during thyroidectomy, or (b) mistaking a response from masseter and temporalis muscles while seeking a facial nerve response during acoustic tumor surgery adjacent to the root entry zone of the trigeminal nerve.

A false-negative error occurs when a response from the nerve of interest is missed. There are multiple causes of such an error. Long-lasting neuromuscular blockade and topical anesthetics can abolish or impair EMG responses. Not understanding that monitoring is disabled during electrocautery can result in the nerve being burned and yet no response will be detected during cautery. The experienced surgeon learns that when cautery must occur in close proximity to a nerve, it should be done at the lowest possible setting and then the *nerve should be electrically stimulated immediately following cautery (or other risky maneuver) to confirm that it has not been injured.*

Incorrect setup of electrodes or monitoring parameters can result in both false negative and false-positive errors. Errors with multimodality devices can occur in numerous additional ways that may be difficult to detect because electrodes cannot only be placed in the wrong input of an interface box that may have scores of different input sockets, but software allocation of stimulus and recording pathways can lead to misallocation of the signals. For example, in SEP monitoring, we have seen stimulation of the left leg when the right arm was the intended target. Similarly, during ABR recording, software misallocation may inadvertently lead to the sound signal being conveyed to the right ear transducer, when the left ear is the intended side. These and other details are addressed later in the chapter.

FACIAL NERVE MONITORING

Clinical Application

Although the indications for facial nerve monitoring are expanding, its benefit has been most apparent during resection of acoustic neuromas given the high incidence of postoperative facial palsy prior to the use of monitoring. These benign tumors typically originate from the superior vestibular nerve in the internal auditory canal. The proximity of the adjacent facial nerve accounts for its routine involvement by tumor displacement or microscopic infiltration. Most clinicians prefer an EMG-based system using intramuscular needle electrodes to maximize recording sensitivity and specificity. The high sensitivity of electromyographic facial nerve monitoring allows electrical stimulation of the nerve to be supplemented by identifying low amplitude mechanical-evoked potentials caused by blunt surgical trauma. The specificity of EMG monitoring reduces the chance for false-positive errors that can occur with a motion detector-based system. Sugita and Kobayashi[8] reported on one case in which the facial nerve was inadvertently cut because stimulation of the trigeminal nerve resulted in contraction of the muscles of mastication. The motion detector was not able to differentiate between this movement versus contraction of the facial musculature.

Retrospective studies indicate improved facial nerve outcome with intraoperative monitoring particularly with large acoustic tumors.[12–15] Although a controlled, prospectively randomized study would be most convincing, such a study is unlikely to take place because most of today's surgeons who have adopted monitoring believe that there is an unequivocal benefit and are reluctant to withhold this modality from their patients. It is surprising that after years of reluctant acceptance, some now refer to the analogy that there has never been a controlled study for skydiving with and without parachutes . . .

Because the incidence of nerve injury in chronic ear surgery is markedly less than that seen in acoustic neuroma surgery, it is more difficult to show if injury could have been avoided with monitoring due to the need for an extremely large sample size. In a recent survey conducted to identify facial nerve IOM practice in the United States in this setting, the authors found that although 75% of the 223 respondents had access to monitoring, only 32% thought that it was a requirement.[16] The standard of care is often defined as what the average provider would have done under similar circumstances. Those who performed more otologic surgeries than other types of surgeries were more likely to use the monitoring for chronic ears.

The use of monitoring in middle ear and mastoid disease, especially in the setting of revision surgery, is justified anatomically. Noss et al[17] retrospectively reviewed 262 cases and found that while a dehiscent facial nerve was visualized during 10% of the primary surgeries and in 20% of the revision surgeries, an electrophysiological dehiscence was detected through the use of stimulation in 53% of the primary surgeries and in 96% of the revision cases. A stimulation threshold of <1 volt was concluded to be a more useful criterion of dehiscence than clinical observation under an operating microscope. The cost-effectiveness of intraoperative facial nerve monitoring in both primary and revision surgeries for middle ear and mastoid disease was demonstrated by Wilson et al.[18] The estimated additional cost of $222.73 to $528.00 to the otologic surgery for monitoring and an audiologist/technician was offset by the avoidance of the high management costs of facial nerve paralysis.

Lowry et al[19] surveyed US otolaryngologists to determine the patterns of use of facial nerve monitoring during parotid gland surgery. Of the 1,548 respondents, the more parotidectomies performed per year (>10 and >20), the more likely monitoring was used (79% and 60%, respectively). Four hundred and ninety-two of the 627 (78.5%) surgeons who responded to a query on the type of monitoring used, reported using intraoperative monitoring without the use of nerve stimulators, whereas 21.5% used nerve stimulators only without EMG monitoring. There was no statistically significant association between the use of monitoring in current practice and a history of inadvertent permanent facial nerve injury. The authors concluded that there was a growing trend of facial nerve monitoring during parotid surgery despite the lack of any published prospective, randomized clinical studies to examine the efficacy of its use in this setting.

An interesting corollary is the gradual acceptance of pulse oximetry in anesthesia. At first many anesthesiologists and nurse anesthetists were reluctant to accept "yet another gimmick" that would take away from the "art" of anesthesiology. Many took pains to vocally indicate that it was not a standard of care. However, as pulse oximetry has become less expensive, widely available and a useful real-time measure to assess oxygenation, it has indeed become a standard of care, even though no controlled study has a shown a statistical difference in outcomes. Like pulse oximetry, we predict that the use of intraoperative neuromonitoring will increase simply because it provides "critical information of key structures at risk in the operative field." Neuromonitoring has become accepted in many surgical fields including brain, spine and thyroid. One of the last remaining fields that we predict will finally adopt monitoring is in pelvic surgery where the risks of impotence and incontinence during prostatectomy, hysterectomy and colorectal oncologic surgery remain problematic.

Setup and Recording Technique

Long-acting muscle relaxants should be avoided. Although low doses may not have a significant effect on the response to electrical stimulation, they diminish the ability to monitor small amplitude responses associated with mechanical evoked potentials of the facial nerve. Therefore, judging depth of paralysis using a "Train of Four" peripheral nerve stimulator at a relatively high current setting is not an accurate measure of the facial nerve's ability to respond to minor surgical trauma.

Figure 11–2 demonstrates the recording electrode montage. Needle electrodes are preferred to surface cup electrodes because the former are less likely to be displaced during surgery and because they are more sensitive to low amplitude responses. A close pair of needle EEG-type electrodes are inserted subdermally into the orbicularis oris at the nasolabial groove and into the lateral orbicularis oculi. The electrodes are inserted parallel and close to each other but should not be in contact. In the past, the electrodes were placed closed to the globe under the brow itself. There is adequate orbicularis oculi contraction above the brow to justify placement in this safer area away from the eye without compromising responses. A separate needle (white) electrode is placed subdermally near the sternum to serve as a return or anode electrode for the monopolar stimulator. Another needle electrode is inserted subdermally near the sternum as a ground (green = ground) for the two recording channels, between the sensor electrodes and anode electrodes. Separate return electrodes are not required for bipolar stimulators. Recording electrode wires should be kept distant from stimulators and electrosurgical cables to prevent electrical artifact. Twisting or braiding the recording electrodes can also reduce artifact.

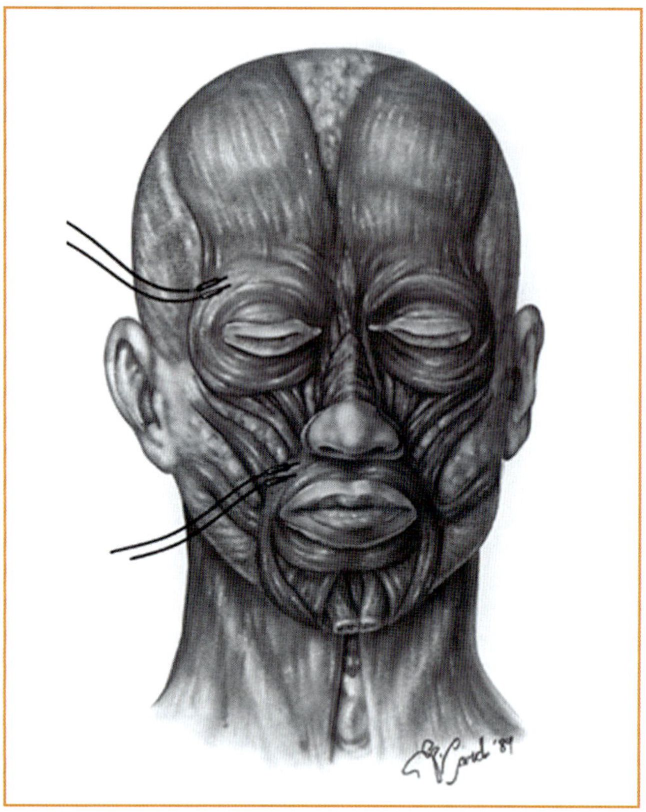

Figure 11–2. EMG recording montage used for two-channel facial nerve monitoring. Close electrode pairs are inserted at the nasolabial and orbicularis oculi regions. (Reprinted with permission[23])

A uniform protocol for electrode set-up should be developed to ensure consistency in channel allocation. For example, we routinely connect blue EMG electrodes from orbicularis oculi to channel 1 and red electrodes from the nasolabial region to recording channel 2. Our simple mnemonic, "Blue eyes, Red lips, and Green ground" has become a de facto protocol in many centers. Once the electrodes have been placed in the face, they must then be securely taped into position and correctly plugged into the patient interface box. Incorrect placement may either lead to confusion or to an inability to stimulate or record appropriately. Some devices such as the NIM use our longstanding color coding as labels to match our "Blue eyes, Red lips, Green ground" mnemonic. The blue electrodes are prelabeled as channel 1, the red electrodes are prelabeled as channel 2, the green as ground, and the white as pickup. The stimulator should always be placed in the cathode (black) position and the pickup electrode placed in the anode (white). Another helpful mnemonic we use is "RAP" (Red Anode Positive) and "BNC" (Black Negative Cathode). Electrode impedances are tested to assure that there are no faulty electrode wires that might cause a loss in electrical continuity. Furthermore, if impedances are too high or are poorly balanced, electrical interference from other devices within the room may be increased. Individual electrode impedances should usually be less than or equal to 5 kOhm with interelectrode imbalances less than 1 kOhm.

There are many devices available with which to perform EMG monitoring. These are preferred to the motion-detector devices in our practice. We have had the greatest experience with the Nerve Integrity Monitor (NIM) and thus its usage will be discussed in the remainder of this chapter. In some centers, multimodality monitoring systems are used to perform facial nerve monitoring in certain centers where dedicated monitors are not available. These multimodality systems allow for the monitoring of up to 32 channels but the increased complexity may lead to error unless operated consistently by well-trained individuals. Furthermore, multimodality devices rarely include built-in cautery suppression and stimulus artifact suppression to allow direct auditory feedback to the surgeon. Consequently, the surgeon remains dependent on a well-trained and very attentive technologist.

Prior to surgery, a functioning recording setup can usually be confirmed by tapping on the facial muscles adjacent to the recording electrodes, which will generate an artifactual response that can be heard through the monitor's loudspeaker. Some devices such as the NIM allow a more sophisticated systems check by measuring the current flow obtained when the electrical stimulator is placed on any soft tissue in the operative field, but this requires that *stimulation is used in every case*. This current flow test will be ineffective if the stimulator is simply placed on skin (or dry bone) due to high impedance.

Care should be taken to assure that the ground pad of a monopolar electrosurgical unit is securely attached to the patient. This reduces the risk of shunting electrocautery energy into the recording electrodes and recording device.

The NIM includes a special muting detector probe that serves to activate a "speaker-muting" circuit during electrocautery. This prevents broadcasting the disruptive sound created by electrosurgical units through the loudspeaker. There are four ports on the back of the NIM ranging from "less mute (1)" to "more mute (4)." Our preferred initial setting is 3. A setting of 1 is relatively insensitive and can result in many outbursts from the loudspeaker due to infrequent muting. A setting of 4 will markedly reduce artifact noise but may cause excessive muting even from cautery usage in an adjacent room. The NIM's muting detection circuit is often sensitive enough to detect cautery even when the detector cable remains coiled on the NIM, some distance away from the electrosurgical unit. However, it functions best when it is clamped around both the monopolar and bipolar cautery cables near the site at which they attach into the electrosurgical units. Note that, although the muting circuit prevents a disruptive noise from being sounded through the loudspeaker *during cautery, valid monitoring does not occur at this time*. Thus, if during cautery the surgeon is concerned that electric or thermal energy could have injured the nerve, the nerve should be stimulated again immediately after cautery.

A facial nerve monitoring system should include a loudspeaker to provide direct feedback to the surgeon. The monitor's volume should be set so that the surgeon can hear the acoustically displayed EMG responses above the ambient noise of the operating room. An oscilloscope screen is also helpful in differentiating artifact from true EMG activity. Many types of artifact cannot be differentiated acoustically.

For ear and parotid operations, typical initial settings include a stimulus of 0.5 to 1.5 mA with an event threshold of 100 microvolts. The oscilloscope scale on the monitoring screen is typically set with an amplitude (vertical scale) of 200 microvolts and a time window of 50 microseconds.

In summary, once the setup is complete, the surgeon subsequently confirms functionality of the monitoring system by stimulating soft tissue and assuring current flow. Table 11–1 summarizes this setup.

Stimulation

Electrical stimulation can be an important adjunct to the surgeon's anatomic assessment in locating the facial nerve. Various stimulation techniques have been described by Moller and Janetta (constant-voltage stimulation), Prass and Luders (flush-tip insulation), and Kartush et al (bipolar and insulated stimulus dissectors).[20–23]

Prass designed a flush-tip probe (Xomed-Treace, Jacksonville, FL), with insulation down to the tip to avoid "shunting" of current away from the facial nerve into the CSF of the cerebellopontine angle during acoustic tumor dissection (Figure 11–3). Although insulation flush to the tip will minimize current shunting, the surgeon must use caution that the tiny portion of exposed electrode does indeed make adequate contact with the nerve in order to avoid a false-negative error due to poor contact.

Regarding voltage versus current generators, we prefer to use a constant–current system to minimize the effects of current shunting because impedance changes are dynamically compensated by changes in

Table 11–1. Summary of Facial Nerve Monitoring Setup and Initial Stimulation

Place bipolar electrodes in ipsilateral orbicularis oculi and oris—"blue eyes, red lips." The electrodes should be close to but not touching each other
Place green ground in sternum above white anode electrode
Plug the electrodes into proper channels on the patient interface box.
Ensure that the total impedance is less than 5 kOhm and that the interelectrode impedance in less than 1 kOhm for each electrode pair.
Perform a tap test on the skin surface above the electrodes to elicit an artifactual response (which only tests the *recording* portion of the system).
Adjust the volume of the NIM so that it can be heard above the ambient noise of the OR.
Once the procedure has begun, always check to ensure that current flow is present by using a stimulating probe or KSI instrument to touch muscle, soft tissue, or wet bone. These media conduct nearly 100% of the current due to their low impedance and therefore require less current to elicit a warble tone. If the monitor confirms proper current flow (visually or audibly), then the *stimulating* portion of the system has been appropriately confirmed.
Stimulate the nerve of interest at an early point in the surgery to ensure the functionality of the intraoperative monitoring and to gauge the appropriate stimulation level. Use a higher current (eg, 1.2 mAmp during cholesteatoma or tumor dissection) when exploring for or "mapping" the nerve and a lower current (eg, 0.1 to 0.3 mAmp at the porus) once the nerve has been localized. Then the lowest current that elicits a consistent response should be used during dissection to maximize spatial selectivity. Most modern monitors provide safe, pulsed current so that excessive stimulation of the nerve is virtually never a concern.

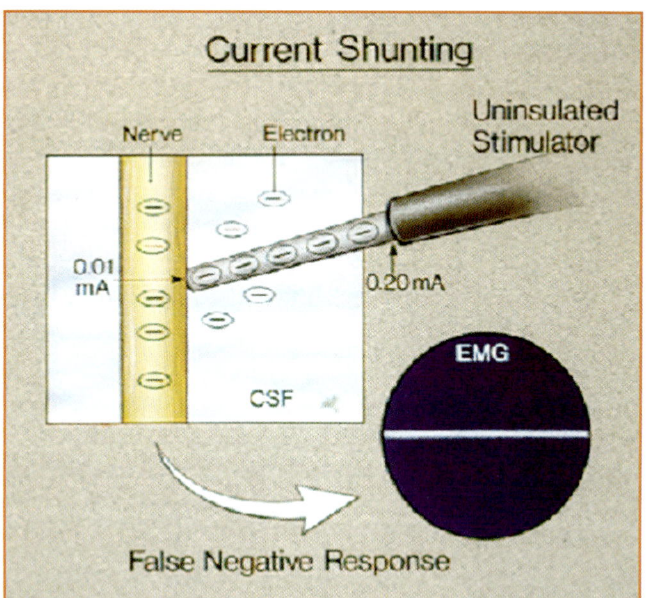

Figure 11–3. Cerebrospinal fluid, blood or soft tissue can *shunt* current away from the nerve which may result in a false-negative error. (Reprinted with permission, courtesy of Jack M. Kartush, MD)

voltage. Stimulation is most effective when the probe is attached to the cathode (black "–" sign) output.

Monopolar stimulation at relatively higher levels (eg, 1 to 1.5 mA) is best used to map the general vicinity of where the nerve is (and where it is not) in regard to tumor mass or cholesteatoma since this electrical configuration allows for some desired spread (volume conduction) of the current beyond the tip of the probe (Figure 11–4).

However, when trying to separate the facial nerve from an immediately adjacent neural structure (eg, the vestibule cochlear complex) or from adjacent soft tissue (tumor or cholesteatoma), a bipolar insulated stimulator is more selective[14,24] (Figure 11–5). Bipolar stimulation helps reduce the chance of a false positive error that can occur if current "jumps" from a monopolar stimulator in contact with the vestibular nerve to the adjacent facial nerve (Figure 11–6). If a bipolar stimulator is unavailable, the possibility of current jump can be minimized by using a monopolar stimulator at the lowest effective current setting. Conventional bipolar stimulators require that

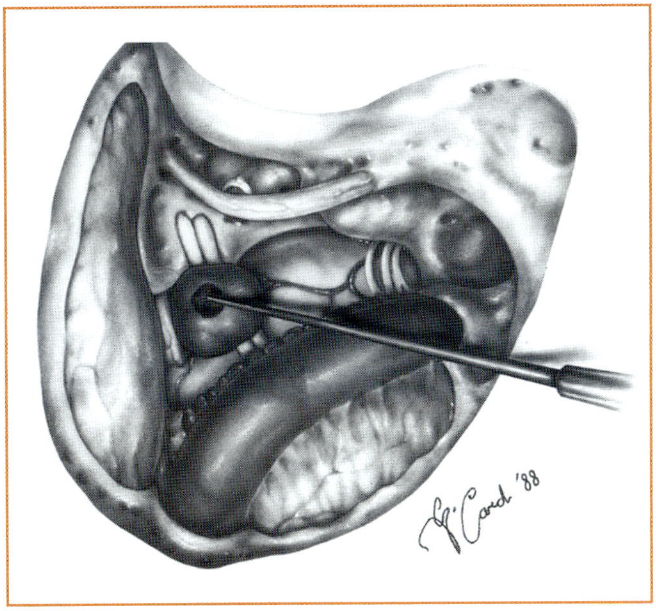

Figure 11–4. Monopolar electrical stimulation in and around acoustic neuroma maximizes sensitivity to tumor mapping. (Reprinted with permission[23])

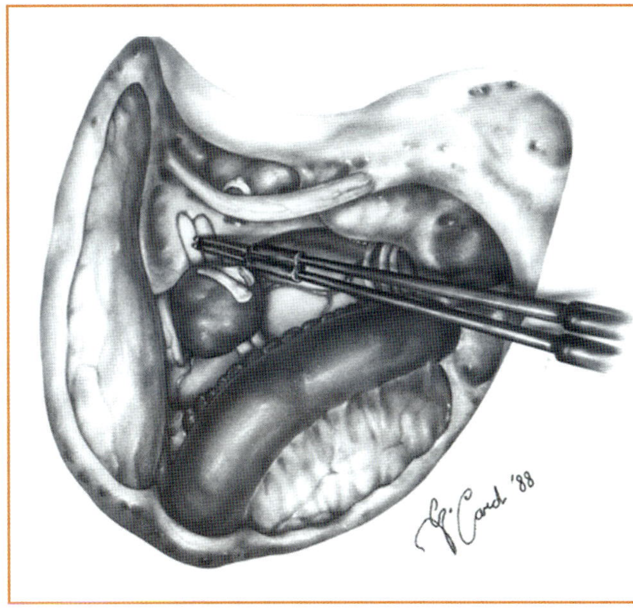

Figure 11–5. Bipolar stimulation maximizes selectivity in differentiating facial nerve from adjacent cochlear, vestibular, and trigeminal nerves. (Reprinted with permission[23])

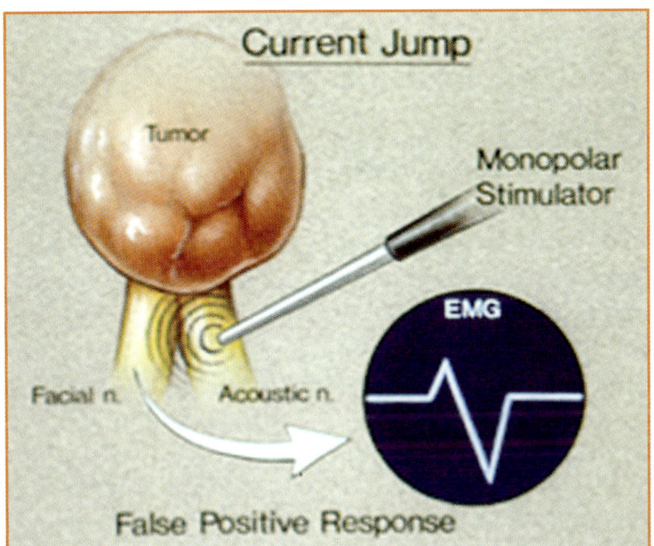

A

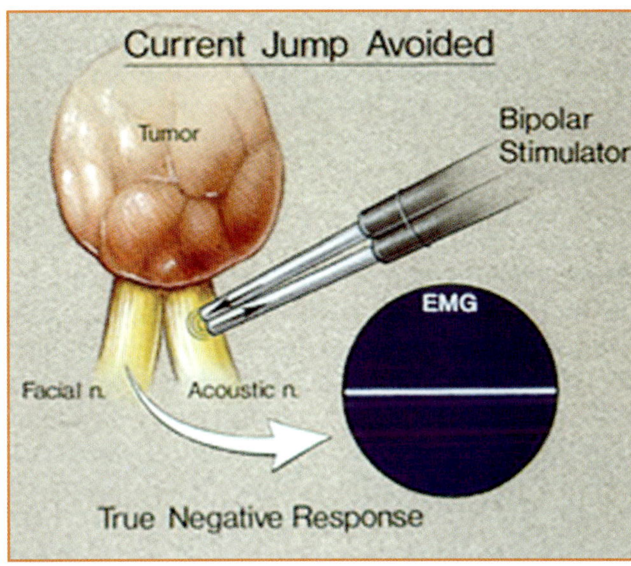

B

Figure 11–6. Spread of current through an adjacent nerve can produce a false-positive error ("current *jump*") (**A**), which can be minimized by the use of (**B**) bipolar stimulation. (Reprinted with permission, courtesy of Jack M. Kartush, MD)

the cathode tip be placed more distally along the motor nerve than the anode in order to achieve the most effective stimulation and to avoid "anodal block." As an alternative, a Kartush concentric bipolar stimulator can be used wherein the cathode is in the center and it is surrounded by a tubular anode.

As discussed earlier, motion detecting monitoring systems can be effective but are more liable to misrepresent stimulation of the trigeminal nerve as a true facial nerve response than EMG systems. Bipolar stimulation helps to further reduce this type of error by minimizing current shunting. Nonetheless, we have found that direct stimulation (0.5 mA) of the trigeminal nerve's pars minor (motor division) can produce such a large electromyographic potential that even EMG recording with close bipolar needle electrodes can pick up this response via volume conduction. This may then be misinterpreted as representing contraction of facial rather than masticatory muscles. One should be aware of the possibility of this false positive error.

Typically, the stimulator is set to a rate of 4 to 5 pulses per second and 100 microseconds pulse duration. Recall that stimulus efficacy is, to some extent, dependent on both current and stimulus duration. Therefore, elevations in stimulus duration beyond 100 microseconds would require lesser current levels to obtain a similar tissue effect.

A very low stimulus current of 0.05 mA is usually sufficient to obtain an adequate electrical evoked facial response when the stimulator is placed in direct contact with the nerve at the cerebellopontine angle (CPA) but may be inadequate to elicit a response more distally along the nerve due to nerve sheath, soft tissue, fallopian canal, etc. If there is intervening tissue or if the nerve has become fatigued because of prolonged dissection, the current intensity may be progressively increased up to 1.0 mA. Although brief, pulsed stimulation 2 to 3 mA has never been shown to cause neural injury, it is rarely needed and may result in an ambiguous response because of excessive current spread through the surrounding tissues. Hughes et al[25] evaluated the safety of electrical stimulation of peripheral nerves. Pulsed, intermittent stimuli can reduce the possibility of electrical injury. In the past, many disposable stimulators used continuous direct current (DC) stimulation, which increased the risk of nerve injury and are thus discouraged. When dissecting in the cerebellopontine angle in an area believed to be distant from the facial nerve (ie, large tumor mass), we set the level of stimulation to 0.4 to 0.8 mA. As soon as the nerve is encountered, the stimulus level is decreased. When surgical dissection is performed adjacent to the facial nerve at the cerebellopontine angle, a setting of 0.05 mA to 0.20 mA is used. However, a higher setting (0.1 mA to 0.5 mA) is used along the tympanic and mastoid nerve segments due to interposition of fascia, periosteum and bone along the nerve. In an unpublished study performed by the senior author (Kartush, 1984), the effects of higher than usual stimulus levels were tested on mouse sciatic nerves, stimulating at 5 mA for 3 minutes at 5 pulses per second with 100 ms duration. After approximately 5 minutes, the amplitude of the response began to decrease. After a 5-minute rest period, however, the nerve then responded normally again. We hypothesized that this was due to the transient depletion of the neurotransmitter acetylcholine at the neuromuscular junction. Consequently, using modern stimulator systems at the ranges described, the surgeon should have no hesitancy in using sufficient current to optimize nerve mapping.

Stimulus Dissecting Instruments

Active monitoring entails frequent use of electric stimulation rather than *passively* awaiting responses after trauma has occurred. Although blunt trauma such as direct manipulation or traction on the facial nerve will usually evoke a facial EMG response, our investigations demonstrate that sharp dissection may evoke little or no response even with complete transection of the nerve. More distal nerves, eg, recurrent laryngeal nerve and spinal nerves, are even less likely to trigger mechanical evoked warning responses. In order to circumvent this problem, insulated stimulating dissection instruments have been designed.[11,24,26] Kartush Stimulating Instruments (KSI; Neurosign, Wales, UK) allow *simultaneous* monopolar stimulation and nerve mapping with sharp surgical dissection (Figure 11–7). Whereas blunt dissection evokes a potential after some degree of nerve manipulation or trauma has already occurred, KSIs alert the surgeon to the proximity of the nerve *before* a cutting maneuver is performed. Unlike dedicated facial nerve probes, however, stimulus dissectors cannot be insulated flush to their tip. In order to allow the instrument an adequate cutting edge, a variable degree of the instrument must remain non-insulated. The area of non-insulation

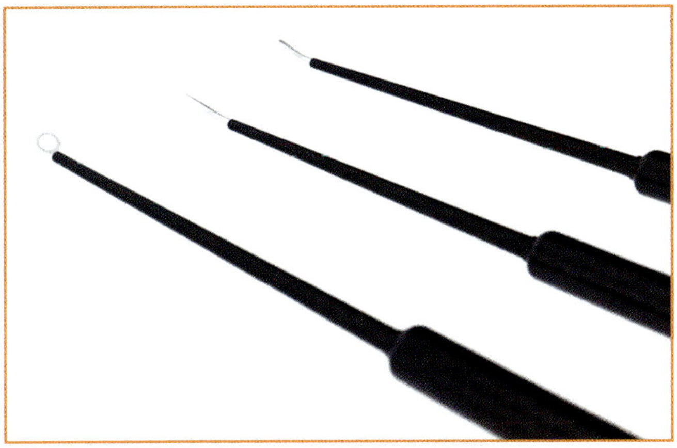

Figure 11–7. A special set of insulated surgical instruments (Kartush Stimulus Instruments) connect directly to the stimulator which allows simultaneous monopolar mapping during sharp surgical dissection. Magstim/Neurosign. (Reprinted with permission, courtesy of Kartush & Magstim/Neurosign)

is dependent upon the instrument. For example, a needle dissector may be almost entirely insulated, whereas a pair of microscissors will require a greater degree of noninsulation in order to allow adequate freedom of movements for its parts.

Therefore, the surgeon using KSIs must be aware of the inherent possibility of current shunting. Fortunately, the near-total insulation of most dissectors precludes shunting under most circumstances. In order to further reduce the possibility of false-negative stimulation particularly during pooling of spinal fluid or blood, the stimulus intensity should be increased (eg, from 0.05 mA to 0.10 mA when working immediately adjacent to nerve; from 0.20 mA to 0.50 mA or more when working at greater distances from the nerve or when the location of the nerve remains uncertain). These principles hold true for middle ear and mastoid surgery; the stimulus intensity should be increased when the nerve is covered by bone, sheath, granulation tissue or cholesteatoma, and then progressively decreased once the nerve has been identified and as dissection proceeds closer to the nerve.

In order to minimize current shunting, some instruments (stimulating round currette) have had their ordinarily large surface area reduced by creating a hole in the center. It is primarily intended to debulk the center of an acoustic neuroma or large cholesteatoma while mapping the position of the facial nerve along capsule. Its small surface area minimizes current shunting. When dissecting relatively distant to the nerve, we use it at a setting of 1.0 mA and aspirate the debulked contents with a 5-gauge suction tip. Stimulus intensity and suction tip size are reduced as dissection proceeds.

Although we had designed insulated self-retaining retractors in the past to avoid the static discharge that two metal instruments may create when they come in contact, the incidence of static artifact has become less common as recording devices have become more sophisticated. Static discharges may be a source of confusion since they are artifacts that the recording device may erroneously signal as an EMG event. A monitoring unit with an oscilloscope is most helpful here to differentiate artifact from actual EMG responses. Static artifact has a typical "spiky" monophasic appearance versus the more rounded, polyphasic response of true EMG.

The concept of stimulating dissection instruments was described over a quarter century ago, but it is only in more recent years that the strategy is being more broadly accepted and applied including the use of stimulating instruments and drills in spinal surgery. Similarly, we have described how impedance changes can help control surgical dissection and drills, eg, automatically stopping a microdrill during cochleostomy based upon changes of impedance from bone to inner ear fluid when current is applied to the round window[27] (Figure 11–8).

Minimizing Neural Trauma

Even after the location of the nerve has been identified, microtrauma associated with dissection may result in significant injury due to prolonged dissection or traction. Fortunately, for facial nerve monitoring, these surgical maneuvers often provoke a mechanically evoked response that alerts the surgeon to possible trauma. Mechanical evoked potentials appear to be a result of rapid neural deformations resulting in ion depolarization that in turn leads to an action potential. The most efficient stimuli include abrupt contact or traction of the nerve. Slower, more progressive traction, however, may

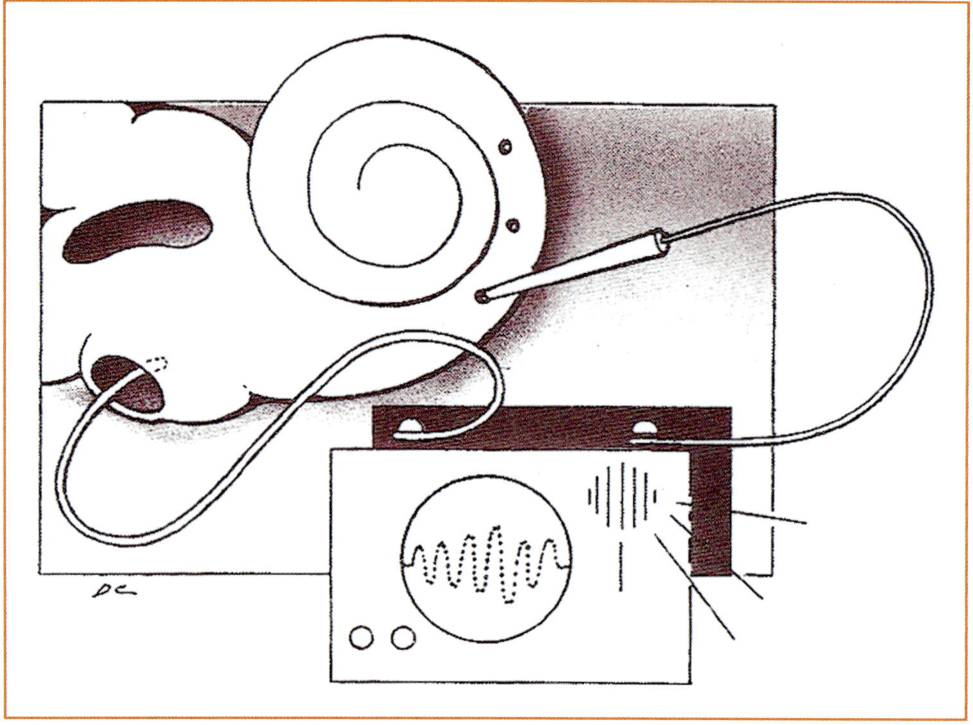

Figure 11–8. Design for cochlear microdrill. Cathodal stimulation occurs through drill with anodal return at round window. As drill penetrates cochlea, electrical impedance between anode and cathode is reduced which turns off drill to minimize cochlear trauma. (Reprinted with permission, courtesy of American Academy of Otolaryngology)

result in little or no response. Traction responses tend to occur as multiple asynchronous potentials, in contrast to the single synchronized potential seen with brief direct mechanical contact. Prass and Luders[9] have categorized these responses as "trains" and "bursts," respectively.

Brief burst potentials result from blunt contact with the nerve and only rarely indicate significant injury (Figure 11–9). In fact following dissection, nerves that readily elicit a burst potential with gentle direct contact often exhibit excellent postoperative function. In contrast, train potentials may indicate some degree of microtrauma (Figure 11–10). Thus, when train potentials occur, we often temporarily cease dissection and relax retractors. If such potentials persist and the surgeon chooses to resume dissection, these potentials can obscure identification of new burst responses. This situation can sometimes be circumvented by temporarily defeating monitoring of nasolabial activity and monitoring only orbicularis oculi activity since this recording site is generally less prone to train potentials. As soon as possible, resume monitoring through both EMG channels to maximize recording sensitivity.

There is tremendous variability between nerves in response to trauma as well as cool irrigation. The occurrence of brief, rare trains of EMG activity during minor, controlled manipulation of the nerve is usually not associated with any postoperative dysfunction. However, prolonged trains (ie, 1 minute or more) often signal trauma. An alternative cause is the patient being "too light" relative to anesthesia, which can cause diffuse muscle movement. In fact, facial monitoring can sometimes serve as an additional warning signal to anesthesia because common signs that the patient may be getting light (ie, tachycardia and elevated blood pressure) may not occur until after the patient begins to move.

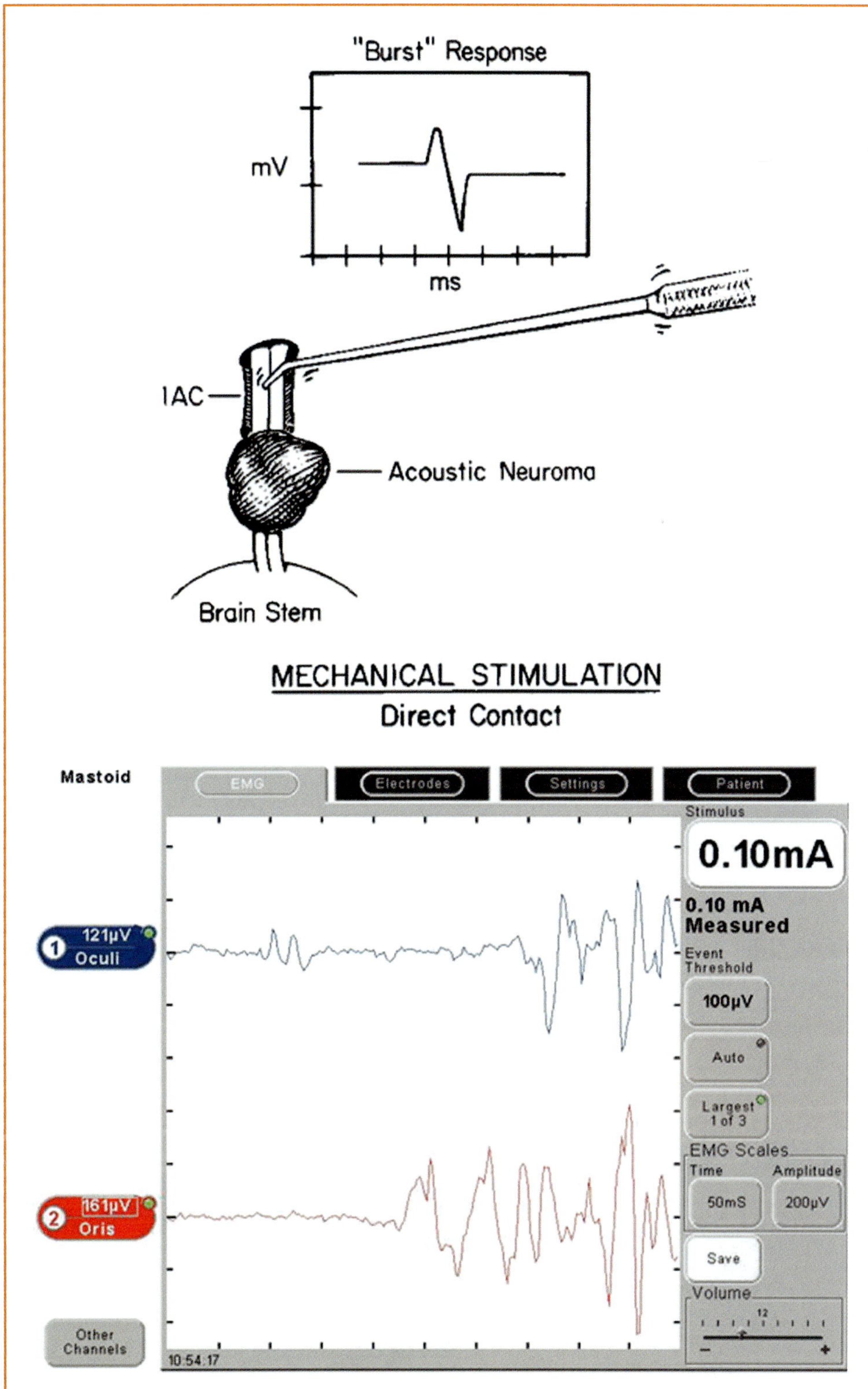

Figure 11–9. Elicitation of "burst" facial evoked response secondary to mechanical manipulation. (Reprinted with permission[23])

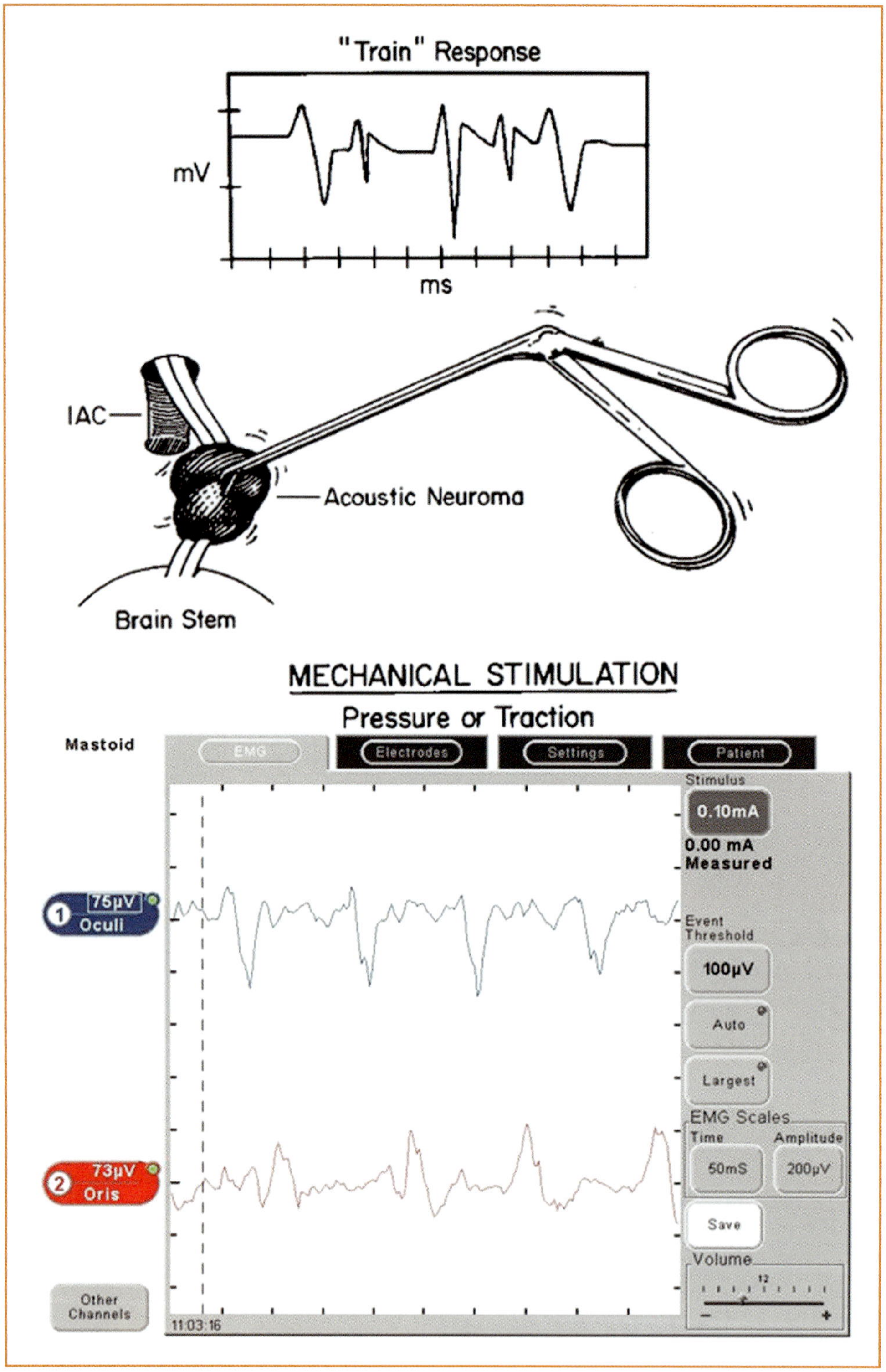

Figure 11–10. Elicitation of "train" facial evoked response secondary to nerve irritation. (Reprinted with permission[23])

When drilling adjacent to the facial nerve, multiple, repetitive responses may occur. While it is possible that this could represent direct trauma to the nerve, in careful, experienced hands, it is more likely due to transmission of vibrations through a thin shell of bone that overlies the nerve called *"drill potentials"* (Figure 11–11). Nonetheless, when it is observed, the surgeon should be cautioned that their drill is adjacent to or on the nerve.

Thermal changes may also evoke train potentials. When this occurs due to cold saline irrigation, it appears to have no association to neural trauma. As the saline gradually warms to body temperature, the asynchronous potentials will subside. Some nerves are hypersensitive to cold irrigation and can benefit by having the irrigation gently warmed in a blood warmer. If thermal-evoked responses are generated during laser surgery, however, they may indicate heating of the nerve and, thus, we temporarily discontinue the laser and irrigate the operative site with cool saline or Ringers solution. If the buildup of heat is slow, there initially may be little or no discrete evoked potentials. Instead, a widened baseline can often be identified in the recorded activity as seen on the NIM display. Because these initial responses to heating may be of low amplitude, and because the NIM is typically set to alarm only when a response is greater than 100 microvolts, the surgeon and/or monitorist must actively look for the silent increase in baseline, or transiently change the baseline alarm to signal at lower response levels.

Electrocautery can be another source of thermal injury. Although bipolar cautery helps to restrict the area of electrical current compared to monopolar cautery, neural injury can still occur due to spread of heat by convection or conduction. Therefore, when cautery is required adjacent to the facial nerve, it should be performed using brief, intermittent applications at the lowest possible power. Since monitoring systems are not effective during periods

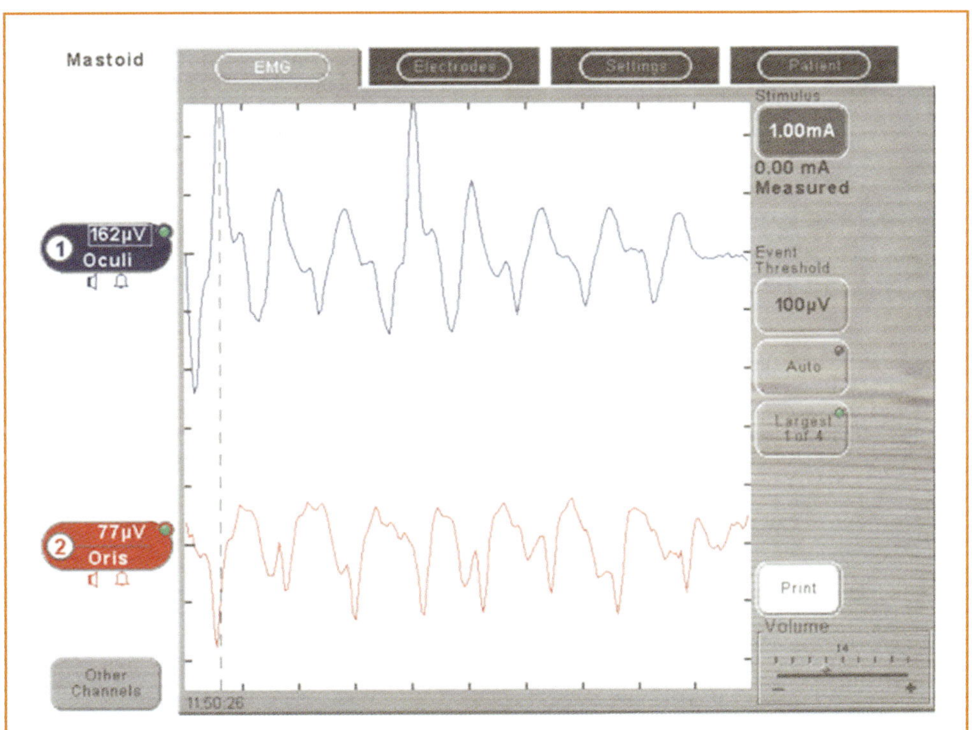

Figure 11–11. Mechanical evoked potentials may sometimes occur even when a thin shell of bone overlies the nerve presumably due to transmission of vibrations through bone. (Reprinted with permission, courtesy of Jack M. Kartush, MD)

of electrocautery, visual observation of facial contractions beneath a sterile transparent drape or palpation of muscle contractures through an opaque drape can be helpful (Figure 11–12).

In summary, in order to obtain maximal benefit from monitoring, burst and train potentials must trigger a troubleshooting algorithm for the surgeon and monitoring team. Depending on the clinical scenario, it may prompt relaxation of retractors, a switch to warmed irrigation, cessation of laser use, or, whenever in doubt, re-testing the nerve electrically to confirm its integrity.

Assessment of Neural Integrity

After dissection is complete, the integrity of the nerve can be assessed by stimulating it at an area *proximal* to the site of dissection. During acoustic neuroma surgery, this stimulation is performed adjacent to the pons at a setting of 0.05 mA. Note that this is a very low current setting used to assess near-threshold stimulation level. Nerves that require elevations in this current intensity to reach response threshold often demonstrate some degree of postoperative weakness. As long as some response is obtained, the continuity of the nerve can be confirmed.

Some patients with normal electrical excitability may nonetheless develop a delayed facial paralysis. At this time, there appears to be no indicator to routinely help predict this phenomenon. It is often helpful to compare the amplitude of the response obtained by stimulation at the proximal nerve to a response obtained distal to the site of surgical dissection. However, rather than assume that these represent a false positive error, it is most likely that, with intracranial surgery, postoperative weakness is due to edema or ischemia. We typically perform decompression of the facial nerve at the meatal foramen during translabyrinthine and middle cranial fossa approaches on the presumption that acoustic tumor patients develop delayed facial palsy due to progressive edema.[28] Of course, one must ensure that the nerve is not injured after the final proximal stimula-

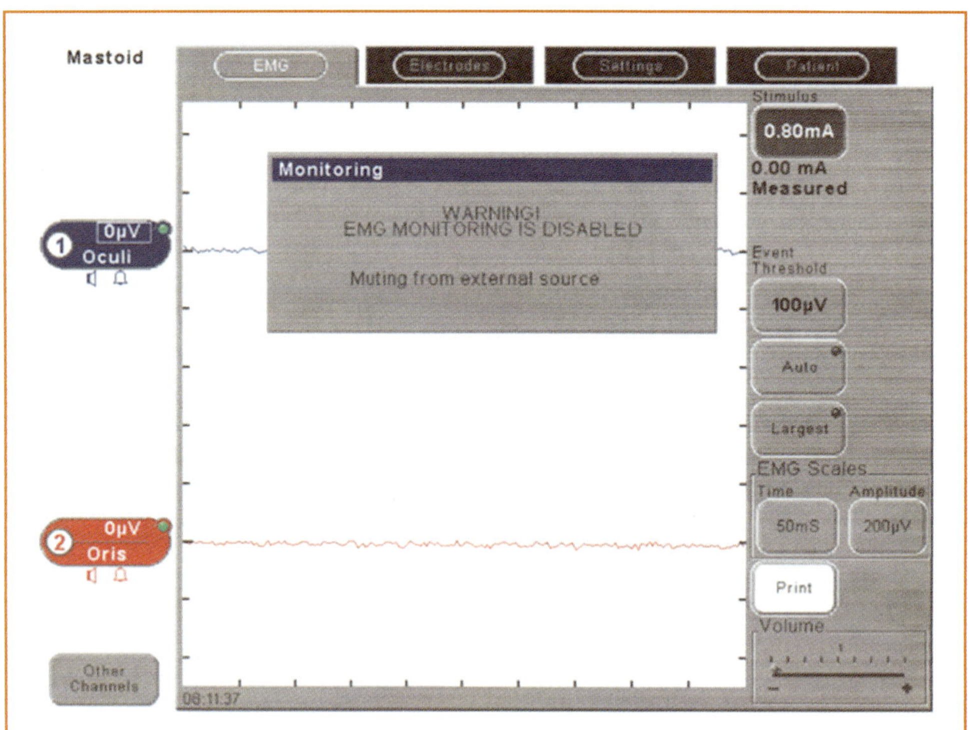

Figure 11–12. The NIM is disabled and muted during electrocautery. (Reprinted with permission, courtesy of Jack M. Kartush, MD)

tion during closure, that is, during fat graft placement. We have also described delayed postoperative facial palsy as a consequence of viral re-activation.[29]

Electrical stimulation of the facial nerve has also been used during surgical decompression for Bell's palsy. Fisch and Esslen[30] described a technique wherein the site of maximal edematous entrapment of the nerve is identified by progressively stimulating along the nerve from distal to proximal until a site of unstimulatable nerve is reached. For this technique to be usable, some fibers must not have undergone Wallerian degeneration.

Interpretation

Intraoperative monitoring can only be effective if the surgeon understands the results of monitoring and is willing to respond appropriately. The presence or absence of facial evoked responses must be interpreted within the context of the surgical procedure. Electrical silence may be a consequence of: (1) the absence of facial nerve stimulation, (2) severe injury precluding depolarization, (3) complete transection of the nerve, or (4) technical problems. When in doubt, electrical stimulation of the facial nerve both proximal and distal to the site of dissection should be performed to assess its integrity. An appropriately functioning system should be confirmed at the start of each case and rechecked intermittently throughout the procedure. Nerves that have been significantly manipulated during dissection may demonstrate "fatigue" wherein responses become more and more difficult to obtain. Under these circumstances, stimulus current intensity may need to be increased. We have encountered an interesting scenario that reduces the reliability of facial nerve monitoring. Following preoperative arterial embolization for glomus jugulare tumors, we have noted a marked decrease in the responsiveness of the facial nerve to both electrical and mechanical stimulation. We believe this phenomenon occurs due to neural devascularization that creates a subclinical neuropraxia and desynchronization. Preoperative electroneurography (ENoG) can sometimes detect such subclinical abnormalities.[22] Table 11–2 lists other possibilities that should be excluded when an expected response does not occur.

Table 11–2. Checklist for Intraoperative Facial Monitoring Problems

Problem	Possible Solution/Cause
Current jump	Lower the current intensity or use bipolar stimulation
Current shunting	Insulated stimulator
Cautery artifact noise	Muting circuit
Cautery precludes monitoring	Visualize or palpate the face
Laser heating effect	Monitor baseline amplitude
Saline cooling	Warm saline with "blood warmer"
Stimulus artifact	Increase "Stimulus ignore" time; exclude an overcharged capacitor
Static discharge	Insulated instruments
No response to stimulation	1. Power off 2. Current intensity too low 3. Current measured too low 4. Electrode impedence too high 5. Electrode disconnect 6. Current shunting 7. Threshold setting too high 8. Volume too low 9. Muscle relaxant used 10. Local anesthetic on nerve 11. "Stimulus ignore" too long 12. Nerve not contacted 13. Other cranial nerve/tissue 14. Nerve injured

Interpretation of burst and train potentials must be performed with great care. The acoustic representation of facial potentials allows the surgeon to interpret these responses in context to the ongoing surgical events. Table 11–3 correlates the cause and acoustic representation of common facial evoked responses using terms coined by Prass and Luders.[21] As the frequency of electrical stimulation is usually set at 4 pulses per second, a uniform machine gun-like response and series of evenly spaced "event" tones are heard. The cause and clinical correlation of burst and train responses have been described in the preceding section. Since surgical traction, high speed drilling and laser heating all create train potentials, the EMG response must be interpreted based on the preceding surgical maneuvers. Consequently, a surgeon trained in intraoperative monitoring is indeed best able to discern the most likely causes of EMG responses. For those without monitoring training, an experienced technologist or neurophysiologist can be an invaluable resource for the surgeon.

The surgeon and monitoring team must be aware that there are a number of EMG responses that may be due to artifact or nontraumatic stimuli (Table 11–4). *Static* discharge between two metal instruments is a common artifact as is detection of stimuli caused by an anesthesiologist's *peripheral nerve stimulator*. Static artifact typically exhibits a much more abrupt electromyographic response regarding onset (rise time) and duration (Figure 11–13). Some devices (such as ultrasonic aspirators) may create low-level artifact or trigger the automatic muting circuitry which may prevent effective monitoring during their use. The use of monopolar electrocautery may occasionally *"charge"* the monitors capacitors that can result in false-positive responses. This artifact can be recognized by: (1) identifying repetitive EMG pulses when the probe is in contact with any soft tissue no matter how distant from the nerve and (2) identifying a *DC shift* of the EMG baseline on the oscilloscope instead of a typical triphasic response (Figure 11–14). If a patient's *depth of anesthesia* becomes too light, facial muscle fasciculations may occur that will generate multiple asynchronous EMG potentials (Figure 11–15). Although these potentials represent true facial muscle activity rather than artifact, they can be misinterpreted as indicators of neural trauma.

A difficult clinical situation may be encountered regarding the desirability of resecting and grafting a facial nerve, which remains in continuity but does not respond to electrical stimulation. Because severe neuropraxic injuries can prevent depolarization just as more severe axonal injuries do, it is currently our practice *not* to resect an apparently intact facial nerve

Table 11–3. EMG and Acoustic Representation of Surgical Stimuli

Stimulus	EMG	Acoustic Representation
Electrical	Precisely timed responses	Machine gun
Mechanical	Single polyphasic response (burst)	Synchronous click
Traction	Multiple asynchronous responses (train)	Popping corn, possibly delayed
Thermal	Initially: widened baseline Later: multiple asynchronous responses	Initially: silent Later: popping corn

Table 11–4. Common Artifacts and Nonsurgical Stimuli

Stimulus	EMG	Acoustic representation
Stimulator charged by prior cautery use	DC offset of EMG baseline even though stimulator placed distant to nerve	Machine gun
Static discharge	Single polyphasic response	Synchronous click
Too little anesthetic (patient "light")	Multiple asynchronous responses	Popping corn
Electrocautery	Multiple asynchronous responses	Silent if muting detector used
Peripheral nerve stimulator	Precisely timed responses	Machine gun

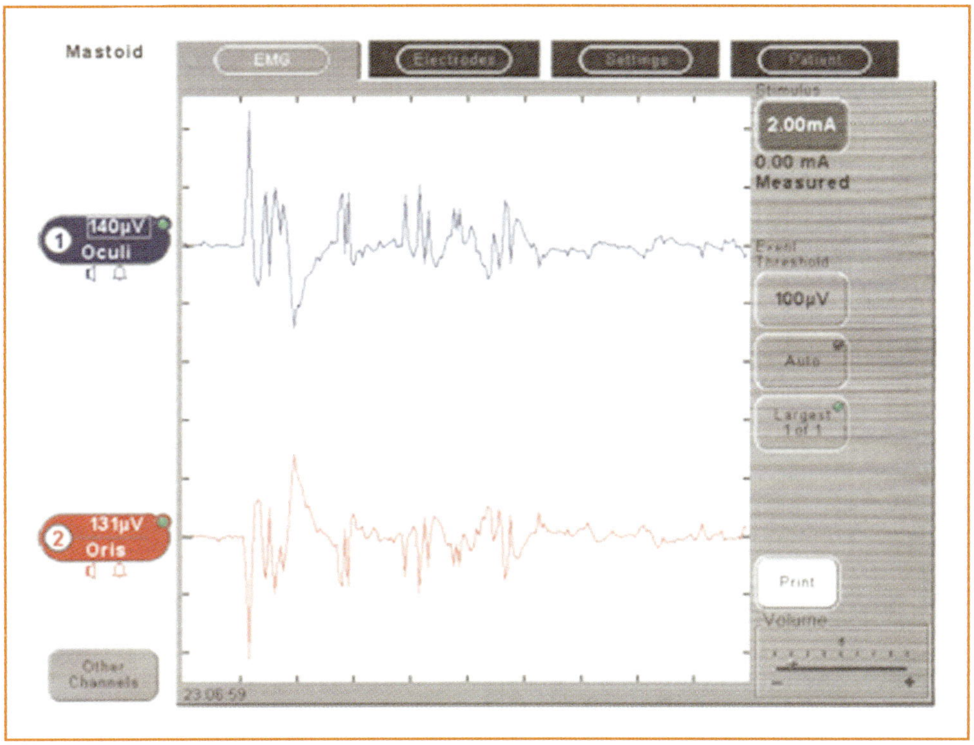

Figure 11–13. Static artifact typically exhibits a much more abrupt electromyographic response regarding onset (rise time) and duration. (Reprinted with permission, courtesy of Jack M. Kartush, MD)

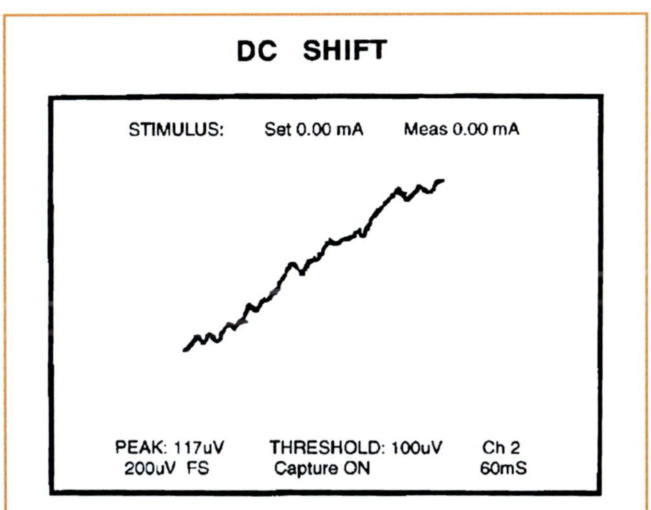

Figure 11–14. A *"charged"* stimulator probe can result in false-positive responses, which can be identified by a *DC shift* of the EMG baseline on the oscilloscope instead of a typical triphasic response. (Reprinted with permission, courtesy of Jack M. Kartush, MD)

solely on the basis of lack of stimulation following surgical dissection. Under these circumstances, the microscopic morphology seen at the time of surgery should be considered in conjunction with preoperative clinical or subclinical abnormalities.

What to Do If the Patient Wakes Up with a Facial Palsy Despite Intraoperative Monitoring?

On rare occasions, the surgeon may be faced with a difficult situation. Having used a facial nerve monitor for a mastoidectomy during which no mechanical evoked potentials were elicited, the patient may awake from anesthesia with a facial palsy. Does this mean that the monitor malfunctioned and the nerve is injured, or does the absence of mechanical evoked potentials mean that there is another cause such as edema?

As noted above, it is not unusual that after acoustic tumor resection, the facial nerve may be

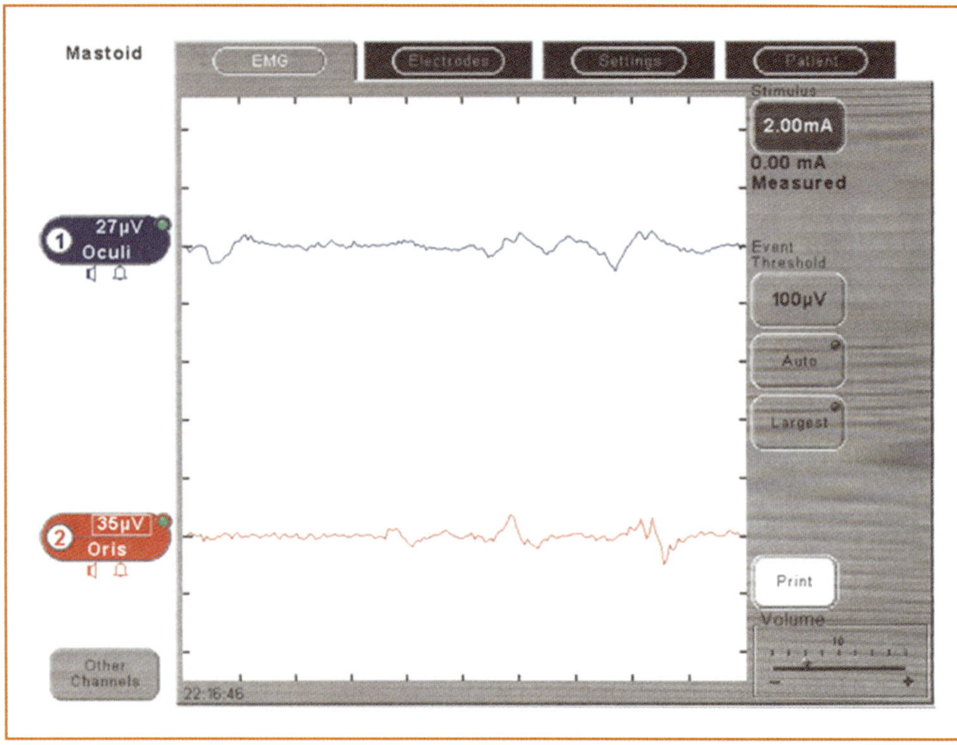

Figure 11–15. Asynchronous EMG potentials in a patient with a light depth of anesthesia. (Reprinted with permission, courtesy of Jack M. Kartush, MD)

ischemic and as edema progresses during closure, the nerve may indeed appear weak when assessed in the recovery room. However, ischemia and edema are *not* expected after mastoid surgery and an immediate postoperative facial palsy must provoke a search for other causes.

Always assure that the facial nerve is accurately assessed at the earliest possible time postoperatively to rule out immediate versus delayed facial palsy. If the patient is very sedated postoperatively and the facial assessment is compromised, note it and then re-assess shortly afterwards. Even though the House-Brackmann facial grading system was not intended for this purpose, most clinicians will grade the facial function using this system. A detailed assessment of the facial nerve should be documented and the time noted. There are two common pitfalls in assessing acute facial palsy. First, in children, their excellent skin, soft tissue, and muscle tone may make a complete paralysis seem incomplete; therefore, do not mistake tone for movement. Seek unequivocal movement of facial muscles. Second, the eye closes due to two mechanisms: (a) contraction of orbicularis oculi from the facial nerve, and (b) relaxation of the levator muscle by the oculomotor nerve. Thus, if the only "movement" seen is a slow, partial closure of the upper eyelid, this may represent relaxation of the levator muscle and should not be misconstrued as an "incomplete facial palsy." If in doubt, hold up the upper eyelid and then ask the patient to close their eye as hard as possible: if there is no visible contraction of orbicularis oculis, the paralysis may be total.

If an immediate facial palsy is noted, it is appropriate to wait a few hours to assure that local anesthetic (either injected or topically affecting the nerve through a perforated tympanic membrane) has had time to wear off. Although some textbooks indicate that mastoid packing should be removed on the chance that it is compressing the facial nerve, we have never seen this help; and unless the nerve were to be dramatically dehiscent throughout a few centimeters of its course, it is hard to imagine that this is a cause.

As noted, in the setting of a routine mastoidectomy, facial edema is an unlikely cause for facial palsy and the possibility of direct nerve injury must be seriously considered. If one focuses only on edema as a cause, it may lead to detrimental delays in treatment.

If intraoperative monitoring was used, the possibility for an error in monitoring must be determined. Firstly, was the monitoring surgeon or technician properly trained? All of the potential pitfalls already discussed must be considered. Also, if stimulating dissecting instruments or some other stimulator were used, was there confirmation of proper function of the monitoring equipment with confirmed current flow? Was there a documented response to stimulation of the nerve at any time during the surgery? This highlights the importance of *routine electric stimulation,* which can confirm both current flow and a response. This ensures that both the device and setup were correct, and also excludes the effects of neuromuscular blockade and injected or topical local anesthetic. Note that if xylocaine simply contacts a dehiscent facial nerve coming through a perforated tympanic membrane, it may cause a temporary facial palsy that makes monitoring useless. If an electrical response was never obtained during the case, the surgeon cannot know with certainty that monitoring was accurate, and consequently surgical re-exploration should be highly considered.

If there is a significant or total facial palsy that is being carefully followed postoperatively without exploration, an ENoG may be useful 2 to 3 days after surgery once Wallerian degeneration has occurred. Little or no response to electric stimulation should again be a strong indicator for surgical exploration and one should consider consulting a surgeon who is experienced in repairing injured facial nerves. A CAT scan should also be considered for postoperative facial palsy if re-exploration is being deferred. Many times in the past, the legal consequence of an iatrogenic facial nerve injury was considered *res ipsa loquitur*, Latin for "it goes without saying," meaning that malpractice was "obvious." Nowadays, inadvertent nerve injury may indeed be defensible particularly in the setting of a very diseased ear, tumors, or anomalous anatomy, but only if prompt, appropriate steps to address the injury are demonstrated postoperatively.

Methods to Minimize Errors in Surgery Involving the Facial Nerve

Specific techniques to minimize errors are critical to performing safe surgery, beyond the use of monitoring.[31] When injecting the external auditory canal with local anesthetic in the presence of a large perforated tympanic membrane, consider covering the perforation with saline-soaked Gelfoam in order to prevent the xylocaine from contacting the facial nerve because it may cause a transient conduction blockade of the facial nerve, which would render the monitor temporarily useless. Similarly, overzealous xylocaine injection at the mastoid tip region should be avoided. Placing the postauricular incision posterior to the mastoid tip in children and avoiding electrocautery use inferiorly reduces the risk to the facial nerve, which is most superficial as it exits the stylomastoid foramen. Proper drilling techniques are also essential. Copious irrigation to avoid thermal injury, drilling parallel to important structures, and using the appropriate size and type of burr are critical. The orientation of drilling should be chosen in anticipation of which structures could be injured in case of an inadvertent skip of the burr. Based on which side of the burr is in contact with bone, the surgeon should know which direction it will most likely slip toward. Natural anatomic protection (ie, bone) should be preserved and the removal of natural protection, if necessary, should be delayed for as long as possible. For example, completing the labyrinthectomy portion of a translabyrinthine approach prior to removal of the incus and opening of the facial recess protects the facial nerve from potential injury from a skipping bur.

INTRAOPERATIVE AUDITORY BRAINSTEM RESPONSES (ABR)

Monitoring cranial nerve VIII during microvascular decompressions, vestibular neurectomies, and resections of acoustic neuromas and other skull base tumors where hearing is at risk, is a common practice. The auditory brainstem response consists of a series of waves primarily occurring within 10 milliseconds of the stimulus onset. These far-field responses are generated from the cochlear nerve and the auditory nuclei of the brainstem. In the clinical setting, standard electroencephalographic disk electrodes are placed on the vertex (Cz), both earlobes or mastoids (A1 and A2), and the forehead (Fpz). The vertex electrode is the positive input to the amplifier, the earlobe/mastoid inputs are negative, and the forehead serves as the ground. The setup for intraoperative ABR is similar to recordings performed in the clinic, with a few modifications to compensate for the setting. An in-the-ear earphone is required to keep the surgical field clear but must still be able to produce a high-quality acoustic stimulus. Plastic tubing to conduct sound into the ear from a nearby transducer is often employed to reduce stimulus artifact. A recording electrode may also be placed adjacent to this tubing to enhance wave I. Another recording electrode is placed between the forehead and vertex, and a ground electrode is placed in the scalp as well. Subdermal needles are preferred for the same reasons as previously stated for facial nerve monitoring. A narrower band-pass than is commonly used in the clinic is utilized for recording in the operating room to decrease the sensitivity to interference. Trained personnel other than the surgeon is required to monitor these readings intraoperatively.

Recording the cochlear nerve action potential with an electrode on the nerve in the cerebellopontine angle is another option. The advantage here is nearly real-time feedback of neural change, but with the caveat that the electrode may be easily displaced or obstruct the surgeon's view. Furthermore, with large tumors, the auditory nerve may not be accessible until some tumor is resected. Lastly, an electrode that is firmly attached to the cochlear nerve leads to the potential risk of stretch or avulsion if the electrode wire is inadvertently pulled.

RECURRENT LARYNGEAL NERVE MONITORING

Setup

Recurrent laryngeal nerve (RLN) monitoring is being increasingly used during thyroidectomy, parathyroidectomy and during skull base procedures where CN X is at risk. Initially, RLN monitoring was performed by placing needle electrodes laryngoscopically or transcutaneously into the vocal folds. Difficulties in achieving this accurately and safely led to a search for alternative means.

RLN monitoring is now often performed by attaching a recording electrode to an endotracheal tube (ETT). The intent is to place the electrodes as close to the vocal folds as possible to measure the EMG with surface electrodes rather than intramuscular needle electrodes. A commonly used design made by Medtronic has factory installed electrodes along the lateral surface of the tube (Figure 11–16). These tubes were initially criticized for being too flexible to which the company responded by stiffening the tube with a reinforcing wire, The current iteration of this tube is susceptible to this internal wiring kinking or unraveling within the lumen of the tube and thus requires special precautions to avoid airway obstruction, as detailed below. If the wire delaminates, it can cause airway obstruction. By convention, the red electrode is placed to contact the right vocal fold and blue is for the left side. The colored band encircling the endotracheal tube must be at the level of the vocal folds. The average tube depth for the Medtronic endotracheal tubes is between 22 to 24 cm at the incisors for most patients. The endotracheal tube must be of the appropriate size and correctly aligned for accurate monitoring to occur. As with all EMG monitoring, long-acting paralytics must not be administered by anesthesia nor should topical viscous lidocaine be used during intubation.

Other options include electrodes that are taped onto conventional endotracheal tubes such as Rea's

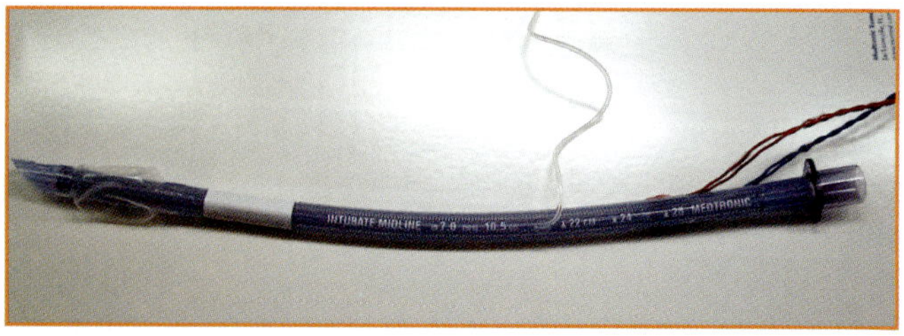

Figure 11–16. Medtronic laryngeal monitoring endotracheal tube. (Reprinted with permission, courtesy of Jack M. Kartush, MD)

design by IOM Solutions/Neurovision and those by Magstim/Neurosign (Figures 11–17 and 11–18). These systems are similar to the Medtronic laryngeal monitoring endotracheal tube but are of lower cost and, because there is because no concern of disrupting a reinforcing wire, do not have the associated disadvantage, such as the inability to suction through the tube or place a tube exchanger through it. These stick-on electrodes must be properly placed on the endotracheal tube, usually about 1 to 2 cm above the cuff. During long cases, it is possible for the adhesive to become less adherent resulting in slippage from the tube. Transiently straightening the normally curved tube can allow better placement of the electrode without buckling. Current experience indicates that placement of the stick-on electrodes works best posteriorly rather than anteriorly. This probably relates to the fact that the EMG response is greater posteriorly near the posterior cricoarytenoid muscles rather than the smaller tensor muscles intrinsic to the cords themselves.

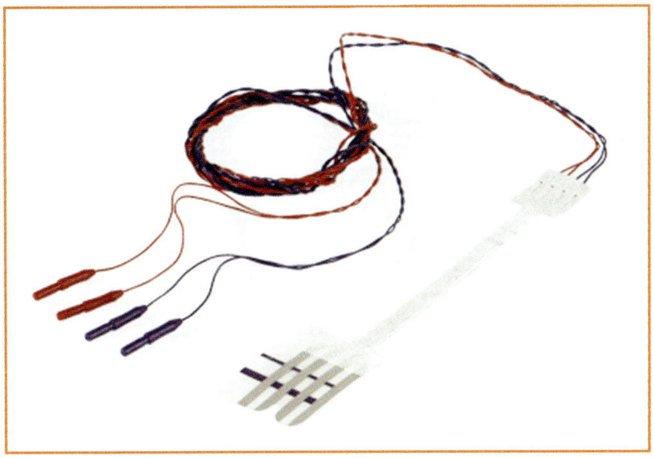

Figure 11–17. IOM Solutions two-channel laryngeal surface electrodes (Ventura, CA).

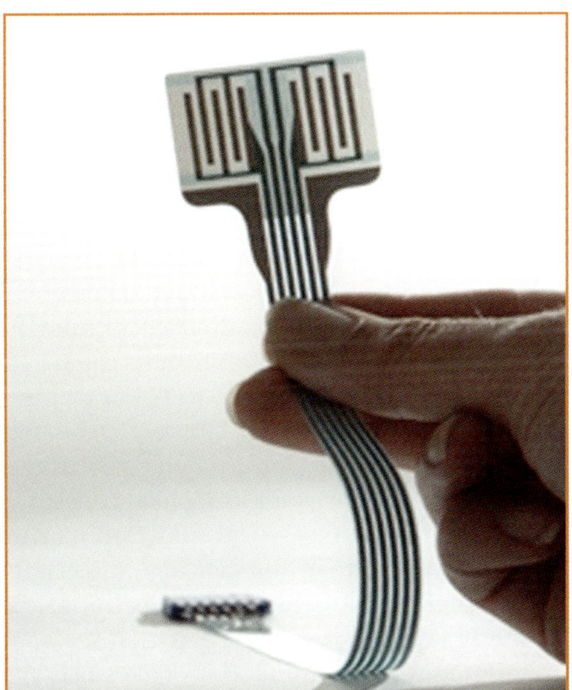

Figure 11–18. Magstim Neurosign (Wales, UK). Original laryngeal surface electrodes.

Laryngeal electrodes that are flush against the endotracheal tube yield a circular surface in the midst of a triangular glottic inlet. This geometric mismatch may lead to poor contact of the electrode to the vocal cords and in turn cause false negative errors due to failure to record laryngeal responses. To the end, a new self-optimizing laryngeal electrode has been designed to gently fill the glottis space atraumatically: Lantern Laryngeal Electrode (Neurosign) (Figure 11–19).

All current endotracheal tube electrodes should have confirmation of their position at the vocal cords by direct laryngoscopic visualization using a laryngoscope, fiberoptic scope, or newer iterations such as the Glidescope (Verathon). If the head must be rotated or hyperextended such as with thyroid surgery, it is best to re-inspect the glottis following repositioning to determine if the electrodes are still adjacent to the cords.

The typical threshold for most recurrent laryngeal nerves is 0.4 mA with maximal responses at around 0.8 mA. Based on these characteristics, the initial current setting for thyroidectomies and parathyroidectomies is typically 1.0mA. Once a brisk response has been elicited, the current can be decreased. Depending on stimulus location, the response latency from the RLN may be less than 2 msec. Therefore in order to prevent filtering the response as well as the stimulus artifact, the stimulation suppression filter should be lowered from the default 3.1msec down to approximately 2.35 msec when using the NIM.

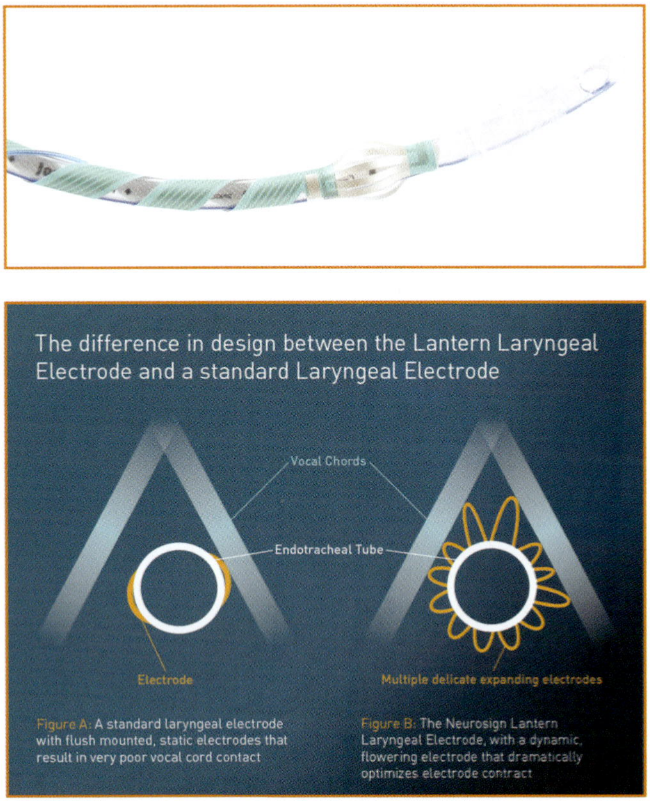

Figure 11–19. Lantern Laryngeal Electrode. New self-optimizing electrode atraumatically improves the electrode to vocal fold contact. Magstim Neurosign.

Pitfalls and Tips

Unfortunately, all of the currently available means to record the RLN response are limited by false positive and negative errors which the careful surgeon and technologist must be aware of in order to minimize the risk of interpretive errors. Electrode-to-Vocal fold contact is key: if the endotracheal tube with attached electrodes is too deep, too shallow, rotated, or too small to contact the vocal folds, false negative errors may occur. Currently, there appears to be a 15% incidence of false negative responses with surface laryngeal electrodes. Randolph et al have noted that suspected false-negative errors can be cross-checked by directly palpating the laryngeal twitch response in the tracheoesophageal junction.[32] If a laryngeal twitch can be palpated despite absence of an EMG response, a technical problem should be assumed.

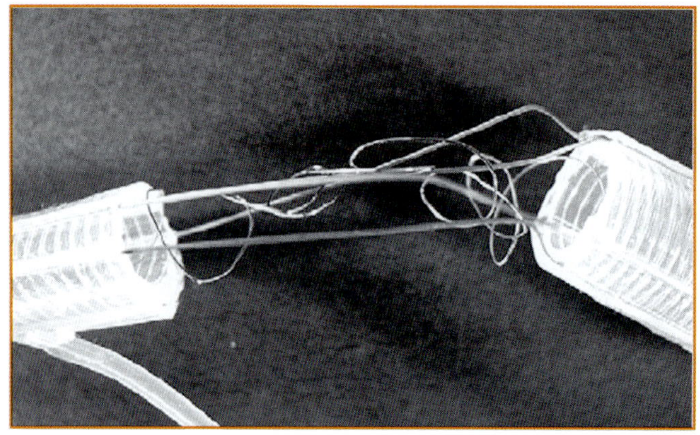

Figure 11–20. The reinforcing wire within the current Medtronic monitoring tube can unravel causing airway obstruction. Consequently, special care must be taken with this tube to prevent wire delamination including use of a bite-block to prevent the patient from biting down on the tube as well as avoidance of suctioning and tube exchangers. (Reprinted with permission[33])

Biting down on the electrodes, prolonged use of the monitoring ETT or damage from suctioning can cause delamination of the wires[33] (Figure 11–20). Medtronic recommends bite blocks to prevent the patient from biting down on the endotracheal tube. A noisy baseline may indicate a cuff leak (ie, from 15 mV to 80 mV), particularly when there is a corresponding EMG response synchronized with ventilation. In contrast, if there is a large baseline shift, it may indicate that the patient's anesthesia may be "light."

It is not widely known that the Medtronic monitoring endotracheal tube has a larger outer diameter than the average endotracheal tube of the same numbered size (which represents the ID, internal diameter), the intent being to try and improve contact with the vocal folds. However, this fact in conjunction with the absence of half sizes, may lead to the use of overly large endotracheal tubes, which can result in inadvertent vocal fold trauma during intubation. To optimize the efficacy and safety of this and other endotracheal tube electrodes, users are strongly advised to familiarize themselves with the manufacturers recommendations for use.

Monitoring cannot detect nerve injury from direct cautery. However, gradual thermal injury in the CPA from adjacent laser use can increase the baseline. Electrocautery should never be used simultaneously with the nerve stimulator because current can travel back through the stimulator and into the monitoring device. Devices like the Harmonic Scalpel (Ethicon Endo-Surgery, Blue Ash, OH) may provide some benefits in thyroid surgery because it does not cause electrical interference and has minimal thermal spread. Because myelinated extracranial nerves, such as the recurrent laryngeal nerve, are less likely to elicit mechanical evoked responses, it is important to use frequent electrical stimulation to map nerve location and confirm functionality after cautery or stretch. The stimulating dissecting instruments allow for simultaneous monitoring and dissection and are even more important in this setting. Increases in nerve threshold may be due to microtrauma, the presence of overlying tissue, wet field, desiccation. or a malpositioned endotracheal tube.

Another potential source of false negative error with RLN monitoring relates to where the nerve is stimulated after dissection. Because Wallerian degeneration takes time, an accurate assessment of nerve integrity must be performed by stimulating the nerve *proximal* to the area of dissection. During acoustic tumor surgery, this is typically easy to achieve; that is, if most of the dissection was at the porus, a final check of integrity must place the stimulator on the nerve near the pons. In thyroid surgery, a not uncommon error we have seen is to stimulate near Berry's ligament, whereas the injury may be missed if it was more proximal. For this reason, assessment of the RLN's integrity may be best made by stimulating very proximally on the RLN, or even at the *vagus* nerve.

False negative error may occur due to an improper "stimulus ignore period." This intentional silencing of the NIM prevents the surgeon from hearing responses created by the stimulus artifact. However, it needs to be set appropriate to the anticipated conduction time based on the distance between we are the nerve is stimulated and the muscle that is being recorded. To prevent inadvertent filtering of a *response* rather than just stimulus artifacts, the stimulation suppression filter should be lowered from approximately the default 3.1 msec (eg. otologic procedures) to approximately 2.35 msec when using the NIM during thyroid or parathyroid surgery (Figure 11–21).

A false positive error at the larynx may occur when the pharyngeal constrictors are inadvertently stimulated. As in the example with trigeminal vs. facial nerve stimulation, the large muscle response may be carried to the laryngeal surface electrodes and misinterpreted as an RLN response. This error appears to be increased if the endotracheal tube has been inserted a bit deep, past the vocal folds, as well as when high levels of stimulation are used that create volume conducted responses or artifact.

LOWER CRANIAL NERVE MONITORING

Monitoring of cranial nerves X through XII can be performed during resections of glomus jugulare tumors and other skull base masses. Because the motor component of CN IX is limited mainly to the stylopharyngeus muscle, which is located deep in the neck, it is extremely difficult to monitor. Placement of an electrode in the soft palate to monitor CN IX is a common misconception given that CN V and X provide motor innervation to this area. CN X is monitored peripherally through detection of EMGs via the recurrent laryngeal nerve. To monitor CN XI, electrodes can be placed in the trapezius or sternocleidomastoid muscles. However, because the muscle response is so large and apparent via visualization or movement of the head and neck, it can often be monitored via electric stimulation without intramuscular needle electrodes. Electrodes placed in the lateral aspect of the anterior third of the tongue are used to monitor CN XII.

CONCLUSION

The benefits of facial nerve monitoring during CPA surgery have made it a standard of care as evidenced by its widespread acceptance and results in the literature. Monitoring is also increasingly being used in otologic, parotid, and thyroid surgery but the low incidence of nerve injury in these procedures make monitoring's efficacy more difficult to assess. It is important that stimulation be done at least once during a case in order to confirm the integrity

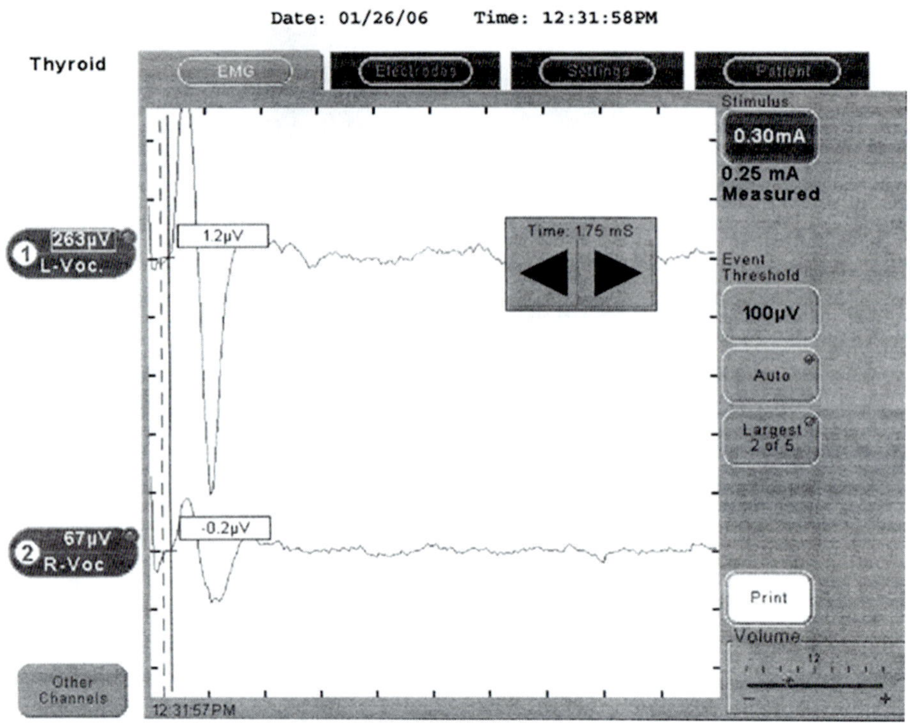

Figure 11–21. Stimulation of the RLN nerve close to the larynx (eg, Berry's ligament) may result in a response with a very brief latency, for example, less than 3 ms. Stimulus filters are helpful in ignoring stimulus artifact but if not used judiciously, can result in masking of both stimulus *and* response, causing a false-negative error. In this case, the response peak occurred at 1.75 ms but was detected because the technologist shortened the stimulus filter's time window from the factory default of 3.1 ms. (Reprinted with permission, courtesy of Jack M. Kartush, MD)

of the monitoring system. *Active* monitoring entails frequent use of electric stimulation rather than *passively* awaiting responses after trauma has occurred. Stimulating dissection instruments are a useful adjunct to detect the location of nerves prior to a mechanical insult. Surgeons as well as technologists must become trained to understand the correct setup and appropriate interpretation of monitoring data because "Poor monitoring is worse than no monitoring."

REFERENCES

1. National Institutes of Health. *Consensus statement: acoustic neuroma.* Presented at the NIH Consensus Development Conference, Bethesda, MD, 1991.
2. Krauze F. *Surgery of the brain and spinal cord.* In First English ed. New York, NY: Rebman; 1912:738–743.
3. Olivecrona H. Analysis of results of complete and partial removal of acoustic neuromas. *J Neurol Neurosurg Psychiatry.* 1950;13(4):271–272.
4. Parsons RC. Electrical stimulation of the facial nerve. *Laryngoscope.* 1966;76:391–406.
5. Jako G. Facial nerve monitor. *Trans Am Acad Ophthalm Otolaryngol.* 1975;69:340–342.
6. Hilger J. Facial nerve stimulator. *Trans Am Acad Ophthalm Otolaryngol.* 1964;68:74–76.
7. Delgado TE, Buchheit WA, Rosenholtz HR, Chrissian S. Intraoperative monitoring of facial muscle evoked responses obtained by intracranial stimulation of the facial nerve: a more accurate technique for facial nerve dissection. *Neurosurgery.* 1979;4:418–420.
8. Sugita K, Kobayashi S. Technical and instrumental improvements in the surgical treatment of acoustic neurinomas. *J Neurosurg.* 1982;57(6):747–752.

9. Prass RL, Luders H. Acoustic (loudspeaker) facial electromyographic monitoring: Part 1. Evoked electromyographic activity during acoustic neuroma resection. *Neurosurgery*. 1986;19(3):392–400.
10. Silverstein H, Smouha EE, Jones R. Routine intraoperative facial nerve monitoring during otologic surgery. *Am J Otol*. 1988;9(4):269–275.
11. Kartush JM, Prass RL. Facial nerve testing—electroneurography intraoperative monitoring. In: Johnson J, Blitzer A, Ossoff R, Thomas JR, eds. *American Academy of Otolaryngology-Head and Neck Surgery Instruction Courses, Vol. I.* St. Louis, MO: CV Mosby Co; 1988:231–247.
12. Harner SG, Daube JR, Beatty CW, Ebersold MJ. Intraoperative monitoring of the facial nerve. *Laryngoscope*. 1988;98(2):209–212.
13. Hammerschlag PE, Cohen NL. Intraoperative monitoring of facial nerve function in cerebellopontine angle surgery. *Otolaryngol Head Neck Surg*. 1990;103(5 pt 1):681–684.
14. Dickins JR, Graham SS. A comparison of facial nerve monitoring systems in cerebellopontine angle surgery. *Am J Otol*. 1991;12(1):1–6.
15. Kwartler JA, Luxford WM, Atkins J, Shelton C. Facial nerve monitoring in acoustic tumor surgery. *Otolaryngol Head Neck Surg*. 1991;104(6):814–817.
16. Greenberg JS, Manolidis S, Stewart MG, Kahn JB. Facial nerve monitoring in chronic ear surgery: US practice patterns. *Otolaryngol Head Neck Surg*. 2002;126(2):108–114.
17. Noss RS, Lalwani AK, Yingling CD. Facial nerve monitoring in middle ear and mastoid surgery. *Laryngoscope*. 2001;111(5):831–836.
18. Wilson L, Lin E, Lalwani A. Cost-effectiveness of intraoperative facial nerve monitoring in middle ear or mastoid surgery. *Laryngoscope*, 2003;113(10):1736–1745.
19. Lowry TR, Gal TJ, Brennan JA. Patterns of use of facial nerve monitoring during parotid gland surgery. *Otolaryngol Head Neck Surg*. 2005;133(3):313–318.
20. Moller AR, Jannetta PJ. Preservation of facial function during removal of acoustic neuromas. Use of monopolar constant-voltage stimulation and EMG. *J Neurosurg*. 1984;61(4):757–760.
21. Prass R, Luders H. Constant-current versus constant-voltage stimulation. *J Neurosurg*. 1985;62(4):622–623.
22. Kartush JM, Niparko JK, Graham MD, Kemink JL. Electroneurography: preoperative facial nerve assessment for tumors of the temporal bone. *Otolaryngol Head Neck Surg*. 1987;97(3): 257–26L.
23. Kartush JM. Electroneurography and intraoperative facial monitoring in contemporary neurotology. *Otolaryngol Head Neck Surg*. 1989;101(4):496–503.
24. Kartush JM, Niparko JK, Bledsoe SC, Graham MD, Kemink JL. Intraoperative facial nerve monitoring: a comparison of stimulating electrodes. *Laryngoscope*. 1985;95(12):1536–1540.
25. Hughes G, Chase S, Dudley A, Sismanis A. Safety of electrical stimulation of peripheral nerves. Potentials. In: Portmann M, ed. *The Facial Nerve*. Paris: Masson Publishers; 1985:381–384.
26. Kartush JM, LaRouere MJ, Graham MD, Bouchard KR, Audet BV. Intraoperative cranial nerve monitoring during posterior skull base surgery. *Skull Base Surg*. 1991;1:85–92.
27. Kartush J. Cochlear implant surgery. In: Kartush JM, *Cochlear Implantation*. Alexandria, VA: American Academy of Otolaryngology-HNS; 1994:53-70.
28. Kartush JM, Graham MD, LaRouere MJ. Meatal decompression following acoustic neuroma resection: minimizing delayed facial palsy. *Laryngoscope*. 1991;101(6 pt 1): 674–675.
29. Gianoli G, Kartush J. Delayed facial palsy after acoustic tumor resection: The role of viral activation. *Am J Otol*. 1996;17:625–629.
30. Fisch U, Esslen E. Total intratemporal exposure of the facial nerve. Pathologic findings in Bell's palsy. *Arch Otolaryngol*. 1972;95(4):335–341.
31. Hamill NJ, Kartush JM. Errors in facial nerve surgery. In: Yanagihara N, Murakami S, eds. *New Horizons in Facial Nerve Research and Facial Expression*. The Netherlands: Kugler Publications; 1998:317–322.
32. Randolph GW, Kobler JB, Wilkins J. Recurrent laryngeal nerve identification and assessment during thyroid surgery: laryngeal palpation. *World J Surg*. 2004;28(8):755–60. Epub 2004 Aug 3.
33. Evanina EY, Hanisak JL. Case study involving suctioning of an electromyographic endotracheal tube. *AANA J*. 2005;73:112.

Index

D

E

F

G

H

I

M

N

O

P

R

S

T

U

V

W

Z